THE MAYO CLINIC MANUAL OF
NUCLEAR MEDICINE

THE MAYO CLINIC MANUAL OF
NUCLEAR MEDICINE

Edited by

Michael K. O'Connor, Ph.D.

Associate Professor of Radiologic Physics
Mayo Medical School
Consultant Physicist
Department of Diagnostic Radiology
The Mayo Clinic
Rochester, Minnesota

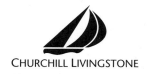

CHURCHILL LIVINGSTONE

New York, Edinburgh, London, Madrid, Melbourne, San Francisco, Tokyo

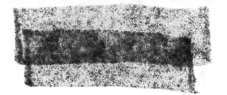

Library of Congress Cataloging-in-Publication Data
The Mayo Clinic manual of nuclear medicine / edited by Michael K.
  O'Connor.
        p.   cm.
     Includes bibliographical references and index.
     ISBN 0–443–07765–7
     1. Nuclear medicine —Handbooks, manuals, etc. 2. Nuclear
medicine—Technique. I. O'Connor, Michael K. II. Mayo Clinic.
     [DNLM: 1. Radionuclide Imaging—methods. 2. Radionuclide Imaging—
instrumentation. 3. Nuclear Medicine—standards. 4. Quality
Control.   WN 203 M 473 1996]
R896.7.M39   1996
616.07′575—dc20
DNLM/DLC
for Library of Congress   96–11649
                                                                         CIP

Published and distributed in the United States of America by Churchill Livingstone, 650 Avenue of the Americas, New York, NY 10011. Distributed in the United Kingdom by Churchill Livingstone, Robert Stevenson House, 1–3 Baxter's Place, Leith Walk, Edinburgh EH1 3AF, and by associated companies, branches, and representatives throughout the world.

Accurate indications, adverse reactions, and dosage schedules for drugs are provided in this book, but it is possible that they may change. The reader is urged to review the package information data of the manufacturers of the medications mentioned.

Nothing in this publication implies that Mayo Foundation endorses the products mentioned.

The Publishers have made every effort to trace the copyright holders for borrowed material. If they have inadvertently overlooked any, they will be pleased to make the necessary arrangements at the first opportunity.

Acquisitions Editors: *Michael J. Houston and Miranda Bromage*
Assistant Editor: *Ann Ruzycka*
Production Editor: *Paul Bernstein*
Production Supervisor: *Laura Mosberg Cohen*
Desktop Coordinator: *Jo-Ann Demas*
Cover Design: *Jeannette Jacobs*

Printed in the United States of America

First published in 1996   7   6   5   4   3   2   1

Contributors

Timothy F. Christian, M.D.

Assistant Professor of Medicine, Mayo Medical School; Consultant, Division of Cardiovascular Diseases, Department of Internal Medicine, The Mayo Clinic, Rochester, Minnesota

Douglas A. Collins, M.D.

Instructor in Radiology, Mayo Medical School; Senior Associate Consultant, Division of Nuclear Medicine, Department of Diagnostic Radiology, The Mayo Clinic, Rochester, Minnesota

Lee A. Forstrom, M.D., Ph.D.

Assistant Professor of Radiology, Mayo Medical School; Consultant, Division of Nuclear Medicine, Department of Diagnostic Radiology, The Mayo Clinic, Rochester, Minnesota

Raymond J. Gibbons, M.D.

Professor of Medicine, Mayo Medical School; Consultant, Division of Cardiovascular Diseases, Department of Internal Medicine; Co-Director, Nuclear Cardiology Laboratory, The Mayo Clinic, Rochester, Minnesota

Mary F. Hauser, M.D.

Assistant Professor of Radiology, Mayo Medical School; Consultant, Division of Nuclear Medicine, Department of Diagnostic Radiology, The Mayo Clinic, Rochester, Minnesota

Joseph C. Hung, Ph.D.

Associate Professor of Radiology, Mayo Medical School; Consultant, Division of Nuclear Medicine, Department of Diagnostic Radiology, The Mayo Clinic, Rochester, Minnesota

Todd D. Miller, M.D.

Associate Professor of Medicine, Mayo Medical School; Consultant, Division of Cardiovascular Diseases, Department of Internal Medicine, The Mayo Clinic, Rochester, Minnesota

Brian P. Mullan, M.D.

Assistant Professor of Radiology, Mayo Medical School; Spokesperson and Consultant, Division of Nuclear Medicine, Department of Diagnostic Radiology; Co-Director, Nuclear Cardiology Laboratory, The Mayo Clinic, Rochester, Minnesota

Michael K. O'Connor, Ph.D.

Associate Professor of Radiologic Physics, Mayo Medical School; Consultant Physicist, Department of Diagnostic Radiology, The Mayo Clinic, Rochester, Minnesota

Gregory A. Wiseman, M.D.

Assistant Professor of Radiology, Mayo Medical School; Consultant, Division of Nuclear Medicine, Department of Diagnostic Radiology, The Mayo Clinic, Rochester, Minnesota

Preface

The Mayo Clinic Manual of Nuclear Medicine is designed for physicians and technologists as a practical guide to the performance of many of the more common procedures in nuclear medicine. We have placed a strong emphasis on the technical aspects of each procedure, providing detailed descriptions of the parameters for data acquisition and analysis. In order to make the manual more useful, duplication of the details of some procedures has been retained. This was done to eliminate the need for technologists or physicians to have to skip back and forth between different sections of the manual for complete details of a given procedure.

This manual is a close reflection of the nuclear medicine practice at the Mayo Clinic. The process of updating and expanding the manual forced us to critically review many of our procedures and led to many changes in how we practice nuclear medicine. We realize that for many procedures, there is no standard method of performing the procedure; rather, a number of different methods can be used to achieve the same end result. Hence, we do not make any claims that the techniques and data analysis described in this manual are the only methods of performing the procedures; rather, this manual should be viewed as a detailed description of one possible way to perform these procedures. The individual circumstances of a given laboratory will generally require that the procedures be modified to suit the practice style of that laboratory.

Critical review of how procedures are performed should always be an ongoing process in every laboratory and is even more important in the current health care environment as we strive to maintain quality while reducing the time and effort required to perform our procedures. We hope that physicians and technologists will find *The Mayo Clinic Manual of Nuclear Medicine* a useful aid in this review process and in the performance of their practice.

Michael K. O'Connor, Ph.D.

Acknowledgments

This book is the cumulative effort of the physicians and technologists in the section of Nuclear Medicine at the Mayo Clinic. In particular, we wish to thank Tim Hardyman, Dan Mack, Gary Truex, Michelle Rank, and Tim Valley for their help in revising and updating many of our procedures. Their input was invaluable, and their technical know-how is evident in many of the finer details of the procedures. We also wish to thank Vicki Krage for secretarial help in typing the many revisions of this book.

Contents

Instrumentation and Radiopharmaceutical Quality Control

Clinical Procedures

5. Endocrine System

Gregory A. Wiseman

6. Gastrointestinal System

Brian P. Mullan

7. Genitourinary System   367

Mary F. Hauser and Douglas A. Collins

8. Infection—Bone   425

Lee A. Forstrom

9. Respiratory System   459

Douglas A. Collins and Mary F. Hauser

10. Tumor Imaging Procedures   489

Gregory A. Wiseman

1

Instrumentation Quality Control

Michael K. O'Connor
Joseph C. Hung

Gamma Camera Planar System—Daily and Weekly Quality Control

Introduction

Gamma camera quality control (QC) can be implemented in a large number of ways in a department. The procedures described here were developed with the goal that daily QC should be simple and quick to perform and should evaluate both the detector and the collimator. For these reasons, ^{57}Co sheet sources are preferred for measurement of system uniformity. Although refillable sheet sources are less expensive, a large number of technical problems are inherent in their use, including leaking, warping of the plastic, poor mixing, and air bubbles.[1–3] These problems make refillable sheet sources unsatisfactory for daily use. Extrinsic measurements are preferred to intrinsic measurements, because they include evaluation of the collimator, do not involve removal of the collimator with the attendant risk of damage to the crystal, and are quicker to perform.[2]

On planar systems, flood images are usually evaluated in a subjective manner. Whereas this is adequate on a daily basis, it is useful on a weekly basis to obtain some quantitative index of system uniformity. The weekly QC procedure measures the integral uniformity of the flood image. It also measures system linearity and resolution. A large number of test phantoms have been designed to measure resolution and linearity, including the 4-quadrant bar phantom,[4] the parallel line equal spacing (PLES) phantom,[4] the BRH test phantom,[5] the orthogonal hole phantom,[6] and the Hine-Duley phantom.[7] Although many of these phantoms can be used intrinsically or extrinsically, the preference should be for intrinsic measurement whenever possible. This eliminates the possibility of moiré fringe patterns that are due to interplay of the bar pattern with the hole pattern of the collimator.[8,9] The basis for selecting the most appropriate test pattern is that gamma camera linearity is linked more closely to uniformity and requires more frequent evaluation than resolution.[10,11] Hence, where possible the PLES phantom is used for all weekly checks of linearity and resolution. These checks are performed intrinsically on single-head systems and extrinsically on dual-head systems, because of the logistic difficulties of performing intrinsic measurements on many dual-head systems. *Note:* On large 50–60 cm field-of-view systems, a suitably sized PLES phantom may not be obtainable. In such cases, a large 4-quadrant bar phantom should be used.

Purpose

The procedures described here are designed for single- or dual-head systems that do not perform tomographic acquisitions. The following describes the QC procedures that must be performed on a planar (non-single photon emission computed tomography [SPECT]) gamma camera system on a daily and weekly basis. These procedures perform the following functions:

1. Check for contamination of detector or surrounding areas (daily).
2. Qualitative check of system uniformity and sensitivity (daily).
3. Quantitative check of system uniformity (weekly).
4. Qualitative check of system linearity and resolution (weekly).

Instrument Specifications

Gamma camera:	Single- or dual-head planar system
Collimator:	Any low-energy collimator
Energy setting:	Background check and ^{99m}Tc procedures—140 keV, 15–20% energy window
	^{57}Co procedures—122 keV, 15–20% energy window
Analog formatter:	Spot views—70-mm (9 on 1) format, 8 × 10 film
Computer system:	Acquisition requirements—static (64 × 64 and 256 × 256 word mode matrix)
	Processing requirements—measurement of image uniformity or region of interest (ROI) analysis
Additional items:	5–10 mCi (185–370 MBq) ^{57}Co sheet source—solid disk impregnated with ^{57}Co
	150–200 μCi (5.55–7.40 MBq) point source of ^{99m}Tc in a volume of 0.1 ml or less
	PLES or 4-quadrant bar phantoms with 2–4 mm bar spacing (intrinsic measurements) or 4–6 mm bar spacing (extrinsic measurements)

Daily Procedure: Background Check

1. *Single-head system:* Ensure that all nearby sources are shielded, and rotate the detector head to face the floor.
   Dual-head system: Detector orientation is not critical, because opposing detectors self-shield each other from nearby sources of radiation.
2. Set a 15–20% energy window around the 140-keV photopeak of ^{99m}Tc. Acquire a 5-minute background image. No hard copy is required at this point.
3. Record the background counts in the QC logbook for that system. Figure 1-1 shows the layout of a typical QC logbook sheet.
4. On a standard 40-cm field-of-view system equipped with a low-energy collimator, the 5-minute background count should be in the range 5–10 kct (normal range should be established for each laboratory).
5. If counts are above this level, check the area for unshielded sources and repeat the measurement. On a single-head system, rotate the detector head to face up in case the floor is contaminated. Record the 5-minute background image on analog formatter, with the image intensity set to maximum, and on computer (64 × 64 matrix). Discrete areas of activity on the background image are generally caused by contamination of either the collimator or the crystal. If background count is still high, repeat the measurement again with a different collimator. This should determine whether the contamination is on the crystal or the collimator.
6. If contamination is present, check the energy spectrum to identify the radioisotope. Decontaminate the appropriate areas with a suitable radioactive decontaminant, and repeat the background check until it is within normal limits.

Single Head System : _____

	Quality Control for Week beginning :						
Day	Background cts / 5 min	Tc-99m kcps	Energy Spectrum	Acquisition Time seconds	Integral Unif (%)	Resolution Linearity	Initials
Mon							
Day	Background cts / 5 min	Co-57 Source	Energy Spectrum	Acquisition Time seconds	Uniformity	Collimator	Initials
Tues							
Wed							
Thurs							
Fri							

Dual Head System : _____

	Quality Control for Week beginning :						
Day	Bkd cts / 5 min head 1 / head 2	Co-57 Source	Energy Spectrum	Acquisition Time seconds	Integral Unif (%) head 1 / head 2	Resolution Linearity	Initials
Mon	/		/		/	/	
Day	Bkd cts / 5 min head 1 / head 2	Co-57 Source	Energy Spectrum	Acquisition Time seconds	Uniformity	Collimator	Initials
Tues	/		/		/		
Wed	/		/		/		
Thurs	/		/		/		
Fri	/		/		/		

Figure 1-1. Sample forms for recording results of daily and weekly QC on a single- or dual-headed planar imaging system.

7. If the contamination cannot be removed or the cause of the high background is unclear, it may be necessary to contact the medical physicist, the service engineer, or the radiation safety officer to assist in evaluating the problem.

Procedure: System Calibration

Many manufacturers require that some type of energy calibration be performed on a daily or weekly basis. This calibration may be internal to the system itself and require no external radiation source, or it may require removal of the collimator for intrinsic measurement with ^{99m}Tc or ^{57}Co point sources. Because of the various methods used by manufacturers, no attempt is made here to describe these procedures, and the manufacturer's instructions should be followed. These calibrations should always be performed before checking the accuracy of the photopeak setting or before proceeding with any measurement of uniformity or resolution.

Daily Procedure: Image Uniformity and Sensitivity

1. *Single-head system:* Place a ^{57}Co sheet source on the collimator as shown in Figure 1-2. *Dual-head system:* For opposing dual-head detector systems, bring both detectors as close together as possible. Place a ^{57}Co sheet source on the lower detector head as shown in Figure 1-3.

2. Ensure that the count rate does not exceed 20 kcps per detector head (*Note:* On some dual-head systems, the same electronic system processes events from both heads. In such cases, the combined count rate from both detectors should not exceed 20 kcps). For a 40-cm field-of-view system, optimum activities are 5 mCi (185 MBq) ^{57}Co for an all-purpose collimator and 10 mCi (370 MBq) ^{57}Co for a high- or ultrahigh-resolution collimator.

3. Check the energy spectrum and ensure that a 15–20% energy window is peaked on the main photopeak at 122 keV. *Note:* A shift of more than 1–2 keV in photopeak location is often an indication of a system malfunction.

4. When the system is peaked, acquire a static acquisition on analog formatter and on computer (256 × 256 word mode matrix). Total counts acquired should be 2 Mct per detector for a 30–40 cm field-of-view system and 3–4 Mct per detector for a 50–60 cm field-of-view system. If system hardware permits disabling of the energy or uniformity correction modules, then acquire the flood images both with and without these corrections enabled.

5. Obtain a hard copy of the flood image(s) on analog formatter, video, or laser imager.

6. Record the ^{57}Co sheet source number, the collimator used, and the time for image acquisition in the QC logbook (see Fig. 1-1). System sensitivity can be determined by noting acquisition time. This time should be similar to that of previous acquisitions (within 5%), allowing for a gradual decay in source activity over time. Furthermore, for dual-head systems, the acquisition times for the 2 detectors should be within 5% of each other.

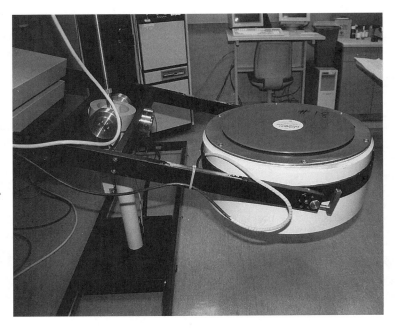

Figure 1-2. ^{57}Co sheet source in place for measurement of extrinsic uniformity.

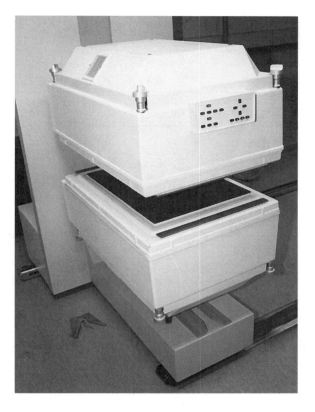

Figure 1-3. ^{57}Co sheet source in position on the lower detector for measurement of extrinsic uniformity. Ensure that it is properly centered over the active field of view.

7. Check that the flood image is uniform, and place the appropriate sticker on the QC hard copy. **The sticker should be dated and initialed by the technologist who performed the quality control.** Three different types of stickers are available, as shown in Figure 1-4. This method requires that the technologist review the film and ensures accountability for decisions taken with respect to image quality.

8. If any problems are noticed during the daily QC procedure, contact the support personnel (service engineer, physicist, etc.) for assistance in resolving the problem.

Weekly Procedure: Intrinsic/Extrinsic Uniformity

Acquisition: Single-Head System

1. Remove the collimator and rotate the detector head so that it faces up. If required by the manufacturer, place a lead masking ring over the exposed crystal, as shown in Figure 1-5. This is designed to shield the edges of the crystal, thereby eliminating "edge packing" artifacts.

2. If no masking ring is required, cover the exposed crystal with an absorbent sheet.

3. Tape a 150–200 µCi (5.55–7.40 MBq) ^{99m}Tc point source to a plastic rod and attach the rod to an IV pole. *Note:* If the point source is in a syringe with a needle attached, it should not be oriented with the needle pointing down, because the needle then can act as a collimator and introduce an artifactual cold ring into the uniformity image.

4. The point source should be positioned over the center of the crystal at a distance of at least 4 times the field of view (e.g., at 200 cm for a 50-cm field-of-view gamma camera), as shown in Figure 1-6.

```
┌─────────────────────────────────────────┐
│  SYSTEM:                    DATE:        │
│  Q.C. CHECK - SATISFACTORY    GREEN      │
│  SIGNED:                                 │
└─────────────────────────────────────────┘
```

```
┌─────────────────────────────────────────┐
│  SYSTEM:                    DATE:        │
│  Q.C. POTENTIAL PROBLEM    YELLOW        │
│  SIGNED:                                 │
└─────────────────────────────────────────┘
```

Figure 1-4. Sample stickers used for daily QC measurements.

```
┌─────────────────────────────────────────┐
│  SYSTEM:                    DATE:        │
│  Q.C. PROBLEM        RED                 │
│  SIGNED:                                 │
└─────────────────────────────────────────┘
```

5. Ensure that the count rate does not exceed 20 kcps. If necessary, increase the source-to-collimator distance to decrease the count rate to an acceptable level (less than 20 kcps).

6. Check the energy spectrum, and ensure that a 15–20% energy window is peaked on the main photopeak at 140 keV. *Note:* A shift of more than 1–2 keV in photopeak location is often an indication of a system malfunction.

7. When the system is peaked, acquire a static acquisition on analog formatter and on computer (256×256 word mode matrix). Total counts acquired should be 3 Mct for a 30–40 cm field-of-view system and 4–5 Mct for a 50–60 cm field-of-view system. If system hardware permits disabling of the energy or uniformity correction modules, then acquire the flood images both with and without these corrections enabled.

Acquisition: Dual-Head System

1. For opposing dual-head detector systems, it is often difficult or impossible to orient each detector so that a point source can be positioned at a distance of 4 times the field of view from the face of the detectors. In such cases, uniformity images should be acquired extrinsically using a ^{57}Co sheet source.

2. Bring both detectors as close together as possible. Place a ^{57}Co sheet source on the lower detector head as shown in Figure 1-3. Ensure that the count rate does not exceed 20 kcps per detector head.

3. Check the energy spectrum of each detector, and ensure that a 15–20% energy window is peaked on the main photopeak at 122 keV. *Note:* A shift of more than 1–2 keV in photopeak location is often an indication of system malfunction.

4. When the system is peaked, acquire a static acquisition on analog formatter and on computer (256×256 word mode matrix). Total counts acquired should be 3 Mct per detector for a 30–40 cm field-of-view system and 4–5 Mct for a 50–60 cm field-of-view system. If system hardware permits disabling of the energy or uniformity correction modules, then acquire the flood images both with and without these corrections enabled.

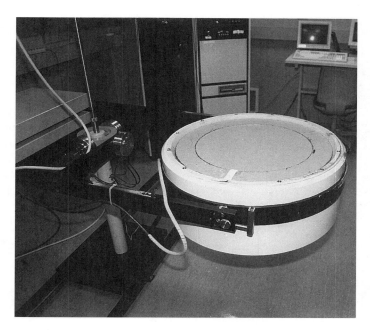

Figure 1-5. Jumbo field-of-view system with collimator removed and masking ring in position for measurement of intrinsic uniformity.

Analysis: Single-/Dual-Head Systems

1. Obtain a hard copy of the flood image(s) on analog formatter, video, or laser imager.
2. On computer, measure image uniformity. Some manufacturers provide software for the measurement of integral and differential uniformity. If no suitable software exists, follow steps a–e to measure integral uniformity:
   a. Compress the image from 256 × 256 to 64 × 64 matrix (if this is not possible, uniformity images should be acquired in a 64 × 64 matrix).
   b. Smooth the image with a standard 9-point smooth function.
   c. Draw an ROI to fit inside the uniformity image, as shown in Figure 1-7. Use a circular ROI for circular field-of-view systems and a box ROI for rectangular field-of-view systems. Irregular or freehand ROIs should be used for rectangular field-of-view systems with clipped corners.
   d. Determine the minimum and maximum counts inside the ROI.
   e. Compute the integral uniformity (IU) from the following equation:

$$IU = \frac{Maximum\ Count - Minimum\ Count}{Maximum + Minimum\ Count} \times 100\%$$

3. Record the integral uniformity and the time for image acquisition in the QC logbook (see Fig. 1-1).
4. Check that the flood image is uniform, and compare the value for integral uniformity with those obtained previously. Integral uniformity should be within ±1% of the previous value. Place the appropriate sticker on the QC hard copy. **The sticker should be dated and initialed by the technologist who performed the quality control.** Three different types of stickers are available, as shown in Figure 1-4.

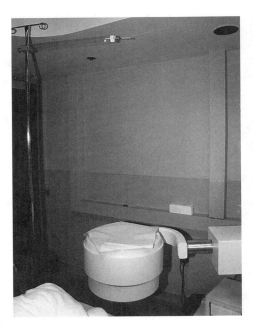

Figure 1-6. Point source in position for measurement of intrinsic uniformity. Exposed crystal has been covered with absorbent sheet to protect against spills.

5. If any problems are noticed during measurement of uniformity, contact the support personnel (service engineer, physicist, etc.) for assistance in resolving the problem.

Weekly Procedure: System Linearity/Resolution

Acquisition: Single-Head System

1. Measurement of intrinsic linearity/resolution uses the same arrangement of point source to detector as used for measurement of intrinsic uniformity.
2. Following acquisition of the intrinsic uniformity images, place a PLES bar phantom on top of the detector head, as shown in Figure 1-8. The bar phantom should have 3-mm wide lead bars with 3-mm spacing between them.

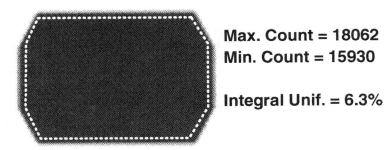

Max. Count = 18062
Min. Count = 15930

Integral Unif. = 6.3%

Figure 1-7. ROI drawn inside flood image for measurement of integral uniformity. Maximum, minimum counts, and integral uniformity are shown.

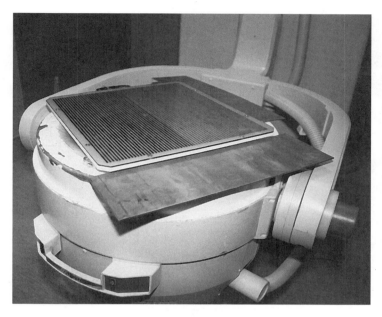

Figure 1-8. PLES phantom in position on top of detector head. Note use of lead strips to shield exposed crystal.

3. The bar phantom should be oriented at an angle of 45° between the x- and y-axis of the detector. In this way, a single image provides adequate assessment of both x and y linearity.
4. If the bar phantom does not completely cover the crystal face, place lead sheets over any region of exposed crystal (see Fig. 1-8).
5. Acquire a static acquisition on analog formatter and on computer (256 × 256 word mode matrix). Total counts acquired should be 3 Mct for a 30–40 cm field-of-view system and 4–5 Mct for a 50–60 cm field-of-view system.

Acquisition: Dual-Head System

Measurement of intrinsic resolution is even more difficult to perform than intrinsic uniformity, because the detector must be face up unless a mechanism is available for securing the bar phantom to the detector face. Hence, the following procedure is limited to an extrinsic measurement of linearity/resolution.

1. Measurement of extrinsic resolution/linearity uses the same arrangement as described for measurement of extrinsic uniformity on a dual-head system.
2. Following acquisition of the extrinsic uniformity images, place a PLES or 4-quadrant bar phantom between the ^{57}Co sheet source and the collimator, as shown in Figure 1-9. The PLES phantom should have 5-mm wide lead bars with 5-mm spacing between them. The 4-quadrant bar phantom should have lead bars 4–6 mm wide.
3. If 2 bar phantoms are available, it is possible to acquire simultaneously images of both phantoms by using the arrangement shown in Figure 1-10. In this arrangement, foam blocks are placed between the ^{57}Co sheet source and the bar phantoms. The detector heads are brought together until they lightly compress the bar phantoms.
4. The bar phantoms should be oriented along the x- or y-axis of the detector.

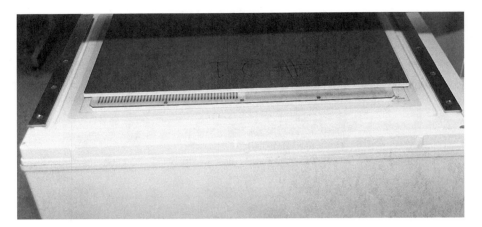

Figure 1-9. Measurement of extrinsic resolution on a dual-head system. Bar phantom in position on collimator with ^{57}Co sheet source on top. *Note:* For illustrative purposes, the sheet source has been displaced to one side to show the bar phantom.

5. Acquire static images on analog formatter and on computer (256 × 256 word mode matrix). Total counts acquired should be 3 Mct per detector for a 30–40 cm field-of-view system and 4–5 Mct per detector for a 50–60 cm field-of-view system.
6. Following acquisition, rotate the bar phantom(s) by 90° and repeat step 5.

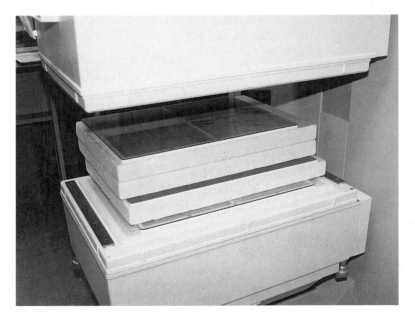

Figure 1-10. Simultaneous measurement of extrinsic resolution on both detector heads. Bar phantoms are placed on top and bottom with the ^{57}Co sheet source in between. Foam pads are used to separate the phantoms and permit detectors to be brought close to the bar phantoms.

Image Review: Single- and Dual-Head Systems

1. Obtain a hard copy of the bar phantom image on analog formatter, video imager, or laser imager.
2. Orient the hard copy so that the bar phantom image is viewed at an angle of 70°–90° to the eye. Check that the images of the bars are straight (good linearity).
3. Record in the QC logbook whether the linearity and resolution are acceptable (Fig. 1-1). Place the appropriate sticker on the QC hard copy.
4. If any problems are noticed during the measurement of system linearity, contact the support personnel (service engineer, physicist, etc.) for assistance in resolving the problem.

Interpretation

Uniformity

A large number of factors can contribute to nonuniformities in the flood images. These include defects or cracks in the collimator; damage to the crystal (cracks, hydration, etc.); noisy, defective, or out-of-tune photomultiplier tubes; failure of the preamplifiers or other electronic components of the pulse arithmetic circuitry; defects in the analog formatter; defective ADCs in the computer; corruption of the energy, linearity, or uniformity correction maps; and problems with the film processor. Uniformity is the most important variable of gamma camera performance, because it is affected adversely by most types of system malfunction.

It generally is accepted that nonuniformities of 15% or less are difficult to perceive by a visual inspection of the hard copy.[12] Most modern gamma cameras achieve nonuniformities of 5% or less, with older systems in the range of 10–15%. Generally, the flood images should show good uniformity, and individual photomultiplier tubes should not be visible. If flood images were obtained both with and without uniformity correction, the uncorrected image should not show gross nonuniformities (e.g., single or multiple cold areas), because this may result in the uniformity correction process introducing artifactual hot or cold regions into clinical studies.

Although major nonuniformities are easily detected from the daily flood image, subtle degradation in uniformity over time is detected best by quantitative measurement of uniformity. It should be noted that values for integral and differential uniformity reflect both system nonuniformities and statistical noise in the flood data. For a 3–5 Mct flood, the measured values of integral and differential uniformity on average are 1–2% larger than the same values calculated from a high-count (20–30 Mct) flood image.[13] Likewise, the measured values fluctuate by about ±1% from week to week, and these variations should be kept in mind when determining whether a significant change in system performance has occurred.[13]

Sensitivity

[57]Co sheet sources are an easy way of determining system sensitivity provided that the same [57]Co sheet source and collimator are used on successive days. Variations in acquisition times that are due to decay and statistical fluctuations should not exceed 1–2 seconds for a 5-minute acquisition. Variations larger than this are attributable to variations in system sensitivity. These should not exceed 5% (15 seconds for a 5-minute acquisition).

Linearity

When viewed at an angle, the PLES image should show straight lines, at most with some distortion at the edges. Wavy lines generally indicate poor linearity correction, which also should be evident as an increase in the measured values of integral and differential uniformity.

Additional Notes

^{57}Co sheet sources are often contaminated with small amounts of ^{58}Co and ^{56}Co. These two isotopes have short half-lives (77.3 and 71 days, respectively) compared with that of ^{57}Co, but they emit high-energy gamma rays (greater than 500 keV). Some gamma cameras are particularly sensitive to these high-energy gamma rays and, consequently, may show nonuniformities in the flood images.[14] The impact of these high-energy gamma rays can be minimized by raising the sheet source 10–15 cm off the collimator face and/or by using a medium- or high-energy collimator. These effects diminish with time and are usually insignificant by 6–8 months after the date of manufacture.

References

1. Newcomer K, Chapman D, Garcia E, et al. Uniformity correction circuitry: the effects of extraneous acquisition errors (abstract). J Nucl Med Tech 1980; 8: 125.
2. Graham LS. Quality assurance of Anger cameras. In "Physics of Nuclear Medicine—Recent Advances," eds Rao DV, Chandra R, Graham MC. American Association of Physicists in Medicine, New York, 1984, pp 68–84.
3. English RJ, Polak JF, Holman BL. An iterative method for verifying systematic nonuniformities in refillable flood sources. J Nucl Med Tech 1984; 12: 7–9.
4. Quality control for scintillation cameras. U.S. Dept. of Health, Education and Welfare, HEW Publications FDA 76-8046, 1976.
5. Paras P, Hine GJ, Adams R. BRH test pattern for the evaluation of gamma-camera performance. J Nucl Med 1981; 22: 468–470.
6. Hine GJ. An ortho test pattern for quality assurance of gamma cameras. Nuclear Associates Pamphlet No. 265K, Washington D.C.
7. Anger HO. Testing the performance of scintillation cameras. Lawrence Berkeley Laboratory Report 2027, University of California, Berkeley, 1973.
8. Yeh E-L. Distortion of bar-phantom image by collimator. J Nucl Med 1979; 20: 260–261.
9. Brown PH, Royal HD. Re: Distortion of bar-phantom image by collimator (letter to the editor). J Nucl Med 1979; 20: 1100–1101.
10. Brookeman VA. Imaging instrumentation quality control. In "Quality Assurance in Nuclear Medicine," eds Hamilton DR, Herrera NE, Paras P, Rollo FD, MacIntyre WJ. U.S. Dept. of Health and Human Services, HHS Publication FDA 84-8224, 1984, pp 160–166.
11. Laird EE, Allen W, William ED. Gamma camera computer system quality control for conventional and tomographic use. In "Quality Control of Nuclear Medicine Instrumentation," ed Mould RF. Hospital Physicists Association, London, 1983, pp. 101–110.
12. Cohen G, Kereiakes JG, Padikal TN, Ashare AB, Saenger EL. Quantitative assessment of field uniformity for gamma cameras. Radiology 1976; 118: 197–200.
13. Young KC, Kouris K, Awdeh M, Abdel-Dayem HM. Reproducibility and action levels for gamma camera uniformity. Nucl Med Commun 1990; 11: 95–101.
14. Cranage RW, Peake JC. The effect of high energy impurities on measurements of gamma-camera resolution and uniformity using ^{57}Co flood sources (letter to the editor). Br J Radiol 1979; 52: 81–82.

SPECT System–Daily and Weekly Quality Control

Introduction

Modern SPECT systems typically have nonuniformities of between 4% and 7%. These nonuniformities can generate ring artifacts in tomographic data; hence, all SPECT systems apply an additional correction to the raw image data, called "uniformity," "flood," or "sensitivity" correction, before data reconstruction. This correction is designed to decrease system nonuniformities to a level low enough so that any ring artifacts generated from residual nonuniformities in the system are less than image noise and, thus, not visible in the reconstructed data. However, image noise in the reconstructed data varies significantly with the type of study; hence, a low-count ^{111}In SPECT study is far noisier than a high-count ^{99m}Tc liver SPECT study. Therefore, a ring artifact that may be clearly visible in a ^{99m}Tc liver SPECT study may not be visible in a ^{111}In SPECT study. This implies that greater nonuniformities can be tolerated for some types of clinical studies than for others.[1] Rather than worrying about how good the system uniformity must be for different types of studies, it is simpler to correct system nonuniformities to a level that will ensure no visible ring artifacts in even the highest count clinical studies. In general, it has been found that a 30-Mct flood image provides sufficiently good correction of system nonuniformities for all current clinical studies. The application of the "uniformity" correction map typically decreases system nonuniformities to between 1% and 3%. It should be noted that this level of correction may not be adequate for some types of phantom studies; e.g., a Jaszczak phantom with 10 mCi (370 MBq) ^{99m}Tc may give 50–70 Mct over a 30-minute SPECT acquisition, and in such studies, ring artifacts may be noted even though the system uniformity is adequate for clinical studies.

The validity of the "uniformity" correction map can be checked by acquiring a flood image, applying the "uniformity" correction map to it, and then assessing the nonuniformities remaining in the flood image. Young et al.[2] studied the reproducibility of uniformity measurements on SPECT systems from flood images acquired with 2, 5, 10, and 30 Mct. They found that measurements of both integral and differential uniformity showed substantial errors at low pixel counts and gave artificially high estimates relative to values obtained with the 30-Mct data. Unfortunately, it is too time-consuming to acquire a 30-Mct flood image on a daily basis; hence, some compromise must be established to decrease QC time to an acceptable level and still permit a check of the validity of the "uniformity" correction map. One possible solution is to acquire a 7–8 Mct flood image in a 64×64 matrix, correct the flood image with the "uniformity" correction map, and then compress the corrected image into a 32×32 matrix. The counts per pixel are now increased by a factor of 4 and are similar to those that would be achieved with a 30-Mct flood image in a 64×64 matrix. Although this method may underestimate nonuniformities spanning 1–2 pixels, such minor variations are generally eliminated in the filtering process during SPECT reconstruction.

A second requirement of SPECT systems is accurate center of rotation (COR) correction. Fortunately, COR is generally a very stable variable, particularly on modern SPECT systems. Changes in COR may occur during a major service or recalibration of the detector head or may result from a mechanical problem with the gantry. It should be measured on a weekly basis for each detector head.

Purpose

These procedures are designed for single-, dual-, or triple-head tomographic systems. The following describes the QC procedures that must be performed on a SPECT system on a daily and weekly basis. These procedures perform the following functions:

1. Check for contamination of detector or surrounding areas (daily).
2. Quantitative check of system uniformity (daily).
3. Measurement of COR (weekly).
4. Qualitative check of system linearity and resolution (weekly).

Instrument Specifications

Gamma camera:	Single-/dual-/triple-head SPECT system
Collimator:	Any low-energy collimator
Energy setting:	Background check and ^{99m}Tc procedures—140 keV, 15–20% energy window ^{57}Co procedures—122 keV, 15–20% energy window
Computer system:	Acquisition requirements—SPECT (64 × 64 word mode matrix), static (256 × 256 and 64 × 64 word mode matrices) Processing requirements—measurement of image uniformity and system COR
Additional items:	5–10 mCi (185–370 MBq) ^{57}Co sheet source—solid disk impregnated with ^{57}Co 150–200 µCi (5.55–7.40 MBq) point source of ^{99m}Tc in a volume of 0.1 ml or less PLES or 4-quadrant bar phantoms with 2–4 mm bar spacing (intrinsic measurements) or 4–6 mm bar spacing (extrinsic measurements)

Daily Procedure: Background Check

1. *Single-head system:* Ensure that all nearby sources are shielded, and rotate the detector head to face the floor.
   Dual-/triple-head system: Detector orientation is not critical, because detectors partly self-shield each other from nearby sources of radiation.
2. Set a 15–20% energy window around the 140-keV photopeak of ^{99m}Tc. For each detector head, acquire a 5-minute background image. No hard copy is required at this point.
3. Record the background counts in the QC logbook for that system. Figure 1-11 shows the layout of a typical QC logbook sheet for SPECT.
4. On a standard 40-cm field-of-view system equipped with a low-energy collimator, the 5-minute background count should be in the range of 5–10 kct (normal range should be established for each laboratory).

Single Head SPECT System : _____

	Quality Control for Week beginning :							
Day	Background cts / 5 min	Tc-99m kcps	Energy Spectrum	Acq. Time sec	Integral Unif (%)	Center of Rotation	Resolution Linearity	Initials
Mon								
Day	Background cts / 5 min	Co-57 Source	Energy Spectrum	Acq. Time sec	Integral Uniformity (%)		Collimator	Initials
Tues								
Wed								
Thurs								
Fri								

Dual Head SPECT System : _____

	Quality Control for Week beginning :							
Day	Bkd cts / 5 min head 1 / head 2	Co-57 Source	Energy Spectrum	Acq. Time sec	Int Unif (%) H 1 / H 2	COR H 1 / H 2	Resolution Linearity	Initials
Mon	/		/	/	/	/	/	
Day	Bkd cts / 5 min head 1 / head 2	Co-57 Source	Energy Spectrum	Acq. Time sec	Integral Unif (%) head 1 / head 2		Collimator	Initials
Tues	/		/	/	/			
Wed	/		/	/	/			
Thurs	/		/	/	/			
Fri	/		/	/	/			

Triple Head SPECT System : _____

	Quality Control for Week beginning :							
Day	Bkd cts / 5 min H 1 / H 2 / H 3	Co-57 I.D.	Energy Spectrum	Acq. Time sec	Int Unif (%) H 1 / H 2 / H 3	COR H 1 / H 2 / H 3	Resolution Linearity	Initials
Mon	/ /		/ /	/ /	/ /	/ /	/ /	
Day	Bkd cts / 5 min H 1 / H 2 / H 3	Co-57 I.D.	Energy Spectrum	Acq. Time sec	Integral Unif (%) head 1 / head 2		Collimator	Initials
Tues	/ /		/ /	/ /	/ /			
Wed	/ /		/ /	/ /	/ /			
Thurs	/ /		/ /	/ /	/ /			
Fri	/ /		/ /	/ /	/ /			

Figure 1-11. Sample forms for recording the results of the daily and weekly QC on a SPECT system.

5. If counts are above this level, check the area for unshielded sources and repeat the measurement. On a single-head system, rotate the detector head to face up in case the floor is contaminated. Record the 5-minute background image on computer (64 × 64 matrix). Discrete areas of activity on the background image are generally caused by contamination of either the collimator or the crystal. If background counts are still high, repeat the measurement with a different collimator. This should determine whether the contamination is on the crystal or the collimator.

6. If contamination is present, check the energy spectrum to identify the radioisotope. Decontaminate the appropriate areas with a suitable radioactive decontaminant, and repeat the background check until it is within normal limits.

7. If the contamination cannot be removed or the cause of the high background counts is unclear, it may be necessary to contact the medical physicist, the service engineer, or the radiation safety officer to assist in evaluating the problem.

Procedure: System Calibration

Many manufacturers require that some type of energy calibration be performed on a daily or weekly basis. This calibration may be internal to the system itself and require no external radiation source, or it may require removal of the collimator for intrinsic measurement with ^{99m}Tc or ^{57}Co point sources. Because of the various methods used by manufacturers, no attempt is made here to describe these procedures, and the manufacturer's instructions should be followed. These calibrations should always be performed before checking the accuracy of the photopeak setting or proceeding with any measurement of uniformity or resolution.

Daily Procedure: Image Uniformity

1. *Single-Head System:* Place a ^{57}Co sheet source on the collimator, as shown in Figure 1-2.
   Dual-Head System: For opposing dual-head detector systems, bring both detectors as close together as possible. Place a ^{57}Co sheet source on the lower detector head, as shown in Figure 1-3.
   Triple-Head System: Each detector head will have to be evaluated separately as if it were a single-head system.

2. Ensure that the count rate does not exceed 20 kcps per detector head (*Note:* On some multidetector systems, the same electronic systems are used to process events from all heads. In such cases, either turn off the detectors not being evaluated or limit the combined count rate from the detectors to less than 20 kcps). For a 40-cm field-of-view system, optimum activities are 5 mCi (185 MBq) ^{57}Co for an all-purpose collimator and 10 mCi (370 MBq) ^{57}Co for a high- or ultrahigh-resolution collimator.

3. Check the energy spectrum, and ensure that a 15–20% energy window is peaked on the main photopeak at 122 keV. *Note:* A shift of more than 1 or 2 keV in photopeak location often indicates a system malfunction.

4. When the system is peaked, acquire a static acquisition on computer (64 × 64 word mode matrix). Total counts acquired should be 7–8 Mct per detector. The flood images should be acquired without uniformity correction.

5. Apply a 9-point smooth to the flood image, and compress the smoothed image into a 32 × 32 matrix to improve count statistics. This increases the counts per pixel by a factor of 4 and gives similar count statistics to those achieved with a 30-Mct flood in a 64 × 64 matrix.

6. Measure integral and differential uniformity for the uncorrected 32 × 32 matrix image. If the computer system does not have any software for calculation of uniformity, follow steps a–c for measurement of integral uniformity:
   a. Draw an ROI to fit inside the uniformity image, as shown in Figure 1-7. Use a circular ROI for circular field-of-view systems and a box ROI for rectangular field-of-view systems. Irregular or freehand ROIs should be used for rectangular field-of-view systems with clipped corners.
   b. Determine the minimum and maximum counts inside the ROI.
   c. Compute the integral uniformity (IU) from the following equation:

$$IU = \frac{\text{Maximum count} - \text{Minimum count}}{\text{Maximum count} + \text{Minimum count}} \times 100\%$$

7. Apply uniformity correction to the original flood image, and repeat steps 5 and 6 for the corrected image.
8. Record the acquisition time and the uniformity of the uncorrected and corrected flood images in the QC logbook (see Fig. 1-11). Visually inspect both the uncorrected and the corrected images, and note the integral and differential uniformity values. Integral uniformity should be within ±1% of the previous value and should be less than 5% over the useful field of view. Differential uniformity (if measured) should be less than 3%.
9. Place the appropriate sticker on a hard copy of the QC results (image and ROI analysis). The sticker should be dated and initialed by the technologist who performed the quality control. Three different types of stickers are available, as shown in Figure 1-4. This method requires the technologist to review the hard copy, and it ensures accountability for decisions taken with respect to image quality.
10. If any problems are noticed during the daily QC procedure, contact the support personnel (service engineer, physicist, etc.) for assistance in resolving the problem.

Weekly Procedure: System Center of Rotation

1. Tape a 150–200 µCi (5.55–7.40 MBq) ^{99m}Tc point source to the end of the SPECT imaging table, as shown in Figure 1-12. *Note:* The point source must be clear of the table. Do not place the point source on the table, because table attenuation at 90° and 270° may corrupt the COR measurement.
2. The position of the point source in the field of view is not critical. However, it must be positioned so that it stays within the field of view at all angles of rotation. If the manufacturer requires a zoomed acquisition for the COR study, carefully check that the point source is within the zoomed field of view at all angles.
3. Set the detector head to a scan radius of 20 cm. For a single- or a dual-head system with head tilt, use a bubble level to check that the detector head is level.
4. Check that the point source is secure and unlikely to shift during acquisition (a common cause of apparent COR changes!) and that the gantry can rotate around the point source without touching anything.
5. Set up the SPECT acquisition. Many manufacturers have a predefined protocol for the COR acquisition. If none is available, use the following acquisition variables: 128 × 128 word mode matrix, 60–64 views, 5 seconds per view. If clinical studies routinely use a noncircular orbit pattern (e.g., body contouring, elliptical, peanut orbit), then the COR study should be acquired using a similar orbit. Following acquisition, the data should be corrected

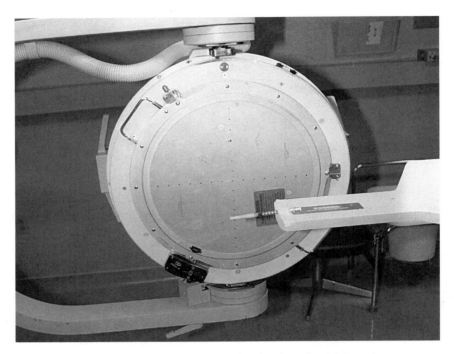

Figure 1-12. Point source taped to headrest for COR study.

for COR shifts introduced by the type of orbit and then analyzed as for a conventional COR study.

6. Analyze the COR study using the software supplied by the manufacturer. This software should show the variations in the COR value as a function of image number or angle (Fig. 1-13). Note that it takes 2 opposing images (e.g., 6° and 186°) to calculate a single COR value. Hence, a 60-image study yields 30 estimates of COR. The software should also show any apparent changes in the y position of the point source with rotation (Fig. 1-14).

7. Check that the COR does not vary by more than 0.5 pixels over 360° (this corresponds to about 1–2 mm for a 40-cm field-of-view system) and lies within 0.5 pixels of the previous value. The absolute value for the COR should be in the range of 63–66 pixels.

8. Check that the y center of mass of the point source does not vary by more than 1 pixel over 360°.

9. If any problems are noticed during the COR procedure, contact the support personnel (service engineer, physicist, etc.) for assistance in resolving the problem.

Weekly Procedure: System Linearity/Resolution

Acquisition: Single-Head/Triple-Head System

1. Remove the collimator, and rotate the detector head so that it faces up. If required by the manufacturer, place a lead masking ring over the exposed crystal, as shown in Figure 1-5. This is designed to shield the edges of the crystal, thereby eliminating "edge packing" artifacts.

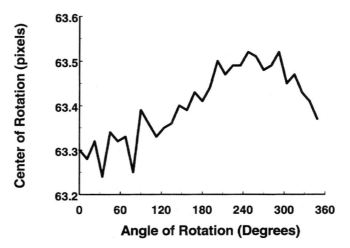

Figure 1-13. Example of a COR curve showing variation of approximately 1/4 pixel (1.0 mm) over 360°.

2. Place a PLES bar phantom on top of the detector head, as shown in Figure 1-8. The bar phantom should have 3-mm wide lead bars with 3-mm spacing between them.
3. The bar phantom should be oriented at an angle of 45° between the x- and y-axis of the detector. In this way, a single image provides adequate assessment of both x and y linearity. If the bar phantom does not completely cover the crystal face, place lead sheets over any region of exposed crystal (see Fig. 1-8).
4. Tape the 150–200 μCi (5.55–7.40 MBq) ^{99m}Tc point source to a plastic rod, and attach the rod to an IV pole. *Note:* If the point source is in a syringe with a needle attached, it should not be oriented with the needle pointing down, because the needle then can act as a collimator and introduce an artifactual cold ring into the image.
5. The point source should be positioned over the center of the PLES phantom at a distance of at least 4 times the field of view (e.g., at 200 cm for a 50-cm field-of-view gamma camera).
6. Ensure that the count rate does not exceed 20 kcps. If necessary, increase the source-to-detector distance to decrease the count rate to an acceptable level (less than 20 kcps).

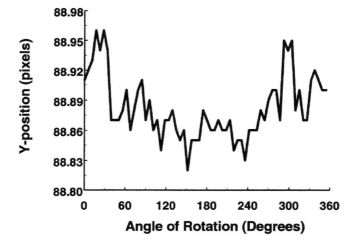

Figure 1-14. Example of the y movement of a point source during a COR study.

7. Acquire a static acquisition on computer (256 × 256 word mode matrix). Total counts acquired should be 3 Mct for a 30–40 cm field-of-view system and 4–5 Mct for a 50–60 cm field-of-view system. For a triple-head system, where gantry geometry permits intrinsic measurement, it will be necessary to repeat these steps for each detector head.

Acquisition: Dual-Head/Triple-Head Systems

Measurement of intrinsic resolution is more of a problem to perform on many multihead systems. Hence, the following procedure has been designed for extrinsic measurement of linearity/resolution.

1. Place a PLES or 4-quadrant bar phantom between the ^{57}Co sheet source and the collimator, as shown in Figure 1-9. The PLES phantom should have 5-mm wide lead bars with 5-mm spacing between them. The 4-quadrant bar phantom should have lead bars 4–6 mm wide.
2. On dual-head systems, if 2 bar phantoms are available, it is possible to acquire simultaneously images of both phantoms using the setup shown in Figure 1-10. In this arrangement, foam blocks are placed between the ^{57}Co sheet source and the bar phantoms. The detector heads are brought together until they lightly compress the bar phantoms.
3. The bar phantoms should be oriented along the x- or y-axis of the detector.
4. Acquire static acquisitions on computer (256 × 256 word mode matrix). Total counts acquired should be 3 Mct per detector for a 30–40 cm field-of-view system and 4–5 Mct per detector for a 50–60 cm field-of-view system.
5. Following acquisition, rotate the bar phantom(s) by 90°, and repeat step 4.

Image Review

1. Obtain a hard copy of the bar phantom image on video or laser imager.
2. Orient the hard copy so that the bar phantom image is viewed at an angle of 70°–90° to the eye. Check that the images of the bars are straight (good linearity).
3. Record in the QC logbook whether the linearity and resolution are acceptable (see Fig. 1-11). Place the appropriate sticker (see Fig. 1-4) on the QC hard copy.
4. If any problems are noticed during the measurement of system linearity, contact the support personnel (service engineer, physicist, etc.) for assistance in resolving the problem.

Interpretation

Uniformity

A large number of factors can contribute to nonuniformities in the flood images. These include defects or cracks in the collimator; damage to the crystal (cracks, hydration, etc.); noisy, defective, or out-of-tune photomultiplier tubes; failure of the preamplifiers or other electronic components of the pulse arithmetic circuitry; defects in the analog formatter; defective ADCs in the computer; corruption of the energy, linearity, or uniformity correction maps; and problems with the film processor. Uniformity is the most important variable of gamma camera performance, particularly for tomographic systems, because nonuniformities can lead to the creation of ring artifacts in the reconstructed data. Quantitative analysis of image uniformity is essential because nonuniformities of 10–15% are difficult to perceive by a visual inspection of the hard copy.[3] Most modern SPECT systems achieve integral uniformities of 5–7% in the uncorrected flood images. These values decrease to less than 5% in the uniformity-corrected image. Values of differential uniformity are generally less than 5% in the uncorrected images and should be less than 3% in the corrected images. If the corrected flood image shows values for integral and differential uniformity that are equal to or higher than the uncorrected flood image, the correction map needs to be updated. In our experience, differential uniformity should be kept at 3% or less to ensure artifact-free clinical studies. In multihead systems, higher levels of nonuniformities can be tolerated *if* each detector performs a 360° orbit, thereby averaging out the nonuniformities over the different detector heads.

Center of Rotation

Accurate COR is important for high-quality tomographic studies. Errors in COR of as little as 0.5 pixel in a 128 matrix can lead to degradation in image quality.[4] If a significant change in COR is noted (greater than 0.5 pixels), the COR study should be repeated to confirm that the change was not due to movement of the point source or the imaging table during acquisition. Check also that the COR study was not inadvertently "corrected" for COR variations. Theoretically, the COR should be independent of the collimator. However, a poorly manufactured collimator may have considerable variation in COR across its surface. These variations cannot be corrected for by the standard COR correction method and are not apparent from inspection of planar image quality.

Variations in the y position of the point source during rotation may be due to a failure to level the detector head before acquisition, or it may be due to gantry misalignment. For a tomographic acquisition on a single-head system, the gantry is usually set to 0°, and the detector head is leveled before an acquisition. This assumes that the axis of rotation of the detector head is horizontal. This axis of rotation is determined by the alignment of the gantry. Misalignment of the gantry can be caused by several things. In many older SPECT systems, sagging of the detector arms can occur. This is particularly true in cantilevered systems, as compared with counterbalanced systems. The gantry itself may not be level on the floor, either because of incorrect shimming of the gantry or irregularities in the surface of the floor. Whatever the cause, the consequences are that leveling the detector head results in data being acquired obliquely rather than perpendicular to the axis of rotation. Many of the multihead systems are self-aligned (no head tilt allowed) and should show little or no y shift of the point source with rotation.

Linearity

When viewed at an angle, the PLES image should show straight lines, at most with some distortion at the edges. Wavy lines generally indicate poor linearity correction, which also should be evident as an increase in the measured values of integral and differential uniformity.

Additional Notes

^{57}Co sheet sources are often contaminated with small amounts of ^{58}Co and ^{56}Co. These two isotopes have short half-lives (77.3 and 71 days, respectively) compared with that of ^{57}Co, but they emit high-energy gamma rays (greater than 500 keV). Some gamma cameras are particularly sensitive to these high-energy gamma rays and, consequently, may show nonuniformities in the flood images.[5] The impact of these high-energy gamma rays can be minimized by raising the sheet source 10–15 cm off the collimator face and/or by using a medium- or high-energy collimator. These effects diminish with time and are usually insignificant by 6–8 months after the date of manufacture.

Additional evaluation of uniformity, over and above that performed on a daily basis, is not required for most SPECT systems. Some manufacturers recommend the acquisition of a new uniformity correction map on a weekly or monthly basis, irrespective of system performance. The decision to acquire a new correction map should be based on the measured values of system uniformity rather than on a fixed schedule. Daily measurement of system uniformity allows this decision to be based on measured values of integral or differential uniformity rather than on a fixed time schedule. This can result in significant savings in the time spent on performing QC, because many modern systems have good stability. Hence, it may be necessary only to upgrade the correction maps every few months rather than weekly.

References

1. O'Connor MK, Vermeersch C. Critical examination of the uniformity requirements for single-photon emission computed tomography. Med Phys 1991; 18: 190–197.
2. Young KC, Kouris K, Awdeh M, Abdel-Dayem HM. Reproducibility and action levels for gamma camera uniformity. Nucl Med Commun 1990; 11: 95–101.
3. Cohen G, Kereiakes JG, Padikal TN, Ashare AB, Saenger EL. Quantitative assessment of field uniformity for gamma cameras. Radiology 1976; 118: 197–200.
4. Cerqueira MD, Matsuoka D, Ritchie JL, Harp GD. The influence of collimators on SPECT center of rotation measurements: artifact generation and acceptance testing. J Nucl Med 1988; 29: 1393–1397.
5. Cranage RW, Peake JC. The effect of high energy impurities on measurements of gamma-camera resolution and uniformity using ^{57}Co flood sources (letter to the editor). Br J Radiol 1979; 52: 81–82.

Special Gamma Camera Quality Control Procedures

Introduction

This section describes a number of procedures that are performed monthly or annually on planar and SPECT equipment. Most of these require additional equipment, some of which is commercially available or can be easily manufactured by a hospital engineering department. The following procedures are described next:

1. Measurement of intrinsic resolution
2. Measurement of multiple window spatial registration
3. Check of whole-body uniformity
4. Measurement of rotational uniformity (SPECT)
5. Measurement of tomographic resolution (SPECT)

Some of these procedures require care and attention to detail for optimum results and, thus, are performed best by a physicist or an experienced technologist.

Procedure: Intrinsic Resolution

The spatial resolution of a gamma camera can be measured using either intrinsic or extrinsic techniques; each has its own advantages and disadvantages. Intrinsic measurements involve removal of the collimator, with the attendant risk to the sodium iodide crystal. However, extrinsic measurements may show moiré patterns that are due to interplay of the bar pattern and the lead septa of the collimator.[1,2] Furthermore, small changes in intrinsic resolution may not be detected extrinsically. In considering intrinsic test phantoms, many (such as the BRH,[3] PLES,[4] and orthogonal hole phantom[5]) are designed to give a qualitative image of intrinsic resolution. Quantitative measurements can be obtained with the National Electrical Manufacturers Association (NEMA) phantom[6]; however, this requires very precise alignment of the phantom along the x- and y-axes of the gamma camera to permit accurate estimation of intrinsic resolution. The line resolution pattern (LRP) is designed to be used with or without computer analysis and can provide quantitative estimates of intrinsic resolution without the need for precise alignment of the LRP along the x- and y-axes of the gamma camera.[7]

Principle

The design considerations for the LRP were that it should allow (1) visual determination of intrinsic resolution to an accuracy of 0.5 mm in both x and y directions and (2) determination of intrinsic full width at half maximum (FWHM) and tenth maximum (FWTM) by NEMA technique.[7] A schematic of the LRP is shown in Figure 1-15. The

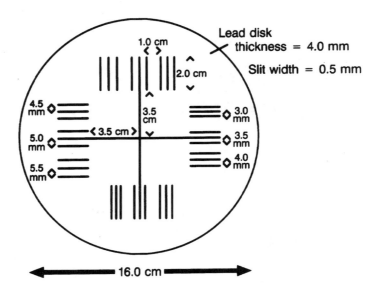

Figure 1-15. Schematic drawing of the LRP phantom.

LRP was designed so that the slit width of 0.5 mm was very much less than gamma camera intrinsic resolution. Under these circumstances, two adjacent slits can be only resolved if the distance between them is greater than the intrinsic resolution of the gamma camera. The LRP is designed with groups of 3 slits whose separation ranges from 3.0 to 5.5 mm in 0.5-mm increments. Thus, a visual inspection of the LRP image allows an estimation of intrinsic resolution to within 0.5 mm. If a more accurate measurement is required, the LRP needs to be positioned precisely, with the long slits aligned with the x- and y-axis of the gamma camera. Quantitative analysis of the LRP image, then, can be performed on computer by obtaining line profiles of the 2 central cross lines and measuring the profile FWHM and FWTM by the NEMA nearest neighboring technique.[6] This analysis yields results in pixels. To convert these to millimeters requires knowledge of the appropriate pixel-to-millimeter calibration factor for the computer acquisition. This factor may be available on the computer, or it can be calculated by measuring the distance in pixels between the 4 corner points of the LRP. These points are 10 cm apart horizontally and vertically.

Instrument Specifications

Gamma camera:	Any planar or SPECT system
Collimator:	No collimator—intrinsic measurement
Energy setting:	140 keV, 15–20% energy window
Analog formatter:	70 mm (9 on 1) format, 8 × 10 film
Computer system:	Acquisition requirements—static (256 × 256 matrix) with zoom of 2–3
	Processing requirements—none
Additional items:	^{99m}Tc point source (2 mCi [74 MBq]) in a volume of 0.1 ml or less
	LRP—This is a 4-mm thick lead disk with very fine slits cut into it. Several commercial companies will cut the pat-

tern shown in Figure 1-15, using high-power water jets (e.g., Jet Edge Ltd.; Minneapolis, MN).

Lead sheets or lead apron to cover exposed crystal

Frequency

This procedure should be performed on a monthly basis.

Method

1. Remove the collimator, and if necessary, position the masking ring on top of the crystal.
2. Place the LRP in the center of the field of view, as shown in Figure 1-16.
3. Mask off exposed crystal with a lead apron and lead sheets (see Fig. 1-16).
4. Tape a 2-mCi (74 MBq) ^{99m}Tc point source to a plastic rod, and attach the rod to an IV stand. Next, the point source should be positioned over the gamma camera at a minimum distance of 50 cm from the crystal face.
5. Check carefully that the point source is directly over the center of the LRP and not displaced to one side.
6. Set a 15–20% energy window, and check that the photopeak is peaked on ^{99m}Tc.
7. Set the zoom factor to 2–3 on the gamma camera or computer (the LRP should fill the field of view).
8. Acquire a static image for 1 Mct on analog formatter and/or on computer (256 × 256 matrix).

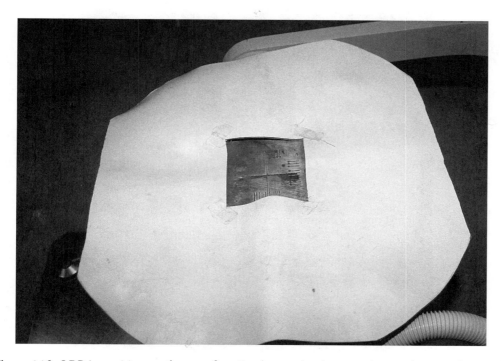

Figure 1-16. LRP in position on detector face. Lead apron has been used to mask areas of exposed crystal.

9. Record the minimum line spacing visible in both the x and y directions. This line spacing should be within 0.5 mm of the system intrinsic resolution.

Interpretation

The LRP is not sensitive to variations in orientation; hence, it does not require precise positioning along x- or y-axis of the detector. Figure 1-17 shows an example of a 1-Mct image of the LRP on a system with a stated intrinsic resolution of 3.3 mm. The 3.5-mm slits are just visible in both x and y directions. The main disadvantage of the LRP is that it measures resolution over only a small portion of the field of view. For this reason it should be used in conjunction with a test pattern (e.g., PLES phantom) that provides some indication of resolution or linearity over the entire field of view.

Procedure: Multiple Window Spatial Registration

Most modern gamma cameras have two or three energy analyzers to permit efficient imaging of multipeak isotopes such as ^{67}Ga. In most clinical studies involving multipeak imaging, the counts from these 2 or 3 energy analyzers are summed to form a composite image. Clearly, it is important that images produced from the different energy analyzers are directly superimposible to avoid loss of image contrast and resolution.

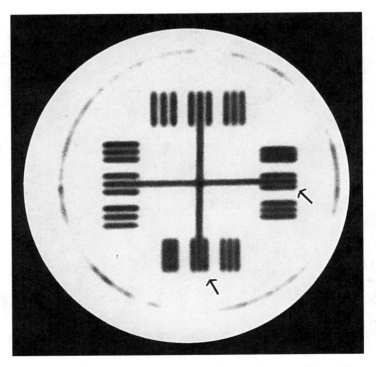

Figure 1-17. Image of the LRP phantom showing the resolution of the 3.5-mm line spacing (arrows) in both x and y directions.

Spatial misregistration can occur by at least two possible mechanisms. Chapman et al.[8] have shown that if the x and y gains from each energy analyzer are not identical, it is possible that an image of a source acquired at one energy level will not directly superimpose on an image of the same source acquired through a different energy analyzer adjusted for a second energy level. The intrinsic properties of a gamma camera are such that the calculation of the x and y positional signals for a gamma ray is energy dependent. All gamma cameras use some type of normalization circuitry to eliminate this energy dependence. Any drift in this normalization circuitry could cause inaccuracies in spatial registration between multiple windows.

Principle

The NEMA protocol for the measurement of multiple window spatial registration (MWSR) is based on the assumption that errors in image registration are minimal in the center of the field of view and become larger as one moves toward the edges of the field of view. A previous study has shown that this assumption is not valid, particularly in modern gamma cameras with linearity correction.[9] Hence, the MWSR protocol used in our laboratory expands on that proposed by NEMA and uses 9 collimated point sources. These sources are collimated using lead holders, as shown in Figure 1-18. Four sources are placed at the 90% of the useful field of view (UFOV), 4 more are placed midway between the 90% UFOV and the center of the crystal, and 1 is placed at the center. Separate images of these 9 sources are acquired at 93 keV and at 296 keV. The 93-keV image is subtracted from the 296-keV image. The degree of misregistration is determined by visual inspection. If necessary, quantitative analysis of the degree of misregistration can be performed using the NEMA technique.[6]

Instrument Specifications

Gamma camera: Any planar or SPECT system
Collimator: No collimator—intrinsic measurement

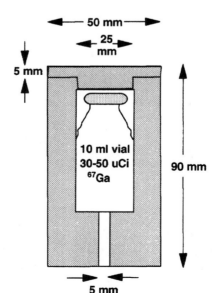

Figure 1-18. Diagram of lead holder used for measurement of MWSR accuracy.

Energy setting: 93 and 296 keV, 15–20% energy window
Analog formatter: 70-mm (9 on 1) format, 8 × 10 film
Computer system: Acquisition requirements—static (256 × 256 matrix)
Processing requirements—image subtraction
Additional items: Nine 10-ml saline vials, each vial should contain 30–50 μCi (1.11–1.85 MBq) ^{67}Ga in 3–5 ml of saline.
Nine lead source holders—the lead holders should have dimensions as specified by NEMA.[6] Holder dimensions are shown in Figure 1-18. (A simple alternative is to obtain lead pots used to supply ^{67}Ga and drill a 5-mm hole in the base.)

Frequency

This procedure should be performed on a monthly basis. *Note:* Whereas many procedure manuals recommend that this test be done on a yearly basis, our experience has been that this variable is very sensitive to any change in photomultiplier gain. Hence, MWSR will be affected by any repairs or updates to the photomultiplier or correction maps on the system.

Method

1. Ensure that the gamma camera is peaked correctly for the 93-keV and 296-keV emissions of ^{67}Ga.
2. For each of the 9 sources, place 30–50 μCi (1.11–1.85 MBq) ^{67}Ga into a 10-ml saline vial, and place the vial into the lead holder.
3. On the gamma camera, set the photopeak to that for the 93-keV peak of ^{67}Ga with a 20% energy window (the energy window for the 296-keV photopeak should be turned off).
4. Remove the collimator, and place the 9 sources on the crystal cover, as shown in Figure 1-19.
5. On computer, acquire a static image with the following variables: 256 × 256 word mode matrix, preset counts = 1 Mct.
6. When the acquisition is finished, change the photopeak setting for the 296-keV peak of ^{67}Ga, and acquire a second static image.
7. Subtract the 93-keV image from the 296-keV image (*Note:* It may be necessary to divide the 93-keV image by a factor of 1.5–2 to prevent oversubtraction). The subtraction image should show a hot doughnut pattern for each source (Fig. 1-20C).
8. Visually inspect the subtracted image for mismatch. Some minor errors in registration will be evident on many systems.
9. Obtain a hard copy of the 93-keV, 296-keV, and subtraction images, and record whether the results were acceptable. For most gamma cameras, the MWSR should be less than 3 mm. Unacceptable results require correction of the energy registration by the service engineer.

Interpretation

The subtraction technique is very sensitive to small errors in registration. Most manufacturers specify MWSR values of 3 mm or less. Figure 1-20 shows examples of the 93-keV and 296-keV images and 2 examples of subtraction images. All points in Figure 1-20C were within 3 mm of each other. The misregistration on the far left side of Figure 1-20D represents a 6-mm misregistration.

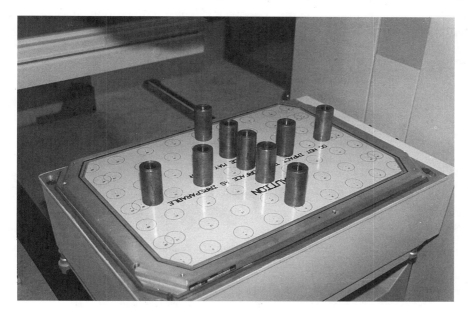

Figure 1-19. Nine lead holders in position on detector face for measurement of MWSR.

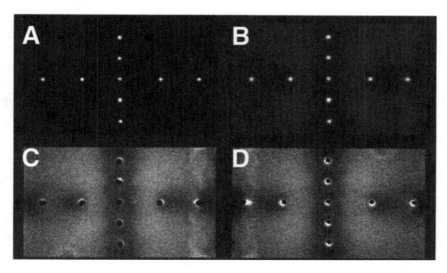

Figure 1-20. Point source images at **(A)** 93 keV and **(B)** 296 keV. Subtraction of A from B results in **(C)** the doughnut appearance shown. **(D)** Misregistration is evident, particularly on the far left side, where the values for MWSR exceeded 6 mm.

Procedure: Whole-Body Uniformity

Whole-body imaging is generally performed with single- or dual-head large field-of-view systems. This procedure checks for smooth and consistent movement of the gantry or imaging table during whole-body acquisition.

Instrument Specifications

Gamma camera:	Single-/dual-head whole-body system
Collimator:	Any type of collimator may be used
Energy setting:	122 keV, 15–20% energy window
Analog formatter:	Whole-body format, 8 × 10 film
Computer system:	Acquisition requirements—whole-body (1,024 × 256 matrix)
	Processing requirements—none
Additional items:	5–10 mCi (185–370 MBq) ^{57}Co sheet source

Frequency

This procedure should be performed on a monthly basis.

Method

1. *Single-Head System:* Orient the detector head to face up. Place a ^{57}Co sheet source on top of the collimator.
   Dual-Head System: Bring the 2 detectors as close together as possible, and place a suitable ^{57}Co sheet source on the lower collimator, as shown in Figure 1-3. *Note:* If the imaging table cannot be removed from the field of view, it may be necessary to perform a second acquisition for the upper detector with the sheet source taped to the detector head.
2. Set a 15–20% energy window around the 122-keV photopeak of ^{57}Co. Check the energy spectrum, and ensure the system is correctly peaked.
3. Set up a whole-body acquisition. Acquisition variables will depend on whether whole-body acquisitions are acquired in continuous mode or as sequential static images. The acquisition mode should be the same as that used for clinical studies. For the continuous mode, set the scan speed at 10 cm/min for a 200-cm scan length. For sequential static images, acquire five images at 4 minutes per image.
4. Whole-body images should be acquired on analog formatter and on computer in a 1,024 × 256 word mode matrix.
5. Results: Check the analog and computer images to ensure that the flood is uniform over the full scan length. Erratic gantry motion will be visible as bands of varying intensity along the length of the whole-body image. Record in the QC logbook whether the whole-body flood images are acceptable.

Interpretation

The whole-body flood images should show the same degree of uniformity as the conventional flood images. Errors in gantry speed or incorrect alignment of sequential static images appear as horizontal bands across the flood image.

Procedure: Rotational Uniformity

On most SPECT systems, the "uniformity" correction map is generated from a flood image acquired with the detector head facing up. It is assumed that this correction map can be applied to images acquired at all angles of rotation. However, in a number of instances, this assumption may not be valid. The photomultiplier tubes in the detector head are heat sensitive; hence, heat generated by the electronics in the head may alter the characteristics of the photomultiplier tubes. If the heat distribution in the head changes as a function of angle, so too can detector uniformity.

Another likely cause of variations in uniformity with angle of rotation is poor optical coupling of a photomultiplier tube to the light guide or crystal. This can cause the tube to decouple slightly at certain angles, leading to a significant change in uniformity with rotation. Photomultiplier tubes are also sensitive to the earth's magnetic field. Their performance characteristics can change with their orientation to the earth's magnetic field, leading to changes in uniformity with rotation. This problem is sometimes seen in older SPECT systems that have inadequate magnetic shielding.

Purpose

This procedure checks for variations in uniformity with rotation. These variations are quantitated and used to determine the suitability of the system for SPECT.

Instrument Specifications

Gamma camera:	Any single- or dual-head SPECT system
Collimator:	Low-energy all-purpose or high-resolution parallel hole collimator
Energy setting:	140 keV, 15–20% energy window
Computer system:	Acquisition requirements—SPECT (64 × 64 word mode matrix)
	Processing requirements—image addition, image filtration, quantitation of image uniformity or ROI analysis
Additional items:	5–10 mCi (185–370 MBq) ^{57}Co sheet source

Frequency

This procedure should be performed every 6 months or after any major repair to the detector head.

Method

1. A ^{57}Co sheet source should be placed on the collimator face and taped to the gamma camera head, as shown in Figure 1-21. (The test can be done with any low-energy parallel hole collimator.)
2. After the sheet source has been taped to the head, check that the detector can be rotated without any slippage of the sheet source relative to the collimator. For detectors with pressure-sensitive panels, it may be necessary to raise the sheet source off the collimator face (by placing supports at the side of the detector) or to inactivate the pressure-sensitive devices.
3. Peak the gamma camera using a 20% energy window centered on the 122-keV emissions of ^{57}Co.

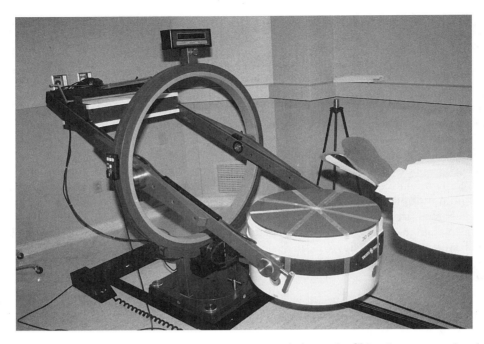

Figure 1-21. Measurement of rotational uniformity. A lightweight ^{57}Co sheet source has been securely taped to the collimator face.

4. The gamma camera/computer system should be set for a SPECT acquisition. Images should be acquired into a 64 × 64 word mode matrix using a step and shoot mode and a circular orbit.

5. The total counts acquired in the study should be 240–300 Mct. These data can be acquired using either a large number of frames with a short time per frame or a small number of frames with a long time per frame. In many cases, the computer acquisition software indicates the minimum number of frames allowed or the maximum time per frame. Once the count rate for the sheet source is known, the number of frames to acquire and the time per frame can be determined with the following equation:

$$300,000 \text{ kct} = \text{No. frames} \times \text{time per frame (sec)} \times \text{count rate (kct/sec)}$$

For example, if the sheet source gives a count rate of 10 kct/sec and 60 frames are acquired, the time per frame should be set to 300,000/(60 × 10) = 5,000 sec = 8.3 min.

6. Because of the long acquisition time, this study should be performed overnight. The count rate, time per frame, and number of frames acquired should be recorded.

7. For studies performed on multihead systems, perform separate acquisitions for each detector head.

8. Following acquisition, sum the raw data to give 8–10 output images. Play back these images in cine mode, adjusting the contrast, to check for gross variations in uniformity with rotation.

9. Quantitative analysis requires measurement of image uniformity. Some manufacturers provide software for the measurement of integral and differential uniformity. If no suitable software exists, follow steps a–f to measure integral uniformity.

a. Smooth each image with a standard 9-point smooth.

b. On each image, draw an ROI to fit inside the uniformity image, as shown in Figure 1-7. Use a circular ROI for circular field-of-view systems and a box ROI for rectangular field-of-view systems. Irregular or freehand ROIs should be used for rectangular field-of-view systems with clipped corners.

c. Determine the minimum and maximum count inside the ROI.

d. Compute the IU from the following equation:

$$IU = \frac{\text{Maximum count} - \text{Minimum count}}{\text{Maximum count} + \text{Minimum count}} \times 100\%$$

e. Repeat the preceding process for all 8–10 images. Note the maximum change in uniformity over the 360° rotation.

f. Using the same ROI, generate a time–activity curve of total counts over the 8–10 images. Record the maximum change in counts (sensitivity) over 360°.

10. Results: Integral uniformity should not vary by more than 2% over the 360° rotation. Sensitivity should not vary by more than 1% over the 360° rotation.

Interpretation

Virtually all systems show some minor changes in uniformity with rotation. Hence, quantitative analysis is important to ensure that such minor changes are interpreted correctly. A change localized to 1 or 2 photomultiplier tubes may indicate a problem with the optical coupling of these tubes. Figure 1-22 shows an example of the analysis of a rotational uniformity study.

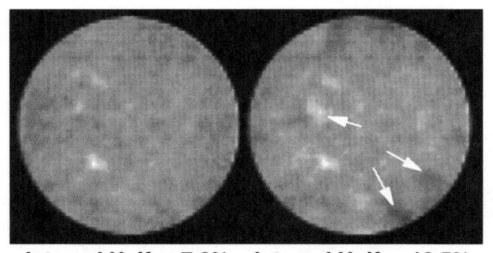

Integral Unif. = 7.6% Integral Unif. = 10.5%

Figure 1-22. Selected images from a rotational uniformity study at 150° and 330°. Focal changes are evident in multiple locations over the field of view (arrows). A 3% change in integral uniformity occurred between the 2 images; this was due to inadequate magnetic shielding of the photomultiplier tubes.

Procedure: Tomographic Resolution

Gamma camera performance is routinely monitored by means of the daily and weekly QC procedures that are performed on all SPECT systems. However, because of the complexity of modern SPECT systems, it is important to perform a more comprehensive evaluation of the system every 6 months. This evaluation should check the accuracy of image uniformity, attenuation correction, spatial resolution, and image contrast. Currently, no recommended guidelines for the evaluation of these variables exist (or have been published). An acceptable way of performing such an evaluation is with a Jaszczak phantom (Data Spectrum Corp., Hillsborough, NC). This is a commonly used phantom in tomographic studies. The phantom should contain a hot or cold rod section and cold spheres—this permits measurement of all the variables listed earlier.

Purpose

This procedure checks the overall resolution and uniformity of a tomographic system using the deluxe version of the Jaszczak phantom. Resolution is determined from the hot or cold rod section of the phantom. Contrast is determined from the cold sphere section, and slice uniformity is determined from the uniform water-filled section of the phantom.

Instrument Specifications

Gamma camera:	Any single- or multihead SPECT system
Collimator:	Low-energy ultrahigh-resolution fan-beam or parallel hole collimators
Energy setting:	140 keV, 15–20% energy window
Computer system:	Acquisition requirements—SPECT (128 × 128 word mode matrix). Processing requirements—SPECT reconstruction software, ROI analysis
Additional items:	Jaszczak phantom (deluxe model with hot or cold rods and cold spheres); rods should vary from 4.8 to 12.7 mm in diameter and cold spheres from 9.5 to 31.8 mm

Frequency

This procedure should be performed every 6 months.

Method

Phantom Preparation and Setup

1. Check that the phantom contains the hot or cold rod section and the 6 cold spheres.
2. Fill the phantom with water to within an inch or two of the top. Add 10–15 mCi (370–555 MBq) ^{99m}Tc to the phantom. Mix well, and top up the phantom with water.
3. Place the phantom on the headrest, as shown in Figure 1-23.
4. Use a bubble level to ensure that the phantom is level, and adjust it so that it lies precisely along the axis of rotation of the gamma camera. This step is very important for ensuring optimum image quality in the reconstructed data.

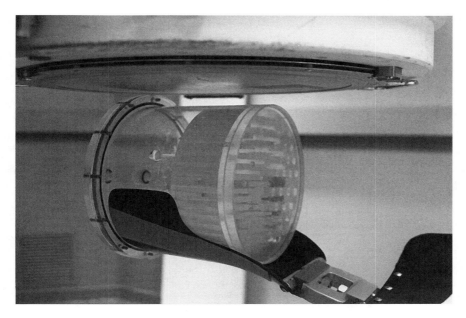

Figure 1-23. Jaszczak phantom secured in position on the headrest of the imaging table. Note the close collimator to phantom separation.

Gamma Camera Acquisition

1. Use the highest resolution collimators available (either high-resolution fan-beam or parallel hole collimators). Check the bubble levels on the detector head(s) to ensure that the heads are level.

2. Adjust the table height until the phantom is at or close to the center of rotation. The detector heads should be able to perform a circular orbit with a separation of 1 cm or less between the collimator surface and the outer rim of the phantom.

3. Set up an acquisition with the following variables: 128 × 128 matrix, 128 views, 30 seconds per view, 360° orbit.

4. Before reconstruction, ensure that uniformity correction and COR correction have been performed or will be performed during the reconstruction process.

5. Data should be reconstructed with little or no smoothing. Reconstruct 1-pixel thick slices through the uniform/cold sphere section of the phantom.

6. Apply attenuation correction using an attenuation coefficient of about 0.12^{-1} cm.

7. Repeat steps 4 and 5 using a slice thickness of 15–20 pixels. The 15–20 pixel thick band should be centered over the rod section of the phantom. *Note:* Because of the high count density in the reconstructed images, the 30-Mct correction map may not correct the image data adequately and some minor ring artifacts may be visible. Whenever possible, a high-count uniformity correction map (120 Mct) should be acquired and used to correct the phantom study.

8. For multidetector systems, reconstruct the data from each detector separately, and check that comparable results are obtained with each detector. The combined results of all detectors should be superior to those of individual detectors.

Data Analysis

1. Resolution: From the 15–20 pixel thick slice through the rod section, record how many segments are completely resolved. Compare the image with that obtained during acceptance testing to verify consistent tomographic resolution.
2. Uniformity: Check the 1-pixel thick slices in the uniform section of the phantom for the presence of ring artifacts.
3. Image Contrast: For each of the cold spheres, determine the transaxial slice that best resolves the sphere and measure the minimum pixel count inside the sphere (Cmin). Now, select a transaxial slice above or below the level of the spheres, and determine the average pixel counts in a uniform section corresponding to the approximate location of the spheres (Cavg). Cold sphere contrast is defined as

$$100 \times \frac{(\text{Cavg} - \text{Cmin})}{(\text{Cavg} + \text{Cmin})}$$

4. Obtain a hard copy of the 15–20 pixel thick slice and slices through the uniform and cold sphere sections of the phantom. Compare the results with those obtained during acceptance testing for any deterioration in system performance.

Interpretation

A single-head SPECT system equipped with a high-resolution collimator should be able to resolve 8–9 mm rods (Fig. 1-24A). Multihead systems equipped with ultrahigh-resolution collimators should be able to resolve 6–7 mm rods. All the cold spheres should be resolved by both single- and multihead systems. Cold sphere contrast is system dependent and should be compared with results obtained during acceptance testing of the system. Transaxial slices through the uniform section of the phantom should show good uniformity, with no ring artifacts (Fig. 1-24B). *Note:* If a 30-Mct uniformity correction map is used to correct the data, some faint ring artifacts may be seen in the reconstructed slices, particularly on single-head systems. These can be eliminated with a 120-Mct correction map.

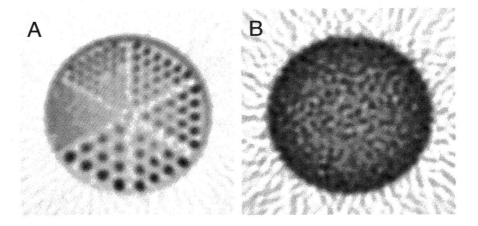

Figure 1-24. (**A**) A 15-pixel thick transaxial slice through the hot rod section of a Jaszczak phantom (model DLX/P). (**B**) A 1-pixel thick slice through the water-filled section. Data obtained from a single-head SPECT system with a low-energy high-resolution collimator.

References

1. Bonte FJ, Graham KD, Dowdey JE. Image aberrations produced by multichannel collimators for a scintillation camera. Radiology 1971; 98: 329–334.
2. Yeh E-L. Distortion of bar-phantom image by collimator. J Nucl Med 1979; 20: 260–261.
3. Paras P, Hine GJ, Adams R. BRH test pattern for the evaluation of gamma-camera performance. J Nucl Med 1981; 22: 468–470.
4. Quality control for scintillation cameras. U.S. Dept. of Health, Education and Welfare. HEW Publications FDA 76-8046, 1976.
5. Hine GJ. An ortho test pattern for quality assurance of gamma cameras. Nuclear Associates Pamphlet No. 265K, Washington D.C.
6. Performance measurements of scintillation cameras, Standard Publication/Nu 1-1994. National Electrical Manufacturers Association, Washington, D.C., 1994.
7. O'Connor MK, Oswald WM. The line resolution pattern: a new intrinsic resolution test pattern for nuclear medicine. J Nucl Med 1988; 29: 1856–1859.
8. Chapman DR, Garcia EV, Waxman AD. Misalignment of multiple photopeak analyzer outputs: effects on imaging. Concise communication. J Nucl Med 1980; 21: 872–874.
9. Kelly BJ, O'Connor MK. Multiple window spatial registration: failure of the NEMA standard to adequately quantitate image misregistration with gallium-67. J Nucl Med Tech 1990; 18: 92–95.

Uptake Probe Quality Control

Introduction

An uptake probe generally consists of a detector (usually a sodium iodide crystal coupled to a single photomultiplier tube), a flat field collimator, and a spectrometer. In the 1960s and 1970s, uptake probes were used extensively for studies of kidney and thyroid function. However, with the widespread availability of gamma cameras, their use is now limited almost exclusively to measurement of thyroid function.

Daily Procedure: System Background and Sensitivity

This procedure checks two aspects of the performance of the uptake probe. It measures room background to ensure that there is no contamination of either the probe or patient couch, and it counts a known standard to ensure that no drift or deterioration in system performance has occurred.

Instrument Specifications

Uptake probe:	This is usually a 2″ × 2″ sodium iodide crystal and photo-multiplier tube assembly.
Collimator:	Flat field collimator; the collimator should meet the International Atomic Energy Agency (IAEA) specifications.[1]
Energy setting:	^{131}I—364 KeV, 20–30% energy window, or the system can be set for integral counting with the lower discriminator set at 300 keV.
Additional items:	Neck phantom—15 cm in diameter and 15 cm in height with hole for standard. Distance from edge of phantom to surface of hole should be 0.5 cm. This phantom should conform to standards proposed by the IAEA.[1]
	5–10 μCi (185–370 kBq) ^{133}Ba standard

Method

1. If the machine was turned off, allow 0.5–1.0 hour for the system to stabilize after being switched on.
2. Record in a logbook the high-voltage setting, photopeak setting, and energy window (or the upper and lower discriminator settings).
3. Position the uptake probe over the patient couch normally used for uptake studies. Acquire a background count for 1 minute. This should be in the range of 50–100 counts. The exact value will depend on the energy window, crystal size, and collimator.

4. Place the ^{133}Ba standard inside the neck phantom, and place the phantom on the patient couch underneath the probe.

5. The uptake probe should be positioned as shown in Figure 1-25, with a probe-to-neck distance of about 25 cm. This distance should be set using the measurement rod (or other similar measuring device) attached to the side of the collimator and should be fixed for *all* uptake studies (both QC and patient).

6. Acquire a 3-minute count over the phantom. Record the counts in the logbook. The standard counts will generally be in the range of 1,000–2,000 counts per minute (cpm)/μCi (27–54 cpm/kBq). Again, the exact value depends on instrument design and settings.

7. Record the counts and compare with previous measurements. The counts should be within 3 standard deviations of the mean count. The mean and standard deviation should be calculated from 10 consecutive daily measurements of the standard.

8. If counts fall outside the expected range, readjust the amplifier gain (high voltage) to ensure that the system is correctly peaked. A change in gain may indicate aging of the photomultiplier tube. A decrease in counts without a change in gain may indicate deterioration in the optical coupling between the crystal and photomultiplier tube.

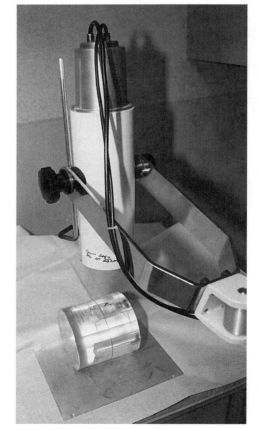

Figure 1-25. Probe positioned over neck phantom containing ^{133}Ba standard.

Reference

1. International Atomic Energy Agency, Vienna 1, Kaerntnerring, Austria. Consultants meeting on the calibration and standardization of thyroid radioiodine uptake measurements, November 28–30, 1960. Br J Radiol 1962; 35: 205–210.

Dose Calibrator Quality Control

Introduction

The dose calibrator is used in nuclear medicine to measure the activity of radiopharmaceuticals before administration to each patient or human research subject. The accuracy of the administered dose depends on the performance of the dose calibrator. In the United States, federal regulations (outlined in 10 CFR 35.50—Possession, Use, Calibration and Check of Dose Calibrator) require that several tests be performed to ensure correct operation of the dose calibrator.[1] These tests check four aspects of the performance of a dose calibrator (i.e., **constancy, accuracy, linearity,** and **geometric dependence**).

Constancy

The constancy check ensures that the dose calibrator gives a consistent reading (±10%) on a daily basis. This check is performed using one of the two reference sources described next.

Accuracy

The accuracy of a dose calibrator can be determined by comparing its reading with the activity of a standard source (with a ±10% error). In the United States, federal regulations require that it be determined with at least two certified reference sources, such as ^{57}Co and ^{137}Cs, whose activities are traceable to the National Institute of Standards and Technology (NIST) and are within 5% of their stated activities.

Linearity

Linearity implies that the dose calibrator read accurately over the entire range of activities used in patients, or in human research subjects. For example, a dose calibrator must be capable of accurately (±10% error) measuring a 30-μCi (1.11-MBq) dose of ^{99m}Tc as well as a 300-mCi (11.1-GBq) dose of ^{131}I.

Geometric Dependence

The measured activity in a dose calibrator varies depending on the volume or configuration of the radionuclide. This variation must be determined and corrections applied for any geometrical error that exceeds 10%.

Tables 1-1 and 1-2 summarize the procedure and record requirements for calibrating a dose calibrator.[1] Table 1-3 lists characteristics and specifications for some suitable reference sources for the calibration of a dose calibrator. ^{137}Cs is similar in photon energy to that of ^{99}Mo, and ^{57}Co has a principal photon energy that is similar to that of ^{99m}Tc. If one uses a dose calibrator just for the measurement of ^{131}I dosages, ^{133}Ba would be a good choice, because it has a photon energy similar to that of ^{131}I.

Table 1-1. Procedure Requirements for the Calibration of Dose Calibrator

Test	Check Source	Frequency	Tolerance	Corrective Action
Constancy	10 µCi (0.37 MBq) ^{226}Ra OR 50–100 µCi (1.85–3.7 MBq) γ-emitter	Beginning of each day of use Adjustment Repair	±10%	Repair or replacement
Accuracy	Two sources (±5% of stated activity) 10 µCi (0.37 MBq) ^{226}Ra 50-100 µCi (1.85–3.7 MBq) γ-emitter At least one source must have photon energy in the range 100–500 keV	Installation Annually Adjustment Repair	±10%	Repair or replacement
Linearity	30 µCi (1.11 MBq) to highest patient or human research subject dose	Installation Quarterly Adjustment Repair	±10%	Arithmetic correction
Geometric dependence	Range and configuration used in clinical practice	Installation Adjustment Repair	±10%	Arithmetic correction

Equipment

Constancy

One of the two reference sources described in Table 1-1 is required.

Accuracy

At least 2 certified reference sources are required. Each reference source should have its activity calibrated to within ±5%, and this calibration should be directly traceable to a standard source at the NIST. Table 1-3 lists possible calibration sources.

Linearity

A ^{99m}Tc source is required with activity equal to or greater than maximum dose administered to a patient or human research subject.

A set of lead-lined tubes (typically 6–8 tubes) is required. These are used to achieve known degrees of attenuation.

Geometric Dependence

30-ml glass vial and 2–20 mCi (74–740 MBq) ^{99m}Tc in a volume of 2 ml
3-ml syringe and 1–10 mCi (37–370 MBq) ^{99m}Tc in a volume of 1 ml

Table 1-2. Record Requirements for the Calibration of Dose Calibrator

	Constancy	Accuracy	Linearity	Geometry
Dose calibrator				
Model No.	✔	✔	✔	✔
Serial No.	✔	✔	✔	✔
Check source				
Identity	✔	✔		
Model No.		✔		
Serial No.		✔		
Activity		✔		
Date of the check	✔	✔	✔	✔
Calculated activity			✔	
Measured activity	✔	✔	✔	✔
				Configuration and activity for each volume
Operator	Initials	Identity	Identity	Identity
Duration of record keeping	3 year	3 year	3 year	Duration of use of the dose calibrator

Table 1-3. Characteristics and Specifications of Reference Sources
for the Calibration of Dose Calibrators

Reference Source	Physical Half-Life	Principal Photon Energy in keV and Abundance (%)	Standard Activity	Minimum Required Activity
^{137}Cs	30 years	662 (85%)	100–250 µCi (3.7–9.3 MBq)	50 µCi (1.85 MBq)
^{60}Co	5.26 years	1,173 (100%) 1,332 (100%)	50–100 µCi (1.85–3.7 MBq)	50 µCi (1.85 MBq)
^{57}Co[a]	270 days	122 (87%)	2–10 mCi (74–370 MBq)	50 µCi (1.85 MBq)
^{226}Ra[a]	1,602 years	186 (4%)	10 µCi (0.37 MBq)	10 µCi (0.37 MBq)
^{133}Ba	7.2 years	356 (69%)	250 µCi (9.3 MBq)	50 µCi (1.85 MBq)

[a]In the United States, these radioisotopes are not subject to NRC licensing; the appropriate state agency should be consulted to determine the requirements for possession of these radioisotopes.

Daily Procedure: Constancy

The constancy check ensures that the dose calibrator can measure a source of constant activity repeatedly within a stated degree of reproducibility over a long period of time. Satisfactory performance of this check indicates that the dose calibrator is operating consistently from day to day. This check should be performed at the beginning of each day of use.[1] This should include weekends if the dose calibrator is used for the measurement of patient dosage. This check should also be performed if the dose calibrator is adjusted or repaired.[1]

Although federal regulations require only one dedicated check source for the constancy testing, one should consider the use of two or more reference sources with different principal photon energies and activities (e.g., ^{57}Co and ^{137}Cs are the two most commonly used check sources for the constancy testing).

Method

1. Assay each reference source using the appropriate dose calibrator setting (i.e., use the ^{137}Cs setting to assay ^{137}Cs).
2. Measure the background activity at the same setting, and subtract it from the measured activity. If an automatic background subtraction circuit is used, confirm that the background was subtracted correctly.
3. For each reference source used, record the net activity (source-background) in the QC logbook for that dose calibrator.
4. Using one of the reference sources (e.g., ^{137}Cs), repeat the preceding procedure for all routinely used radioisotope settings of the dose calibrator (e.g., ^{99m}Tc, ^{201}Tl, ^{111}In), and record the measurements in the QC logbook.

Corrective Actions

1. If the net measured radioactivity of the standard source after decay correction differs by more than ±5% from the expected activity, the person who performs the task should automatically notify the chief technologist, authorized user, or radiation safety officer.
2. If the error exceeds ±10%, the federal regulations state that the dose calibrator must be repaired or replaced.[1]

Yearly Procedure: Accuracy

The purpose of using the dose calibrator is to measure the radioactivity of a radiopharmaceutical drug with a high degree of accuracy. Accuracy means that for a given calibrated reference source, the indicated activity is equal to the radioactivity determined by the NIST or by the supplier, who has compared the reference source to a source that was calibrated by the NIST.[2] The specific requirements for selecting a reference source (i.e., type of radioisotope, amount of calibrated activities, energy levels) are stated in Table 1-1. This test must be performed at the time of installation and on a yearly basis thereafter. It must also be performed after repair or adjustment of the dose calibrator.[1]

Method

1. Assay one of the reference sources by using the appropriate radioisotope setting (i.e., use the ^{57}Co setting to assay ^{57}Co). Allow sufficient time for a stable reading to be obtained.

2. Remove the reference source, and measure background activity. Subtract background from the indicated activity to obtain the net activity. Confirm the proper operation of the automatic background subtract circuit, if it is used.

3. Record the measured activity and the setting used on the dose calibrator (e.g., dial, setting, voltage).

4. Repeat the previous step for a total of 3 independent determinations, and average the activity measured.

5. The average value must be within ±10% of the certified radioactivity of the reference standard after decay corrections.

6. Repeat the preceding steps for at least one other reference source.

7. At the same time that each accuracy test is performed, measure the standard source that is used for the daily constancy test (it need not be a certified reference source) at the setting normally used for that source.

8. Record the settings, reference standard readings, and the respective cross-calibrated readings of the long-lived sources with the accuracy data.

Corrective Actions

1. If the average activity measured does not agree with the certified activity of the reference source within ±5% (mathematically corrected for decay), the person who performed the measurement should notify the chief technologist, authorized user, or radiation safety officer.

2. If the average activity measured does not agree with the certified activity of the reference source within ±10% (mathematically corrected for decay), the dose calibrator needs to be repaired or adjusted according to 10 CFR 35.50.[1]

Quarterly Procedure: Linearity

In the United States, linearity testing is required by the Nuclear Regulatory Commission (NRC) on all dose calibrators at the time of installation and quarterly thereafter. This procedure tests the ability of a dose calibrator to accurately determine activity over a wide range of radioactivity. As stated in the federal regulations,[1] this testing must be performed over a range of radioactivities from 30 µCi (111 kBq) to the highest dose administered to the patient or human research subject, with an acceptable linearity error not exceeding 10%.

In our institution the highest dose administered to a patient for therapeutic purposes is 300 mCi (11.1 GBq) [131]I, and the maximum activity used in the preparation of radiopharmaceutical kits is 600 mCi (22.2 GBq) [99m]Tc. The regulations do not specifically define which radioisotope should be used for the linearity testing. Although the NRC Regulatory Guide 10.8, Revision 2[2] does suggest that ^{99m}Tc should be used as the test source, the question can be raised as to whether it is acceptable to use 300 mCi (11.1 GBq) ^{99m}Tc to perform linearity checks, given a maximum patient therapeutic dose of 300 mCi (11.1 GBq) [131]I. Because of the impracticality of using ^{131}I for linearity evaluation, an adjusted ^{99m}Tc dose can be used to comply with NRC guidelines.[1] We found that an adjusted ^{99m}Tc dose of 430 mCi (15.9 GBq) must be used to replace 300 mCi (11.1 GBq) [131]I for checking the linearity of a dose calibrator.[3]

The two methods for checking the linearity of the dose calibrator are the decay method and the attenuation method. The more accurate one is the decay method,[4] which consists of multiple measurements of the same radionuclide source over an extended time period, typically 2–3 days. The attenuation method uses a series of lead-lined sleeves of varying thickness (Fig. 1-26). These sleeves attenuate the radioactive source to different degrees, thus simulating decay of the source. These two methods are described next.

Decay Method

1. Before performing the linearity check, make sure that the dose calibrator is properly set to zero. Use a reliable and accurate clock or watch to record the time (an error of 10 minutes in the recorded time gives an apparent error in the dose calibrator linearity of 2%).

2. Obtain a ^{99m}Tc source that contains the largest activity routinely administered to a patient or routinely measured in the dose calibrator (e.g., the first elution from a new ^{99}Mo/^{99m}Tc generator).

3. Assay the ^{99m}Tc source in the dose calibrator and subtract background activity to obtain the net radioactivity in mCi (MBq). Record the date, the time, and the measured activity of the ^{99m}Tc source. Repeat this measurement 3 times, and obtain the average value.

4. Repeat this process at 6, 24, 30, 48, 54, 72, and 78 hours thereafter until the activity level of the ^{99m}Tc source has decreased to 30 μCi (111 kBq) or less.

5. Using the 30-hour activity measurement $A_{(30)}$ as a reference point, calculate the predicted activity $A_{(t)}$ at the other specified times (t) using the following decay equation:

$$A_{(t)} = A_{(30)} \times e^{-0.1151\,(t\,-\,30)}$$

6. On semilogarithmic graph paper, label the logarithmic vertical axis in activity (mCi or MBq) and the linear horizontal axis in decay time (hours). At the top of the graph, note the dose calibrator information (i.e., manufacturer, model number, and serial number) and the day and time of the initial assay.

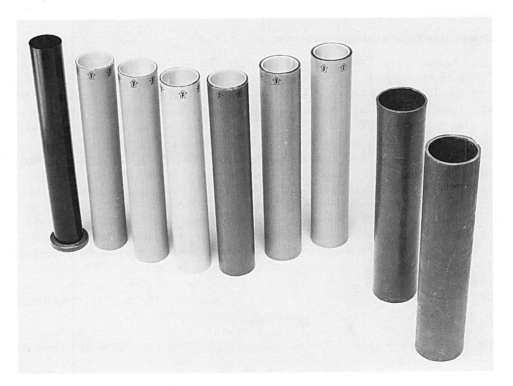

Figure 1-26. Lead sleeve shielding system for dose calibrator linearity testing.

7. Plot the data points and draw a "best fit" straight line through the data points. Figure 1-27 shows an example of a linearity decay graph. The linearity of the dose calibrator is determined by selecting the point that deviates furthest from the best fit line and calculating its deviation according to the following equation:

$$\% \text{ Deviation} = \frac{\text{Measured Activity} - \text{Calculated or Fitted Activity}}{\text{Calculated Activity}} \times 100\%$$

Attenuation Method

The set of lead sleeves should be calibrated before being used. This calibration may be performed by the supplier of the sleeves or as outlined next, using a dose calibrator that has been previously shown to have good linearity.

1. Begin the linearity test as described for the decay method. After making the first assay with the decay method, the lead sleeves can be calibrated as follows: Each measurement must be performed 3 times, and the average value obtained. In addition, the entire calibration must be completed within 6 minutes.
2. The ^{99m}Tc source is placed in the base sleeve, which is not lead lined. Assay the activity of the ^{99m}Tc source in the dose calibrator, and record the results.
3. Put the first lead-lined sleeve (thinnest lining) over the unlined base sleeve, and record the results.
4. Remove lead sleeve 1, and put in lead sleeve 2. Record the measured radioactivity.
5. Repeat this process until all the lead sleeves have been measured.
6. Determine the attenuation (calibration) factors for each lead-lined sleeve by dividing the activity measured in step 1 by the measured activity for the lead sleeve.
7. This procedure needs to be performed only once on a new set of lead sleeves. The lead-lined sleeves may now be used to test a dose calibrator for linearity.
8. Obtain a ^{99m}Tc source that contains the largest activity routinely administered to a patient or human research subject.

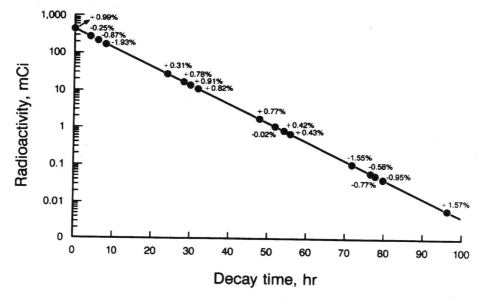

Figure 1-27. Dose calibrator linearity decay graph.

9. Assay the ^{99m}Tc source in the dose calibrator, and subtract the background activity to obtain the net radioactivity in millicuries or megabecquerels. Record the date, time, and measured activity of the ^{99m}Tc source. Repeat this process using each of the lead sleeves. This should be performed as quickly as possible to minimize errors that are due to decay. A maximum of 6 minutes (1% decay) is allowed before decay correction must be applied to the results.

10. Repeat this measurement 3 times, and obtain the average value for each lead sleeve.

11. For each average activity measured, multiply the result by the appropriate calibration factor for each sleeve to obtain the factored activity. See the example in Table 1-4.

12. Add all the products from step 11, and divide the sum by the total number of sleeves to obtain the mean factored activity. The percent deviation for each measurement can then be obtained from the following equation:

$$\% \text{ Deviation} = \frac{\text{Mean Factored Activity} - \text{Factored Activity}}{\text{Mean Factored Activity}} \times 100\%$$

Corrective Actions

1. If the percent deviation exceeds ±5%, the person who performed the measurement should notify the chief technologist, authorized user, or radiation safety officer.

2. If the percent deviation exceeds ±10%, the dose calibrator should be repaired or adjusted. After the repair, the linearity test should be repeated. If the percent deviation still exceeds ±10%, it will be necessary to make a correction table or graph that will allow one to convert from activity measured in the dose calibrator to "true activity."

Table 1-4. Example of Dose Calibrator Linearity Test Report

Tube No	Net Measured Activity (mCi)			Readings Average	× Calibration Factor	= Factored Activity	Percent Error
	1	2	3				
1	61.700	60.800	60.400	60.967	1.000	60.967	-0.36%
2	35.300	34.800	34.500	34.867	1.758	61.296	-0.90%
3	19.300	19.000	18.900	19.067	3.144	59.946	1.32%
4	6.170	6.030	5.990	6.063	10.089	61.173	-0.70%
5	2.590	2.540	2.520	2.550	23.638	60.277	0.78%
6	0.441	0.437	0.434	0.437	140.456	61.426	-1.11%
7	0.131	0.128	0.128	0.129	474.422	61.137	-0.64%
8	0.060	0.060	0.060	0.060	1020.35	61.153	-0.66%
9	0.009	0.009	0.009	0.009	6736.32	59.369	2.27%

Average factored activity = 60.749
Mean + 5% = Upper Limit = 63.787
Mean - 5% = Lower Limit = 57.712
Instrument performance is within the acceptable limits of ± 5% error.

Installation: Geometric Dependence

Geometric dependence means that the indicated activity does not change with volume or configuration. To evaluate these two factors, the Regulatory Guide 10.8, Revision 2,[2] suggests the use of a 3-ml plastic syringe and a 30-ml glass vial for evaluation of source geometry. These were selected because a syringe is normally used for injections, whereas the 30-ml glass vial is similar in size, shape, and construction to the radiopharmaceutical kit vials or generator milking vials.

Method (3-ml Syringe)

1. Place about 2–20 mCi (74–740 MBq) ^{99m}Tc in a volume of 1–2 ml into a vial. The ^{99m}Tc should have a specific concentration of 1–10 mCi/ml (37–370 MBq/ml). Prepare a second beaker or vial with nonradioactive normal saline or water.
2. Draw 0.5 ml of the ^{99m}Tc solution into a 3-ml syringe, and assay the radioactivity. Subtract the background activity, and record the net activity.
3. Remove the syringe from the dose calibrator, draw an additional 0.5 ml of nonradioactive saline or water into the 3-ml syringe, and assay it again. Record the total volume and the net measured activity.
4. Repeat the same process in steps 1–3 until a final syringe volume of 2.0 ml is obtained.
5. The volume that is normally injected is used as the standard volume for purposes of comparison. The readings acquired in the previous steps are compared with those obtained from the standard volume by dividing the standard activity by the activities indicated for each volume. The quotient is the volume correction factor.

Method (30-ml Vial)

1. Place about 1–10 mCi (37–370 MBq) ^{99m}Tc in 1 ml into a 30-ml glass vial. Assay the vial, and record the volume and the net activity.
2. Remove the vial from the calibrator. Using a clean syringe, add 2.0 ml of nonradioactive saline or water. Assay the vial, and again record the volume and net activity.
3. Repeat the process until a 19.0-ml volume has been assayed. The entire process must be completed within 10 minutes.
4. Select a volume that is closest to that normally used when assaying radiopharmaceutical kits or generator vials. This volume is set as the standard volume. For all the other volumes, divide the activity in the standard volume by the measured activity. The quotient in each case is the volume correction factor.

Corrective Action

If any correction factors exceed 10% (i.e., the correction factor is less than 0.9 or greater than 1.1), a correction table must be established so that the indicated activity can be converted to "true activity" (i.e., true activity = indicated activity × correction factor).

References

1. Possession, use, calibration, and check of dose calibrator. U.S. Nuclear Regulatory Commission Rules and Regulations, Code of Federal Regulations, Energy, Title 10, Part 35.50, 1994.

2. Model procedure for calibrating dose calibrator. U.S. Nuclear Regulatory Commission, For the Preparation or Application for Medical Programs, Regulatory Guide, 10.8, Appendix C, 1987.

3. Oswald WM, Herold TJ, Wilson ME, Hung JC. Dose calibrator linearity testing using an improved attenuator system. J Nucl Med Technol 1992; 20: 169–172.

4. Chu RY. Accuracy of dose calibrator linearity test (letter to the editor). Health Phys 1988; 55: 95.

Survey Instrument Quality Control

Introduction

Two types of survey meters are in use in nuclear medicine. They are the Geiger-Müller counter and the ionization chamber. All survey instruments require routine quality control to ensure that they are operating correctly. Furthermore, federal regulations (10 CFR 35.51) require that all survey meters be calibrated before first use, and then annually thereafter and after repair.[1] Specifically, the regulations require the user to comply with the following standards:

Calibrate the instrument as follows:

1. Calibrate all scales with readings up to 1,000 mrem/hr with a radiation source.
2. Calibrate 2 separate readings on each scale.
3. Conspicuously note on the instrument the apparent exposure rate from a dedicated check source as determined at the time of calibration and the date of calibration. (Battery changes are not considered "servicing.")

When calibrating a survey instrument, the licensee should consider a point as calibrated if the indicated exposure rate differs from the calculated exposure rate by not more than 20% and should attach a conspicuous correction chart or graph to the instrument.

A licensee should check each survey instrument for proper operation with the dedicated check source each day of use. A licensee is not required to keep records of these checks.

A licensee should retain a record of each survey instrument calibration for **3 years**. The record must include the following:

1. A description of the calibration procedure
2. Date of the calibration
3. A description of the source used
4. The certified exposure rates from the source
5. The rates indicated by the instrument being calibrated
6. The correction factors deduced from the calibration data
7. The signature of the person who performed the calibration

Yearly Procedure: Calibration of Survey Meters

Method: Survey Meter

1. Place a planchette source on a countertop. This source should contain 0.1–0.5 µCi (3.7–18.5 kBq) ^{57}Co dispersed uniformity throughout a solid 0.5–1 inch disk. Ensure that all other sources of radiation have been removed from the area.
2. Place the survey meter either directly on top of the source (Fig. 1-28) or at a distance of 5 cm.
3. Measure the exposure rate in cpm. Note the source activity and calibration date, and compute its current activity in microcuries (kilobecquerels). Divide the exposure rate by activity

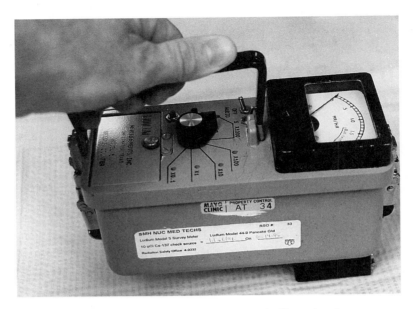

Figure 1-28. Survey meter positioned on top of a ^{57}Co planchette source.

to get the efficiency factor of the meter in cpm per microcuries (cpm per kilobecquerels). This factor should be recorded on a label to be affixed to the detector.

Method: Exposure Rate Meters

1. Each meter with a scale that reads below 1 R/hr should be calibrated at 2 points on the scale located at about 1/3 and 2/3 of full scale.
2. The calibration should be performed with a ^{137}Cs reference source with a strength of about 100 mCi (3.7 GBq) or greater.
3. The activity of the ^{137}Cs reference source should be documented to an accuracy of ±5% by intercomparison with a NIST-calibrated reference source. The radiation exposure from the source should be documented in terms of milliroentgens per hour at 1 m and should be corrected for decay before the calibration procedure.
4. To obtain the appropriate scale reading, position the exposure rate meter at various distances from the ^{137}Cs source. Record the distance and meter reading. The expected reading at each distance can be determined from the inverse square law. For example, at a distance of 30 cm (0.3 m), the expected reading can be calculated from the following equation:

$$R_{0.3} \times (0.3)^2 = R_1 \times (1)^2$$

Corrective Action

1. If the measured and expected exposure rates differ by more than 10% but less than 20%, a calibration chart, graph, or response factor should be prepared and attached to the instrument.
2. If the measured and expected exposure rates differ by more than 20% (or greater than 10%, and the preparation of a correction factor is not desirable), the meter should be repaired or adjusted until the measured readings are within 10% of the expected reading.

Daily Procedure: Constancy Check

Method

1. All survey meters should be checked each day before being used.
2. Place the survey meter in front of a long-lived reference source. Constancy check sources are commercially available from several vendors and usually consist of a plastic disk impregnated with 1–10 µCi (37–370 kBq) ^{137}Cs. The geometric arrangement of both source and survey meter should be noted and should be reproducible on a daily basis.
3. Note the meter reading, and record it on a label placed conspicuously on the surface of the survey meter.
4. On a daily basis, repeat step 2 and note the reading. Verify that the meter gives a reading within 10% of the value documented on the meter. Note that it is very important to maintain the same counting geometry every day.

Corrective Action

1. If the meter reading is not within 10% of the expected value, the meter should be recalibrated.

References

1. Calibration and check of survey instruments. U.S. Nuclear Regulatory Commission Rules and Regulations, Code of Federal Regulations, Energy, Title 10, Part 35.51, 1994.

Radiopharmaceutical Quality Control

Joseph C. Hung

Radiation Tests

Introduction

Quality control (QC) of radiopharmaceuticals has been defined by Briner[1] as "a series of tests, analysis, and observations which establish beyond reasonable doubt the identity, quality, and quantity of a product's ingredients and which will demonstrate that the technology employed in its formulation will yield a dosage form of highest safety, purity, and efficacy." Because radiopharmaceuticals are intended for administration to humans, QC procedures are imperative to ensure the safety of this preparation. Although extensive QC procedures are performed by the manufacturer, the use of cold kits to prepare radiopharmaceuticals with short-lived radionuclides, such as ^{99m}Tc and ^{111}In, requires that quality control tests be conducted on all on-site radiopharmaceutical preparations before dispensing this product for administration to humans.

The routine radiopharmaceutical QC procedures can be divided into two categories: radiation tests and pharmaceutical tests. The radiation tests include radionuclidic purity, radiochemical purity, and assessment of radioactivity. These methods are discussed in detail next.

Radionuclidic Purity

Radionuclidic purity is defined as the fraction of the total radioactivity in a source that is present in the form of the desired radionuclide and is expressed as a percentage. Radionuclidic impurities in radiopharmaceuticals usually arise from (1) the method of radionuclide production and (2) incomplete radionuclide separation during radiochemical processing. Examples of radionuclidic impurities include 60-hour ^{99}Mo impurity in 6-hour ^{99m}Tc, 4-day ^{124}I impurity in 13-hour ^{123}I, and 12-day ^{202}Tl impurity in 73-hour ^{201}Tl. Radionuclidic impurities are significant because they may contribute to an increased radiation dose without adding to the diagnostic information.

Radionuclidic impurity is usually determined by measuring the half-life ($t_{1/2}$) and characteristic energies emitted by each radionuclide. Identification of the gamma-ray energies can be achieved by a sodium iodide scintillation detector or a high-resolution lithium-drift germanium detector (GeLi detector) coupled to a multichannel analyzer.

It is important to remember that radionuclidic purity is constantly changing. If the half-life of the contaminant is much longer than that of the primary radionuclide, its relative contribution will increase with time; for example, ^{201}Tl ($t_{1/2}$ = 73 hours) is contaminated with ^{202}Tl ($t_{1/2}$ = 12 days). Even if contamination is less than 0.5%, the abundant (95%) higher energy gamma ray (439 keV) of ^{202}Tl may substantially affect image quality when low-energy collimation is used. Therefore, radionuclidic purity for short-lived nuclides should be determined immediately before use.

Table 2-1 lists some commonly detected radionuclidic impurities, with their half-lives and major photon energies, and their acceptable limits according to the *United States Pharmacopeia* (23rd rev.) and the *National Formulary* (18th ed.) (USP 23/NF 18). Commercially produced radioisotopes are monitored carefully by the manufacturer for radionuclidic impurities, and it is not necessary that all such radiopharmaceuticals be

Table 2-1. Radionuclidic Purity for Some Commonly Used Radionuclides (USP 23/NF 18)

Radionuclide	Half-Life (Principal Energy)	Purity	Contaminants	Half-Life (Principal Energy)	Acceptable Limits
^{67}Ga	77.9 hr (93 keV) (184 keV) (296 keV)	99% ^{67}Ga			
^{111}In	2.81 days (173 keV) (247 keV)		^{114m}In	50 days (558 keV) (724 keV)	<3 μCi/mCi ^{111}In
			^{65}Zn	243.9 days (1,115 keV)	<3 μCi/mCi ^{111}In
^{123}I	13.3 hr (159 keV)	85% ^{123}I			
^{99m}Tc	6.05 hr (140 keV)		^{99}Mo	66.7 hr (740 keV) (181 keV) (778 keV)	<0.15 μCi/mCi ^{99m}Tc
^{201}Tl	74 hr (60–80 keV) (167 keV)	95% ^{201}Tl	^{200}Tl	26.1 hr (368 keV) (1.21 Mev)	<2%
			^{203}Tl	52.1 hr (825 keV)	<0.3%
			^{202}Tl	12.2 days (439 keV) (522 keV) (961 keV)	<2.7%
^{133}Xe	5.27 days (81 keV)	95% ^{133}Xe			

checked rigorously by the end user. However, it is important that the ^{99}Mo content in the generator eluate be checked before clinical use.

Permissible ^{99}Mo Concentration

In the United States, the Code of Federal Regulations issued by the Nuclear Regulatory Commission (NRC) (10 CFR Part 35.204) states that a licensee may not administer to humans a radiopharmaceutical containing more than 0.15 μCi ^{99}Mo/mCi ^{99m}Tc (equivalent to 0.15 kBq ^{99}Mo/MBq ^{99m}Tc).[2] A licensee that uses ^{99}Mo/^{99m}Tc generators for preparing a ^{99m}Tc radiopharmaceutical should measure the ^{99}Mo concentration in each eluate.

USP 23/NF 18 requires that the amount of ^{99}Mo is not greater than 0.15 kBq/MBq (0.15 μCi/mCi) of ^{99m}Tc per administered dose in the injection at the time of administration. Furthermore, the total amount of other gamma-emitting radionuclidic impurities should not exceed 0.5 kBq/MBq (0.5 μCi/mCi) of ^{99m}Tc, and should not exceed 92 kBq (2.5 μCi) per administered dose at the time of administration.

Characteristics of ^{99}Mo

1. Nuclide: ^{99}Mo$_{42}$
2. Physical half-life: 67 hours
3. Mode of decay: beta negative (100%)
4. Gamma-ray keV (percentage): 181 (7), 740 (12), 780 (4)
5. Common production methods: ^{98}Mo (n, gamma) ^{99}Mo or ^{235}U(n,f)^{99}Mo

Causes of ^{99}Mo Breakthrough

1. Exceeding the ion-exchange capacity of alumina column
2. pH of eluate greater than 7
3. Channeling of disrupted alumina bed
4. Excessive elution

Procedure for Measuring ^{99}Mo Breakthrough

Two methods are used for the measurement of ^{99}Mo breakthrough: the lead cannister method and the CAP-MAC cannister method.

Lead Cannister Method

Most manufacturers of dose calibrators have available ¼-inch thick lead canisters designed for measurement of ^{99}Mo breakthrough.

1. Place the ^{99}Mo assay lead cannister (Fig. 2-1) in the dose calibrator to obtain a background reading.
2. Set the calibrator setting for ^{99}Mo assay.
3. Transfer the generator eluate vial from its lead container to the ^{99}Mo assay cannister, and place it in the dose calibrator. Measure the ^{99}Mo activity.
4. The net activity of ^{99}Mo in the generator eluate is determined by subtracting the background activity from the ^{99}Mo activity of the generator eluate vial.

Note: Because the ^{99}Mo assay lead cannister has a lead wall approximately ¼-inch thick, which effectively absorbs the lower energy gamma rays of ^{99}Mo (180 keV) and ^{99m}Tc (140 keV) and yet permits the passage of approximately one-half of the more energetic ^{99}Mo gamma rays (740 and 780 keV), the net activity of ^{99}Mo has to be multiplied by a factor of 2. Some calibrators automatically correct for this attenuation of the ^{99}Mo assay cannister by incorporating a multiplication factor and displaying the corrected ^{99}Mo activity. Check the instruction manual of the dose calibrator to determine the appropriate correction factor.

CAP-MAC Cannister Method

The CAP-MAC cannister (Fig. 2-2) not only allows the generator to elute directly into the elution vial inside the lead cannister, but it also permits one to measure the ^{99}Mo breakthrough and the total ^{99m}Tc activity in the elution vial without the need to transfer the

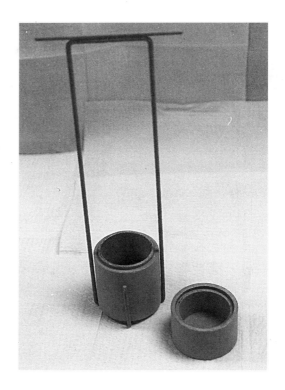

Figure 2-1. Lead cannister and holder for measurement of ^{99}Mo breakthrough.

elution vial into a different lead cannister. The CAP-MAC cannister accommodates 5–20 ml elution vials with different bottom assemblies. Because the CAP-MAC has a thicker wall than the regular ^{99}Mo assay cannister (see Fig. 2-1), the calibration settings for ^{99}Mo assay and for ^{99m}Tc need to be changed. For a ^{99}Mo assay using a Capintec dose calibrator, the correct measurement is 4 times the reading obtained with the calibrator set to 030. The correct calibration setting for ^{99m}Tc is 042 when the elution vial is measured in the CAP-MAC holder with the lead cannister retracted. For dose calibrators other than Capintec, check the instruction manual accompanying the CAP-MAC cannister for the appropriate settings. The CAP-MAC cannister can be obtained from Capintec, Inc., 6 Arrow Road, Ramsey, NJ 07446 (800-ASK-4-CRC).

^{99}Mo Preliminary Setup

1. Place the lever of the CAP-MAC assembly in the lower vertical position (Fig. 2-3, left). While holding the handle, place the lever in the raised vertical position (Fig. 2-3, middle). Slide an empty cannister into the cannister holder by rotating the holder.
2. Gently place the entire CAP-MAC assembly into the well chamber of the dose calibrator.
3. Adjust the background reading of the dose calibrator, and set to zero.
4. Remove the entire CAP-MAC assembly from the dose calibrator chamber well by lifting with the handle.
5. Remove the cannister from the holder by following the procedure in step 1 to slide the cannister out of the cannister holder.

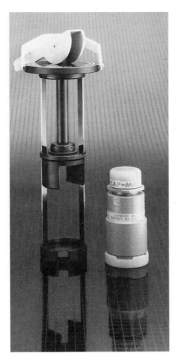

Figure 2-2. Photograph of the CAP-MAC cannister. (Courtesy of Capintec, Inc., NJ.)

6. Remove the cannister base (large yellow plastic piece) by holding it with one hand while turning the cannister counterclockwise.
7. Place the elution vial into the vial holder of the cannister base. The elution vial must be from the manufacturer and be the size indicated on the vial holder.
8. Slide the cannister over the vial, and lock it to the cannister base by turning it clockwise.
9. Remove the cannister cap (small yellow plastic piece), and set it aside.
10. Use the CAP-MAC to elute the generator according to the manufacturer's instructions.
11. When the generator elution is completed, remove the cannister from the generator, and immediately replace the cannister cap.
12. Slide the cannister back into the cannister holder.
13. Lift the lever, and gently lower it to the horizontal position (Fig. 2-3, right).
14. Press down on the lever until the cannister is snugly fit in the cup.

Measurement of 99Mo Breakthrough and 99mTc Activity

1. Lift the complete CAP-MAC assembly by the handle, and slowly lower it into the chamber well of the dose calibrator.
2. If the dose calibrator has a button labeled "Mo assay," press it. If not, set the manual calibration to the appropriate setting for ^{99}Mo.
3. Record the reading displayed on the dose calibrator, and multiply it by 4. This is the ^{99}Mo activity.

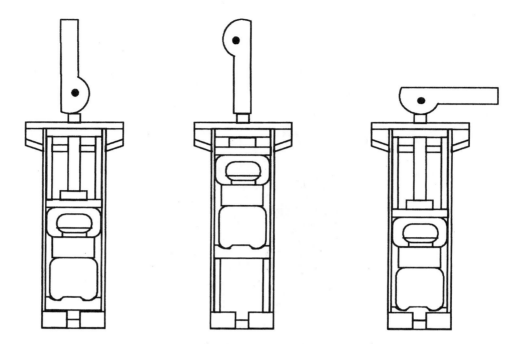

Figure 2-3. Schematic diagram of the CAP-MAC cannister with the lever in the lower vertical position (left), raised vertical position (middle), and horizontal position (right).

4. Open the cannister by holding the handle and rotating the lever counterclockwise until it stops. Move the lever to the raised vertical position (see Fig. 2-3, middle), and let go.
5. If the dose calibrator has a button labeled "^{99m}Tc CAP-MAC," press it. If not, set the manual calibration to the appropriate setting described in the CAP-MAC instruction manual.
6. Record the reading displayed on the dose calibrator. This is the ^{99m}Tc activity.
7. Close the cannister by lowering the lever to the horizontal position (see Fig. 2-3, right).
8. Lock the cannister to the base by holding the handle, pressing down, and rotating the lever clockwise until it stops.
9. Remove the entire CAP-MAC assembly from the chamber well, and remove the cannister from the holder, as described in the previous section.
10. Be sure to reset the background reading of the dose calibrator after removing the CAP-MAC cannister.

Corrective Action

1. A higher reading of ^{99}Mo than expected may be due to radioactive contamination, physical damage to the lead cannister, or improper seal of the CAP-MAC cannister.
2. After correcting any problems with the cannister, if the ^{99}Mo reading still exceeds the maximum limits (i.e., 0.15 µCi ^{99}Mo/mCi ^{99m}Tc), the generator eluate must not be used for studies in patients, and the generator should be returned to the manufacturer. Because ^{99m}Tc decays at a faster rate than ^{99}Mo, the ratio of ^{99}Mo to ^{99m}Tc increases with time. Therefore, the useful shelf life of the ^{99m}Tc eluate is determined by the initial ratio of ^{99}Mo to ^{99m}Tc. Figure 2-4 shows the time limits for the shelf life of ^{99m}Tc eluate based on the ratio of ^{99}Mo/^{99m}Tc activity.

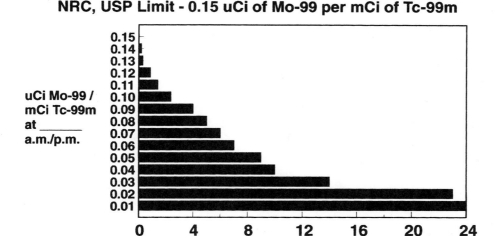

Figure 2-4. Time limits for the shelf life of ^{99m}Tc eluate based on the initial ^{99}Mo/^{99m}Tc ratio of activity.

^{99}Mo/^{99m}Tc Generator Records

In the United States, NRC regulations (10 CFR 35.204) require a licensee to retain a record of each ^{99}Mo concentration measurement for 3 years.[2] The record for each elution or extraction of ^{99m}Tc must include the following information:[2]

1. The measured activity of ^{99m}Tc expressed in millicuries
2. The measured activity of ^{99}Mo expressed in μCi
3. The ratio of the measured activity expressed as μCi ^{99}Mo/mCi ^{99m}Tc
4. The time and date of the measurement
5. The initials of the person who made the measurement

Radiochemical Purity

The radiochemical purity (RCP) of a radiopharmaceutical is the percentage of the total radioactivity in a radioactive drug that is present in the desired chemical form. Radiochemical impurities may arise from competing chemical reactions during the radiolabeling process, decomposition of the final product that is due to radiolysis, the presence of oxidizing or reducing agents, changes in pH or temperature, the presence of the solvent, and exposure to light.

Radiochemical impurities are unacceptable because their distribution in the body differs from that of the radiopharmaceutical, making it difficult to obtain useful information in nuclear medicine studies. High background radioactivity counts that are due to the presence of radiochemical impurities in areas not of primary interest in the study can degrade image quality, interfere with diagnostic interpretation, and expose the patient to unnecessary radiation. Therefore, it is vitally important that radiopharmaceuticals have an acceptable RCP before they are administered.

The three basic sources of information on RCP testing methods are USP 23/NF 18, package inserts, and publications other than USP 23/NF 18. However, because the infor-

Table 2-2. Chromatographic Systems for ^{99m}Tc Radiopharmaceuticals

^{99m}Tc Radiopharmaceutical	Stationary Phase	Mobile Phase	R_f Values			Minimum RCP	Special Instructions	Reference
			Bound ^{99m}Tc	Free ^{99m}Tc	H-R ^{99m}Tc			
^{99m}Tc-albumin (HSA)	Whatman 31ET	Acetone	0.0	1.0	0.0	95	—	3
^{99m}Tc-albumin aggregated (MAA)	Whatman 31ET	Acetone	0.0	1.0	0.0	90	—	4
^{99m}Tc-albumin colloid	ITLC-SG	Methyl acetate	0.0	1.0	0.0	90	a	5
^{99m}Tc-bicisate (ECD)	1. Bakerflex silica gel 1BF	Ethyl acetate	1.0	0.0	0.0	90	—	6
	2. Whatman 17	Ethyl acetate	1.0	0.0	0.0	90	—	7
^{99m}Tc-disofenin (DISIDA)	ITLC-SA	20% NaCl	0.0	1.0	0.0	90	—	8
^{99m}Tc-exametazime (HMPAO)	1. ITLC-SG	Methyl ethyl ketone	0.8–1.0	0.8–1.0	0.0	80	—	9
	ITLC-SG	0.9% NaCl	0.0	0.8–1.0	0.0	80	—	9
	2. Gelman Solvent Saturation Pads	Ether	1.0	0.0	0.0	80	—	10, 11
^{99m}Tc-glucepate (GH)	Whatman 31ET	Acetone	0.0	1.0	0.0	90	—	12
^{99m}Tc-mebrofenin (BrIDA)	ITLC-SA	20% NaCl	0.0	1.0	0.0	90	—	8
^{99m}Tc-medronate (MDP)	Whatman 31ET	Acetone	0.0	1.0	0.0	90	—	4
^{99m}Tc-mertiatide (MAG3)	1. Sep-Pak C18 cartridge	200 proof ethanol 0.9% NaCl 0.001 N HCl 1:1 ethanol/0.9% NaCl	—	—	—	90	b	13
	2. Gelman Solvent Saturation Pads	Chloroform/acetone/tetrahydrofuran (1:1:2, v/v)	0.0	0.5–1.0	0.0	90	—	14
	Gelman Solvent Saturation Pads	0.9% NaCl	0.5–1.0	0.5–1.0	0.0	90	—	14
^{99m}Tc-oxidronate (HDP)	Whatman 31ET	Acetone	0.0	1.0	0.0	90	—	4
^{99m}Tc-pentetate (DTPA)	Whatman 31ET	Acetone	0.0	1.0	0.0	90	—	12
^{99m}Tc-pyrophosphate (PYP)	Whatman 31ET	Acetone	0.0	1.0	0.0	90	—	4

^{99m}Tc-sestamibi (MIBI)	1. Baker Flex aluminum oxide coated, plastic	Ethanol	1.0	0.0	0.0	90	c	15
^{99m}Tc-sestamibi (MIBI)	2. Gelman Solvent Saturation Pads	Chloroform/tetra-hydrofuran (1:1, v/v)	0.8–1.0	0.0	0.0	90	—	16, 17
^{99m}Tc-sodium pertechnetate (^{99m}TcO$_4$)	ITLC-SG	Acetone	—	1.0	1.0	90	—	18
^{99m}Tc-succimer (DMSA)	ITLC-SA	Acetone	0.0	1.0	0.0	85	—	4
^{99m}Tc-sulfur colloid (SC)	Whatman 31ET	Acetone	0.0	1.0	0.0	92	—	4
^{99m}Tc-red blood cells (UltraTag RBC)	—	—	—	—	—	90	d	19, 20

Abbreviations: ITLC-SA, instant thin-layer chromatography-polysilicic acid; ITLC-SG, instant thin-layer chromatography-silica gel; TCL, thin-layer chromatography.

[a](1) Pre-equilibrate the chromatographic developing tank with ethyl acetate for 15–30 minutes. (2) The sample spot should not be greater than 10 mm; allow the spot to dry for 5–10 minutes. (3) The developing time takes approximately 15 minutes.

[b](1) Preparation of Sep-Pak C18 cartridge. The Sep-Pak C18 cartridge is first flushed with 10 ml of 200-proof ethanol and is followed by flushing the cartridge with 10 ml of 0.001 N HCl. The cartridge is then drained by pushing 5 ml of air through the cartridge with a syringe. (2) Sample Analysis. Apply 0.1 ml of ^{99m}Tc-MAG3 to the long end of the cartridge. The cartridge is then eluted successively with 10 ml of 0.001 N HCl and 10 ml of 1:1 ethanol/0.9% NaCl solution. The two fractions of sample eluates and cartridges are collected in separate culture tubes for counting. (3) Counting. The radioactivity of the first sample elution (hydrophilic ^{99m}Tc impurity plus a fraction of H-R ^{99m}Tc), the second sample elution (^{99m}Tc-MAG3), and the cartridge (the remaining H-R ^{99m}Tc plus nonelutable impurities) are assayed in a dose calibrator. The percentages of ^{99m}Tc-MAG3, hydrophilic ^{99m}Tc species, and H-R ^{99m}Tc are calculated by dividing each fraction of radioactivity by the total of activity of both sample liquid fractions and the cartridge.

[c](1) The TLC plate has to be predried in an oven at 100°C for 1 hour. (2) After two drops of ^{99m}Tc-sestamibi sample are applied side-by-side on top of the ethanol wet spot, the TLC plate is placed in a desiccator to allow the spot to dry before the plate is developed in the TLC tank. (3) This TLC system requires about 30 minutes to complete the drying and development.

[d](1) Transfer 0.2 ml of ^{99m}Tc-red blood cells (RBC) to a centrifuge tube containing 2 ml of 0.9% NaCl. (2) Centrifuge the ^{99m}Tc-RBC sample at 150 g for 1 minute. (3) Carefully pipet off the diluted plasma. (4) Measure the radioactivity in the plasma and the RBC separately in a dose calibrator. (5) Calculate the labeling efficiency of ^{99m}Tc-RBC as follows:

$$\% \text{ RBC labeling} = \frac{\text{RBC activity}}{\text{RBC activity} + \text{Plasma activity}} \times 100$$

mation given by these sources is not always complete or practical, it can be difficult to select and perform an adequate RCP test on the prepared radiopharmaceutical. The focus of this procedure manual is RCP testing of radiopharmaceuticals labeled with ^{99m}Tc, because this type of radiopharmaceutical is used extensively in nuclear medicine studies. The RCP testing methods recommended by the manufacturers and/or alternative methods that are better than those recommended are presented in Table 2-2. The RCP testing procedures listed in the USP 23/NF 18 are either impractical in a nuclear medicine laboratory or do not include specific details; therefore, these testing procedures are not included in this manual.

The three radiochemical species in a stannous-reduced ^{99m}Tc-labeled radiopharmaceutical are (1) bound ^{99m}Tc, which is the desired radiochemical species; (2) free ^{99m}Tc, which is technetium in the form of ^{99m}TcO$_4^-$ (because it was not reduced by divalent stannous ions [Sn^{2+}] or was reduced but then oxidized); and (3) hydrolyzed-reduced ^{99m}Tc (H-R ^{99m}Tc), which includes ^{99m}TcO$_2$ (did not react with the chelating agent) and ^{99m}Tc-Sn^{2+} colloid (formed by the binding of reduced ^{99m}Tc to hydrolyzed Sn^{2+}). Free ^{99m}Tc and H-R ^{99m}Tc are radiochemical impurities. Free ^{99m}Tc pertechnetate increases the background activity attributable to uptake in the stomach, gut, and thyroid. H-R ^{99m}Tc complex is a colloidal impurity that localizes in a patient's reticuloendothelial system and interferes with the imaging interpretation.

RCP Analytical Methods

The determination of RCP values usually involves the use of instant thin-layer chromatography (ITLC) and paper chromatography methods or some form of column chromatography, such as the Sep-Pak technique.

Instant Thin-Layer and Paper Chromatography

ITLC and paper chromatography are the methods used most frequently to identify the various radiochemical species in a radiopharmaceutical preparation, especially for ^{99m}Tc-labeled radiopharmaceuticals. In each of these two techniques, a sample of microliter amounts of the radiopharmaceutical is spotted at the end of a chromatographic strip (the stationary phase). Next, the chromatographic strip is placed vertically in a chromatographic chamber (usually a vial or glass tube) that contains an appropriate solvent (mobile phase). The strip is placed in the solvent so that the origin of the spot is not immersed.

The stationary phase may be paper, such as Whatman 31ET or Gelman's Solvent Saturation Pads, or ITLC strips, which are made of glass fiber impregnated with silica gel (ITLC-SG) or polysilicic acid (ITLC-SA). The solvent used as the mobile phase is usually water or an organic chemical. The chromatographic chamber must be covered tightly to maintain a solvent-saturated atmosphere. The electrostatic forces (adsorption and capillary action) of the stationary phase tend to retard the movement of various radiochemical species, whereas the mobile phase carries each radiochemical component according to its partition between the stationary phase and the mobile phase. The partition of each radiochemical species between the stationary and mobile phases is determined by the solubility of the radiochemical species in the mobile phase, which is affected by the polarity of the solvent. Therefore, the electrostatic attractive forces of the stationary phase and the polarity of the mobile phase are the two determining factors in the separation of different radiochemical components in a sample.

Solvent front (S_f) is the location where solvent usually reaches the top of the chromatographic strip, whereas relative front (R_f) is the distance traveled by a given radiochemical component compared with the S_f (Fig. 2-5).

$$R_f = \text{distance from origin to spot center/distance from origin to } S_f$$

The R_f values are determined with known radiochemical species and are used primarily for the identification of different radiochemical components in a given radiopharmaceutical sample.

In general, H-R ^{99m}Tc contaminants remain at the origin ($R_f = 0.0$) because they are particulate matter. A simple RCP chromatography system would allow bound ^{99m}Tc to migrate to the S_f, whereas free ^{99m}Tc and H-R ^{99m}Tc would remain at the origin. The percent RCP for the bound ^{99m}Tc radiopharmaceutical is easily calculated by dividing the radioactivity of the top portion of the strip by the total activity in both sections of the chromatographic strips. Using the so-called single-strip radiochemical purity analysis procedure, it is quite simple to calculate the percent bound of the radiopharmaceutical. However, some other ^{99m}Tc-labeled radiopharmaceutical complexes require a two-solvent dual-strip system to determine the percent RCP of the desired radiochemical form. Because the bound ^{99m}Tc complex is always associated with one of the two radiochemical impurities (i.e., free ^{99m}Tc or H-R ^{99m}Tc) and cannot be isolated by itself, the RCP value of the bound ^{99m}Tc-labeled radiopharmaceutical is determined indirectly. This is accomplished by subtracting the percentage of each radiochemical impurity from 100% to obtain the percentage of bound ^{99m}Tc complex.

Reversed-Phase Chromatography With Sep-Pak C18 Cartridge

To perform reversed-phase chromatography with Sep-Pak C18 cartridges (Waters Chromatography, Millipore Corporation, Milford, MA) for the RCP determination, a series of solvents of decreasing polarity has to be used for the complete separation of different radiochemical species.

1. Condition the Sep-Pak cartridge with 6–10 cartridge hold-up volumes of ethanol, methanol, or acetonitrile.
2. Flush the cartridge with 6–10 hold-up cartridge volumes of 0.001 N HCl, water, or buffer. For most applications, the cartridge should not be allowed to dry out.
3. Load the radiopharmaceutical sample dissolved in a high-polarity solvent.
4. Elute unwanted components with a high-polarity solvent.
5. Elute weakly held components of interest with less polar solvents.
6. Elute more tightly bound components with progressively less polar solvents.
7. When all components are recovered, discard the used cartridge in the appropriate manner.

Figure 2-5. Schematic diagram of chromatographic strip showing the location of the solvent front, S_f, and the relative front, R_f.

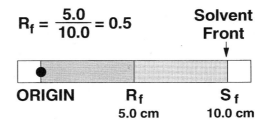

Although the Sep-Pak cartridge can provide a more complete chromatographic separation of the ^{99m}Tc radiochemical species, the solvent elution process, costly cartridge, and lengthy procedure process do not make the Sep-Pak cartridge method ideal for routine use in a busy nuclear medicine department or commercial nuclear pharmacy. Also, technical errors can occur with the use of the Sep-Pak cartridge method. After the radiopharmaceutical loading, the cartridge must be eluted slowly with the appropriate solvent. If not eluted slowly, the ^{99m}Tc compound will remain on the cartridge, producing a false estimation in RCP values. Another disadvantage associated with the use of the Sep-Pak cartridges for RCP determination is the increased radiation exposure to the person performing the RCP procedure. The Sep-Pak cartridge method requires at least 0.1 ml of ^{99m}Tc radiopharmaceutical preparation to be loaded into the cartridge. This volume may contain several millicuries (megabecquerels) of activity.

Currently, the Sep-Pak cartridge method is required only for RCP determination of ^{99m}Tc MAG3. For a regular ^{99m}Tc MAG3 kit preparation, 0.1 ml contains between 0.5 mCi (18.5 MBq) and 2.5 mCi (92.5 MBq) per application. An alternative minipaper chromatographic system using two-strip paper chromatography (see Table 2-2) requires only two 5-µl samples (50–250 µCi; 1.9–9.3 MBq) for the RCP analysis and takes less than 3 minutes to complete the RCP determination for ^{99m}Tc-MAG3.[16]

The Pros and Cons of Counting Instruments for Radiochromatography

Radionuclide Dose Calibrators

The dose calibrator is a common instrument in a nuclear medicine or nuclear pharmacy laboratory. However, the accuracy of the dose calibrator in measuring the low amount of radioactivity that is usually associated with the RCP testing procedure is the primary concern. In general, to use a dose calibrator for the measurement of radioactivity of RCP strips, the chromatographic strip should contain 100 µCi or more of ^{99m}Tc to reduce the error to less than 1%.

Well Scintillation Counters

Although the well counter is an appropriate counting instrument for the RCP chromatographic strips, the counting rate of its detection system is easily exceeded. To avoid exceeding the maximum counting capabilities of the well counter, four different methods are recommended:[21] (1) increasing the distance from the source to the detector; (2) use of an attenuator on the well counter—the most commonly used attenuator is an appropriately sized metal disk or coin placed over the opening of the well counter; (3) decreasing the volume of the radioactive sample; and (4) correcting for instrument deadtime—some well counters are equipped with a device that automatically compensates for high amounts of radioactivity.

Radiochromatogram Scanners

Scanning the chromatographic strip with a radiochromatogram scanner detects and measures the distribution of radioactivity along the intact radiochromatographic strip. Although the radiochromatogram scanner can analyze samples that have a wide range of activities and can calculate the percentage of radioactivity for each activity selected, the procedure is time-consuming and the instrument is expensive.

Gamma Cameras

Although an uncollimated gamma camera may be used as a well counter having two-pi geometry and an elevated background, this method increases the risk of damage to the crystal and/or contamination of the crystal, thus rendering the gamma camera unusable for clinical studies.

Common Errors or Pitfalls Associated With Chromatographic Techniques

Although ITLC and paper chromatographic procedures are easy to perform and are usually trouble-free, several procedural errors and/or artifactual results can occur. Apart from the previously described limitations of the counting instruments, technical variables and artifacts are associated with the use of chromatographic systems. This area has been reviewed by several authors.[18,22–24] The possible causes of the artifacts and errors are summarized in the following list:

1. The radiopharmaceutical sample spot is placed below the initial solvent level in the developing chamber.
2. The chromatographic strips and solvent are too old, causing cross contamination with other ^{99m}Tc radiochemical species.
3. The chromatographic strip is eluted past the S_f line. If the strip is eluted significantly past the S_f line, the cut line must be changed to maintain the same R_f value.
4. Reactions on the chromatographic paper or ITLC media. (Reduced states of ^{99m}Tc are easily oxidized; the spot of radiopharmaceutical should not be dried on the ITLC media or paper strip before it is placed in the solvent; ^{99m}Tc may also bind with the media or strip, which is often the cause of streaking, i.e., inadequate or no separation of free ^{99m}Tc and H-R ^{99m}Tc from the ^{99m}Tc-labeled radiopharmaceuticals.)
5. Uneven spotting or splattering when spotting the radiopharmaceuticals.
6. Interaction with marking compounds used to visualize solvent flow.
7. Grease from fingerprints.
8. The chromatographic strip touches the side of the wet chromatographic chamber.
9. Strip contamination with other radiopharmaceuticals when spotting.
10. The wrong solvent was used, or the mixing of the solvents was poor.
11. The solvent evaporated in the chromatographic chamber; solvent evaporates freely through the vent of the chamber.
12. Contaminated tweezers and scissors.
13. The work surface was not level, too much solvent was in the chromatographic chamber, and the solvent splashed when the strip was immersed; the solvent may wash the spot to the bottom of the chromatogram, thus contaminating the solvent for subsequent chromatograms.
14. The solvent was exposed to the atmosphere for too long, resulting in the evaporation of one solvent in a mixture, hence altering the R_f values.
15. The chromatographic chamber moved after the strip was immersed.

Although air drying of the applied sample spot on the chromatographic strip is generally not desirable because the ^{99m}Tc complex may be oxidized, occasionally it is important that the spot be dried before development in organic solvents such as acetone. Acetone mixes freely with water; hence, radiochemical species that are soluble in water but not soluble in acetone, such as ^{99m}Tc complexes, will streak up the strip from the origin if the spot is wet. If streaking extends into the top half of the strip, the results will be erroneous. This is more likely to occur with the 5-cm ministrips than with the standard 10-cm strips.

Corrective Actions

If a low RCP value is obtained, one should perform the following:

1. Review the RCP testing technique to ensure that the appropriate procedures to avoid errors and artifacts, as described earlier, have been followed. Repeat the RCP testing procedure.
2. If the RCP is still below the acceptable limit, the reconstituted kit should be discarded and another kit prepared.
3. If several kits from the same lot number have failed RCP testing, the manufacturer should be notified.

Assessment of Eluate Radioactivity and Yield From ^{99}Mo Generators

Measurement of the amount of radioactivity of a radiopharmaceutical is usually determined by either the whole-vial assay or counting an aliquot of the radiopharmaceutical in a dose calibrator. Radioactive concentration is usually expressed in terms of specific activity, which is defined as the activity per unit weight of the labeled compound (e.g., mCi/g or MBq/g), or specific concentration, which is defined as the activity per unit volume (mCi/ml or MBq/ml). The value of the radioactive concentration is usually stated on the vial label along with the calibration date and time. Each vial of the radiopharmaceutical should be radioassayed to confirm that it is within ±10% of the stated activity on the label, allowing for decay.

The radioactivity and the radioactive concentration of the ^{99m}Tc eluate can be determined by the whole-vial method and the aliquot method, as described next.

Whole-Vial Method

1. Assay the whole ^{99m}Tc elution vial in a dose calibrator to obtain the total radioactivity. This can be accomplished either by using the CAP-MAC cannister (refer to the preceding section entitled "CAP-MAC Cannister Method" for the detailed operation) or by transferring the elution vial from the lead container to the holder of the dose calibrator.
2. From the total volume eluted, one can determine the specific concentration of the ^{99m}Tc eluate by dividing the total measured radioactivity (millicuries or megabecquerels) by the total volume of ^{99m}Tc eluate (milliliters).

Aliquot Method

1. Withdraw a 1-ml aliquot of ^{99m}Tc eluate into a 1-ml syringe, and assay the syringe in a dose calibrator (this measurement includes radioactivity in the 1-ml ^{99m}Tc volume plus that in the needle and the dead space of the syringe).
2. Expel the 1-ml ^{99m}Tc eluate back into the elution vial.
3. Reassay the syringe to determine the residual activity in the needle and dead space of the syringe.
4. Calculate the difference between the two measurements to determine the radioactivity of ^{99m}Tc eluate per milliliter. This value is the specific concentration of ^{99m}Tc eluate.
5. The total activity of ^{99m}Tc in the elution vial can be obtained by multiplying the specific concentration of ^{99m}Tc eluate by the total volume in the elution vial.

Note: The CAP-MAC method is generally preferred, because it minimizes exposure of the operator to activity in the ^{99m}Tc elution vial. If the CAP-MAC cannister is not available, the aliquot method is preferred over transfer of the whole vial to the dose calibrator, because the operator is exposed to only a small fraction of the total activity. The aliquot method is more accurate in terms of the specific concentration measurement than the whole-vial technique.

Yield of ^{99m}Tc

The practical yield of ^{99m}Tc eluate generally ranges from 75% to 85% of the theoretical value. A generator should be replaced by manufacturer if the ^{99m}Tc yield is below 70%.

Calculation of Generator Yields

The theoretical value of generator yields can be calculated by performing the following four steps:

1. Determination of the present ^{99}Mo radioactivity (Table 2-3).
2. Calculation of the ^{99m}Tc radioactivity fraction as compared with the ^{99}Mo radioactivity (Table 2-4).

Table 2-3. ^{99}Mo Decay Factors[a]

Time (hr)	Decay Factor	Time (hr)	Decay Factor	Time (hr)	Decay Factor
-168	5.76	-48	1.65	36	0.687
-144	4.49	-44	1.58	40	0.659
-124	3.64	-40	1.52	44	0.632
-120	3.49	-36	1.46	48	0.606
-116	3.35	-32	1.40	52	0.581
-112	3.22	-28	1.34	56	0.558
-108	3.08	-24	1.28	60	0.535
-104	2.96	-20	1.23	64	0.513
-100	2.84	-16	1.18	68	0.492
-96	2.72	-12	1.13	72	0.472
-92	2.61	-8	1.09	96	0.368
-88	2.50	-4	1.04	120	0.286
-84	2.40	0	1.00	144	0.223
-80	2.30	4	0.959	168	0.174
-76	2.21	8	0.920	192	0.135
-72	2.12	12	0.882	216	0.105
-68	2.03	16	0.846	240	0.082
-64	1.95	20	0.812	264	0.064
-60	1.87	24	0.779	288	0.050
-56	1.79	28	0.747	312	0.039
-32	1.72	32	0.716	336	0.030

[a]Activity remaining = original activity $\times$ decay factor.

Table 2-4. Amounts of ^{99}Tc Present on Generator Column at Time (t) Post Generator Elution and Expressed as Fraction of Present ^{99}Mo Radioactivity^a

Time (t) (hr)	$\dfrac{A_2}{A_1}$	Time (t) (hr)	$\dfrac{A_2}{A_1}$	Time (t) (hr)	$\dfrac{A_2}{A_1}$
0.5	0.048	10.0	0.614	27	0.890
1.0	0.094	10.5	0.631	28	0.896
1.5	0.138	11.0	0.647	29	0.901
2.0	0.179	11.5	0.662	30	0.905
2.5	0.218	12.0	0.677	32	0.913
3.0	0.255	13.0	0.704	34	0.919
3.5	0.290	14.0	0.728	36	0.924
4.0	0.324	15.0	0.750	38	0.929
4.5	0.356	16.0	0.769	40	0.932
5.0	0.386	17.0	0.787	44	0.937
5.5	0.414	18.0	0.803	48	0.940
6.0	0.441	19.0	0.817	54	0.943
6.5	0.467	20.0	0.830	60	0.944
7.0	0.492	21.0	0.841	66	0.945
7.5	0.515	22.0	0.852	72	0.946
8.0	0.537	23.0	0.861	78	0.946
8.5	0.558	24.0	0.870	84	0.946
9.0	0.578	25.0	0.877	90	0.946
9.5	0.596	26.0	0.884	96	0.946

Note: $\lambda = 0.693/\text{T}\frac{1}{2}$, where T$\frac{1}{2}$ is the half-life in hours. A_2 refers to ^{99m}Tc activity, and A_1 refers to ^{99}Mo activity.

$$\frac{A_2}{A_1} = 0.860\lambda_2 \times \frac{(e^{-\lambda_1 t} - e^{-\lambda_2 t})}{(\lambda_2 - \lambda_1)e^{-\lambda_1 t}}$$

3. Measurement of removed ^{99m}Tc.
4. The fractional ^{99m}Tc generator yield is given by the measured ^{99m}Tc eluate radioactivity (millicuries or megabecquerels) from step 3 divided by the theoretical radioactivity of ^{99m}Tc eluate (millicuries or megabecquerels) from step 2.

Factors That Decrease ^{99m}Tc Generator Yield

1. Fluctuation in the loading of ^{99}Mo radioactivity into the column
2. Formation of channels in the Al_2O_3 column
3. Self-radiolysis
4. Air bubbles, air leaks, improperly functioning tubing, and other mechanical problems

Problems of the ^{99}Mo Generator

^{99m}Tc Eluate—Correct Volume and Low Radioactivity

This may be due to self-radiolysis or to channeling.

Self-Radiolysis Ionization of water, especially in a wet generator column, produces hydrogen peroxide (H_2O_2) and, in the presence of oxygen, hydroperoxy-free radicals ($HO_2\cdot$). Both of these chemical species are strong oxidizing agents and may attack the ^{99m}Tc sodium pertechnetate molecule to form a different chemical species that may have a stronger bond to the generator column. The formation of this chemical compound will undoubtedly decrease the generator yield. The radiolysis of water is also likely to occur in a higher activity ^{99}Mo generator.

Channeling Channeling is a physical defect of a generator column in which the column material bed is disrupted and a channel is created, allowing liquid to pass through without permeating the column material.

Channeling—Correction Method Method 1: Lift the generator and tap sharply against a hard surface several times to settle the contents of the column. Method 2: Carry out several maximum-volume elutions in rapid succession so that the flow of liquid may carry particles of column material into the channel to block it.

^{99m}Tc Eluate—Low Volume and Activity

This may be due to air bubbles, air leaks, improperly functioning tubing, or other mechanical problems. To correct for low volume and low eluate activity, re-eluate the generator, and leave the elution vial in place for 10–15 minutes. If the correct activity and volume are then obtained, proceed with the check for ^{99}Mo and aluminum breakthrough. Otherwise, check the connecting tubes for air locks or air leaks. If there are no discernible problems, there may be a partial blockage within the column itself. In such cases, do not use the generator, and return it to the manufacturer.

References

1. Briner WH. Sterile kits for the preparation of radiopharmaceuticals: some basic quality control considerations. In: "Radiopharmaceuticals," eds Subramanian G, Rhodes B, Cooper J, Sodd V. Society of Nuclear Medicine, New York, 1975, pp 246–253.
2. Permissible molybdenum-99 concentration. U.S. Nuclear Regulatory Commission Rules and Regulations, Code of Federal Regulations; Energy, Title 10, Part 35.204, 1994.
3. Thrall JH, Freitas JE, Swanson D, et al. Clinical comparison of cardiac blood pool visualization with technetium-99m red blood cells labeled in vivo and with technetium-99m human serum albumin. J Nucl Med 1978; 19: 796–803.
4. Zimmer AM, Pavel DG. Rapid miniaturized chromatographic quality-control procedures for Tc-99m radiopharmaceuticals. J Nucl Med 1977; 18: 1230–1233.
5. Microlite package insert. Du Pont Merck Pharmaceutical Co., Billerica, MA, November 1991.
6. Neurolite package insert. Du Pont Merck Pharmaceutical Co., Billerica, MA, November 1990.
7. Budde PA, Hung JC, Mahoney DW, Wollan PE. Rapid quality control procedure for technetium-99m-bicisate. J Nucl Med Technol 1995; 23: 190–194.
8. Zimmer AM, Majewski W, Spies SM. Rapid miniaturized chromatography for Tc-99m ZDA agents: comparison with gel chromatography. Eur J Nucl Med 1982; 7: 88–91.
9. Ceretec package insert. Amersham Corporation, Arlington Heights, IL, November 1990.
10. Jurisson S, Schlemper EO, Troutner DE, et al. Synthesis, characterization, and X-ray structural determinations of technetium(V)-oxo-tetradentate amine oxine complexes. Inorg Chem 1986; 25: 543–549.

11. Hung JC, Taggart TR, Wilson ME, Owens TP. Radiochemical purity testing for [99]Tc[m]-exametazime: a comparison study for three-paper chromatography. Nucl Med Commun 1994; 15: 569–574.

12. Zimmer AM. Re: radiochemical purity of Tc-99m oxidronate. (reply to letter to the editor.) J Nucl Med 1981; 22: 1016.

13. TechneScan MAG3 package insert. Mallinckrodt Medical Inc., St. Louis, MO, November 1992.

14. Hung JC, Wilson ME, Brown ML. Rapid preparation and quality control of technetium-99m MAG3. J Nucl Med Technol 1991; 19: 176–179.

15. Cardiolite package insert. Du Pont Merck Pharmaceutical Co., Billerica, MA, March 1994.

16. Hung JC, Wilson ME, Brown ML, Gibbons RJ. Rapid preparation and quality control method for technetium-99m-2-methoxy isobutyl isonitrile (technetium-99m-sestamibi). J Nucl Med 1991; 32: 2162–2168.

17. Hung JC, Wilson ME, Gebhard MW, Gibbons RJ. Comparison of four alternative radiochemical purity testing methods for [99]Tc[m]-sestamibi. Nucl Med Commun 1995; 16: 99–104.

18. Levit N, ed. Radiopharmacy Laboratory Manual for Nuclear Medicine Technologists. University of New Mexico College of Pharmacy, Albuquerque, NM, 1980, pp 69–80.

19. UltraTag RBC package insert. Mallinckrodt Medical, Inc., St. Louis, MO, January 1992.

20. Chowdhury S, Hung JC. Optimal centrifugation: parameters for labeling efficiency determination of technetium-99m labeled red blood cells (abstract). J Nucl Med Technol 1993; 21: 114–115.

21. Martinez E, Study KT. Scintillation well counter: too much activity? Monthly Scan, July 1980; p 1.

22. Vivian A, Ice RD, Shen V, et al. Procedure Manual. Radiochemical Purity of Radiopharmaceuticals Using Gelman Sepachrom (ITLC) Chromatography. Gelman Sciences, Ann Arbor, MI, 1977; pp 3–56.

23. Williams CC. Re: Radiochemical purity of ^{99m}Tc-oxidronate (letter to the editor). J Nucl Med 1981; 22: 1015–1016.

24. Zimmer AM, Spies SM. Quality control procedures for newer radiopharmaceuticals. J Nucl Med Technol 1991; 19: 210–214.

Pharmaceutical Tests

Introduction

Because radiopharmaceuticals are intended for administration to humans, QC procedures are imperative to ensure the safety of this preparation. Although extensive QC procedures are performed by the manufacturer, the use of cold kits to prepare radiopharmaceuticals with short-lived radionuclides, such as ^{99m}Tc and ^{111}In, requires that QC tests be conducted on all on-site radiopharmaceutical preparations before dispensing this product for administration to humans.

The routine radiopharmaceutical QC procedures can be divided into two categories: radiation tests and pharmaceutical tests. The pharmaceutical tests include visual inspection, particle size, chemical purity (presence of aluminum), and acidity (pH). These methods are discussed in detail next.

Visual Inspection

One should be thoroughly familiar with the normal color and appearance of every radiopharmaceutical (Table 2-5). The difference between ^{32}P-sodium phosphate, which is a colorless clear solution, and ^{32}P-chromic phosphate, which is a bluish green and slightly turbid insoluble suspension, should especially be noted.

Particle Size

Table 2-6 lists the range of particle size for some commonly used particulate radiopharmaceuticals. Microscopic inspection with the use of a light microscope and hemocytometer grid

Table 2-5. Color and Appearance of Radiopharmaceuticals

Radiopharmaceutical	Color	Appearance
^{99m}Tc-MAA	White	Turbid
^{99m}Tc-sulfur colloid	Milky	Slightly turbid
Other ^{99m}Tc-labeled compounds	Colorless	Clear
^{131}I-sodium iodide	Colorless	Clear (turns light amber with time)
^{131}I-OIH	Colorless	Clear
^{32}P-sodium phosphate	Colorless	Clear
^{32}P-chromic phosphate	Bluish green	Slightly turbid
Other non-^{99m}Tc-labeled compounds	Colorless	Clear

Table 2-6. Particle Size of Common Particulate Radiopharmaceuticals

Material	Diameter (nm)
^{99m}Tc-antimony sulfide colloid	3–30
^{99m}Tc-sulfur colloid (thiosulfate)	100–1,000
^{99m}Tc-albumin colloid (Microlite, DuPont)	200–1,000 (80%)
	<200 (15%)
^{99m}Tc-MAA	10,000–90,000 (85%)
	<150,000 (100%)

(Fig. 2-6) may be used to estimate particle size and number. According to USP 23/NF 18, at least 90% of the particles in a ^{99m}Tc-MAA preparation should have a diameter between 10 and 90 μm, and none of the observed particles should have a diameter greater than 150 μm.[1]

Chemical Purity

Chemical purity is a measure of the presence of undesirable chemical species in radiopharmaceuticals. Examples of chemical impurities are aluminum ion (Al^{3+}) in the ^{99m}Tc generator eluate, carrier iodine in radioiodide solution, and trace metals such as iron in ^{111}In-indium chloride solution. Excessive Al^{3+} may induce flocculation of ^{99m}Tc sulfur colloid because Al^{3+} combines with the phosphate buffer in the product to form insoluble aluminum phosphate.[2,3] In bone scanning, liver localization and degradation of image quality have been noted when Al^{3+} concentrations exceed 10 μg/ml ^{99m}Tc-eluate.[4] Carrier iodine can compete with radioiodine in the radioiodination process, resulting in poor labeling efficiency. Trace metals can significantly decrease labeling yield with ^{111}In, especially in OncoScint, OctreoScan, and platelet labeling with ^{111}In-oxine.

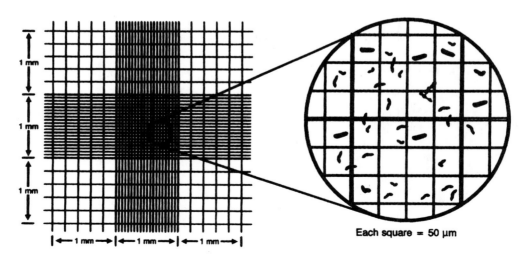

1 mm

1 mm

1 mm

|← 1 mm →|← 1 mm →|← 1 mm →|

Each square = 50 μm

Figure 2-6. Schematic diagram of hemocytometer display for estimation of ^{99m}Tc-MAA particle size and number.

In this procedure manual, only the chemical purity tests for the concentration of aluminum ion (Al^{3+}) are discussed. According to USP 23/NF 18, the concentration of aluminum ion in ^{99m}Tc sodium pertechnetate eluate should not exceed 10 µg/ml.[5] The most commonly used method for checking aluminum breakthrough is the colorimetric spot test.

Procedure for Determining Aluminum Breakthrough

1. Place a small drop (about 10 µl) of ^{99m}Tc eluate on an Al^{3+} test paper strip.
2. A similar size drop of a standard Al^{3+} solution (concentration: usually 10 µg Al^{3+}/ml) is placed next to the sodium pertechnetate ^{99m}Tc spot.
    a. The Al^{3+} ion present in ^{99m}Tc eluate reacts with the indicator of the test paper column.
    b. If the color of the ^{99m}Tc spot is less intense than the standard Al^{3+} spot, the ^{99m}Tc eluate passes the test (i.e., eluate contains less than 10 µg Al^{3+}/ml ^{99m}Tc eluate).
    c. If the intensity of the ^{99m}Tc sample spot is the same or more intense than the aluminum standard spot (i.e., pink color), the ^{99m}Tc eluate fails the test (i.e., the amount of Al^{3+} ion present in the ^{99m}Tc eluate is greater than 10 µg Al^{3+}/ml).

Alumina (Al_2O_3) Bed of the ^{99}Mo Generator

1. The ^{99}Mo generator is constructed with alumina loaded in a plastic or glass column.
2. At a pH of 5–6, alumina is "+" charged.
3. The loading capacity of molybdate (MoO_4^{2-}) on the alumina is approximately 2 mg MoO_4^{2-}/g Al_2O_3.

Causes of Aluminum Breakthrough

1. Improper heat treatment of alumina
2. Presence of alumina fines
3. Acid treatment of alumina

Aluminum breakthrough was a common problem with the older, large-column neutron-activated ^{99}Mo generators. With the present generator technology (i.e., small-column fission ^{99}Mo generators), alumina breakthrough occurs only rarely.

Acidity (pH)

All radiopharmaceuticals have an optimal pH range for stability, and most radiopharmaceuticals are within the pH range of 4–8. However, there are some exceptions:

1. Radioiodine solution should be kept at alkaline pH to prevent volatilization of iodine.
2. Indium chloride solution must be kept quite acid (pH 1–3) for it to remain in solution and to prevent formation of insoluble indium hydroxides.
3. The pH of the prepared ^{99m}Tc-exametazime (^{99m}Tc-HMPAO) is in the range of 9.0–9.8.

References

1. Technetium Tc 99m albumin aggregated injection. In: "United States Pharmacopeia," 23rd ed., and "National Formulary," 18th ed., The United States Pharmacopeial Convention, Inc., Rockville, MD, 1995, pp 1480–1481.

2. Staum MM. Incompatibility of phosphate buffer in ^{99m}Tc-sulfur colloid containing aluminum ion. J Nucl Med 1972; 13: 386–387.

3. Study KT, Hladik WB, Saha GB. Effects of AI^{3+} ion on Tc-99m sulfur colloid preparations with different buffers. J Nucl Med Technol 1984; 12: 16–18.

4. Sodium pertechnetate Tc 99m injection. In: "United States Pharmacopeia," 23rd ed., and "National Formulary," 18th ed., The United States Pharmacopeial Convention, Inc., Rockville, MD, 1995, pp 1486–1487.

5. Zimmer AM, Pavel DG. Experimental investigations of the possible cause of liver appearance during bone scanning. Radiology 1978; 126: 813–816.

3

Central Nervous System

Brian P. Mullan

Brain Imaging–SPECT Study

Summary Information

Radiopharmaceutical

    Adult dose: 20 mCi (740 MBq) ^{99m}Tc ethylcysteinate diamer (ECD) (bicisate) or ^{99m}Tc hexamethylpropyleneamine-oxine (HMPAO).

    Pediatric dose: Based on body surface area, see Appendix A-3.

               Notes: Previously ^{99m}Tc HMPAO injection had to be used within 30 minutes after preparation. A more stable formulation of HMPAO (4–6 hour reconstituted shelf life) has recently been approved by the Food and Drug Administration (FDA).

Contraindications   None.

Dose/Scan Interval   Commence imaging about 10–15 minutes after ^{99m}Tc ECD injection or 1 hour after ^{99m}Tc HMPAO injection.

Views Obtained   Tomographic views of the brain.

Indications

Brain perfusion agents, such as ^{99m}Tc ECD and ^{99m}Tc HMPAO, are useful in the evaluation of patients with various cerebrovascular abnormalities, such as stroke, transient ischemia, and other neurologic disorders (e.g., Alzheimer's disease, epilepsy, Parkinson's disease).[1–3]

Principle

^{99m}Tc HMPAO is a lipophilic agent capable of penetrating the intact blood-brain barrier. In vivo, it displays high instability, reacting within seconds after intravenous injection. On crossing the blood-brain barrier, it loses its lipophilic characteristics and becomes trapped inside the brain.[4] The regional uptake and retention are related to the regional perfusion.[5] The prior formulation of ^{99m}Tc HMPAO was limited by low in vitro stability, which does not affect the recently approved stabilized form.

    Like ^{99m}Tc HMPAO, ^{99m}Tc ECD is retained in the brain as a result of ester hydrolysis. ^{99m}Tc ECD is rapidly eliminated from the body via the kidneys, giving low soft tissue background activity compared with ^{99m}Tc HMPAO. Also, ^{99m}Tc ECD is stable for up to 6 hours after reconstitution.[5]

Patient Preparation

The patients should be kept in a quiet darkened room with their eyes closed before ^{99m}Tc HMPAO or ^{99m}Tc ECD is administered, in order to reduce uptake in the visual cortex.

Instrument Specifications

Gamma camera:	Single-/dual- or triple-head single photon emission computed tomography (SPECT) system
Collimators:	Single-head system—high resolution fan-beam collimator Dual-/triple-head systems, ultrahigh-resolution fan-beam collimators
Energy setting:	140 keV 15–20% energy window
Computer system:	Acquisition requirements—SPECT (128 × 128 matrix) Processing requirements—SPECT reconstruction software optional; quantitative regional uptake program

Imaging Procedure

Ensure that the patient's head is securely restrained in the head holder as shown in Figure 3-1. Even small head movements during the acquisition can cause a noticeable degradation in image quality. *Note:* With fan-beam collimators, it is difficult to determine whether the brain is fully visualized in the field of view, because of distortion of the images. Hence, with the detector head close to the patient's head, move the patient up into the gantry until the shoulders just clear the edge of the detectors, as shown in Figure 3-2. Perform a SPECT study using the following acquisition variables.

Single-Head System

A 128 × 128 matrix (fan-beam collimators) or a 64 × 64 matrix (parallel-hole collimators) 120 views every 3° at 20 seconds per view. Use a 360° circular orbit. For fan-beam collimators, zoom factor = 1. For parallel-hole collimators, set zoom factor = 2, with offset along the y-axis, to the lower part of the detector field of view.

Dual-/Triple-Head System

A 128 × 128 matrix with 120 views every 3° at 15 seconds per view. Use a 360° circular orbit with no zoom. If hardware permits, perform a multiorbit acquisition with 10 orbits, each with 120 views at 1.5 seconds per view.

Computer Analysis

Data Reconstruction

1. Before reconstruction, ensure that uniformity correction and center-of-rotation correction have been performed or will be performed during the reconstruction process.
2. If fan-beam collimators were used, rebin the raw data into a 64 × 64 matrix (this may be done automatically on some systems during reconstruction).
3. Planar data should be prefiltered before back-projection and reconstructed with a Ramp filter. Suggested filters are a Butterworth (order 10–15, cutoff at 0.4–0.6 Nyquist) or Weiner

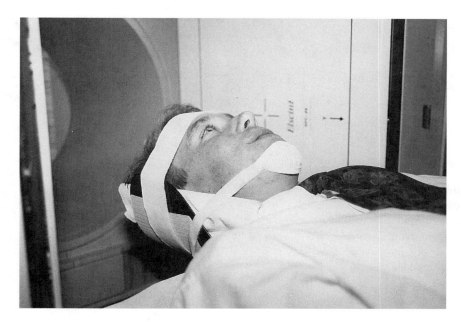

Figure 3-1. Secure restraint of the patient's head for SPECT acquisition.

filter (full width at half maximum [FWHM] = 7–9 mm). Reconstruct planar data into a 64 × 64 matrix. Apply attenuation correction (attenuation coefficient = 0.10–0.12 cm^{-1}).

4. For multiorbit acquisitions, if no patient motion is present, sum all 10 orbits and reconstruct as previously. Otherwise, eliminate bad orbits from summation. The multiorbit function is particularly valuable in seizure patients and children, who are most likely to move during the study. If motion is limited to 3 orbits or less, the remaining orbits may yield acceptable image quality. More extensive motion may require repeat acquisition of the study.

5. Review the sagittal slices, and check that the fronto-occipital plane is horizontal. This plane can be seen best by drawing a line on a midline sagittal slice, as shown in Figure 3-3. If the plane is not horizontal, generate a new set of oblique transaxial slices along this plane, and from these, produce new sagittal and coronal slices. Recheck the new sagittal slices to ensure correct orientation of the tomographic slices.

Semiquantitative Analysis

Note: Software for semiquantitative analysis is not yet standardized on many nuclear medicine computer systems. A common feature of many semiquantitative analysis techniques is the use of the cerebellum as a reference activity against which activities in other regions of the brain are compared.[6,7] The analysis described here requires the ability to generate circumferential profiles from elliptical regions of interest (ROIs). This function is available on many computer systems, as it is commonly used in cardiac analysis software to generate short-axis circumferential count profiles.

Analysis of the transaxial and sagittal images requires as input the oblique transaxial and sagittal data sets generated in the preceding step 5. Analysis of the temporal lobes, which is particularly critical for epilepsy patients, requires oblique transaxial slices whose plane of orientation lies midway between standard transaxial and coronal orientations. These

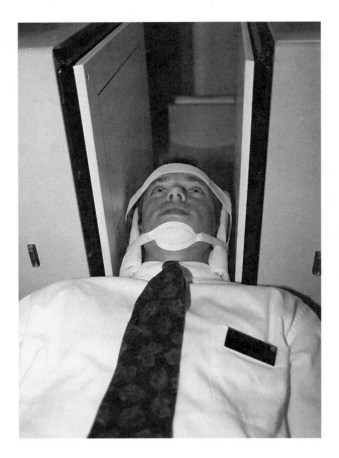

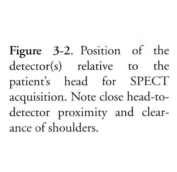

Figure 3-2. Position of the detector(s) relative to the patient's head for SPECT acquisition. Note close head-to-detector proximity and clearance of shoulders.

oblique slices should be oriented to cut through the long axis of the temporal lobes, as shown in Figure 3-4.

1. Display the transaxial data, and select those slices encompassing the cerebellum. Next, place a box ROI over the region of the cerebellum in each slice. Determine and record the highest pixel count in the cerebellum.
2. Select 3 transaxial slices for analysis, showing basal, midventricle, and vertex regions of the brain (Fig. 3-5).
3. Center and rotate 2 elliptical ROIs on a transaxial slice so that the cerebral cortex is located between the 2 ROIs (Fig. 3-6). Exclude the central structures (basal ganglia, thalamus) from the region between the 2 ROIs.
4. For the region between the 2 ROIs, generate circumferential count profiles by obtaining the maximum pixel count every 6° over 360° (60 points). Decrease the 60 points to 20 by obtaining the average of every 3 points (15°). Normalize the results by dividing by the maximum count in the cerebellum. Obtain the left-to-right ratio. Typical results from this type of analysis are shown in Figure 3-6.
5. Repeat steps 3 and 4 for the other 2 transaxial slices.
6. For sagittal analysis, select right and left sagittal slices equidistant from the midline of the brain (Fig. 3-7).
7. On the right sagittal slice, position and rotate the elliptical ROIs until the cortex is enclosed in the upper half of the 2 ellipses, as shown in Figure 3-8.

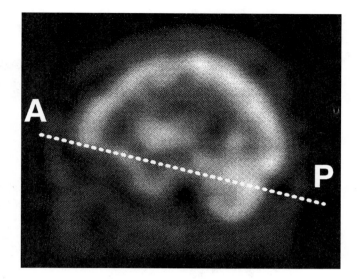

Figure 3-3. Midline sagittal slice showing the correct plane for the transaxial slices. A, anterior; P, posterior.

8. For the region between the two ROIs, generate circumferential count profiles by obtaining the maximum pixel count every 6° over 180° (thirty points). Decrease the thirty points to ten by obtaining the average of every three points (15°). Normalize the results by dividing by the maximum count in the cerebellum.

9. With identical ROIs, repeat this analysis on the left sagittal slice. Normalize the results by dividing by the maximum count in the cerebellum. Obtain the left-to-right ratio. Typical results from this type of analysis are shown in Figure 3-8.

10. For analysis of the temporal lobes, select the oblique transaxial data set generated at the angle shown in Figure 3-4. Position small elliptical ROIs over the right and left temporal lobes, and subdivide them as shown in Figure 3-9. Determine the maximum count in each region, normalize to cerebellum counts, and obtain the left-to-right ratio.

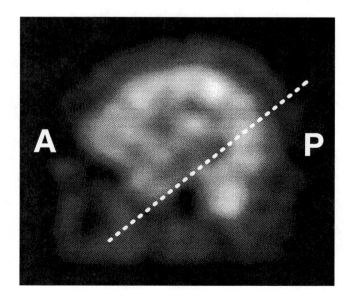

Figure 3-4. Midplane sagittal slice showing the correct plane for the oblique transaxial slices used to evaluate the temporal lobes. A, anterior; P, posterior.

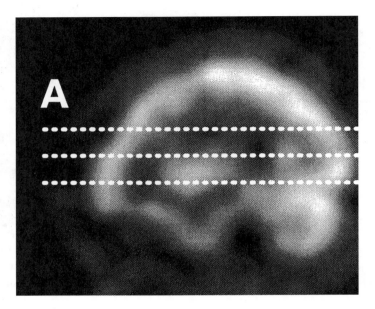

Figure 3-5. Midline sagittal slice showing the location of the 3 transaxial slices selected for analysis. A, anterior; P, posterior.

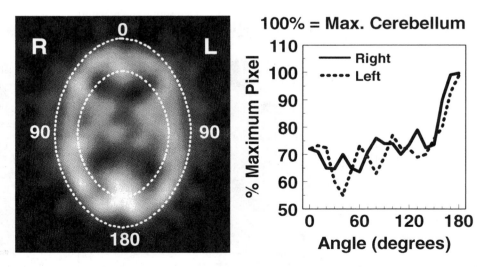

Figure 3-6. Transaxial slice with elliptical ROIs positioned for analysis of cortical activity. Left and right counts, normalized to cerebellum, are shown. R, right; L, left.

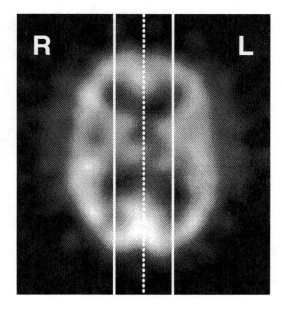

Figure 3-7. Transaxial slice showing location of left and right sagittal slices selected for analysis. R, right; L, left.

Information on Film

On all computer films, ensure that the following information is recorded:

> Patient's name and clinic/hospital number
> Date and time of study after the injection
> Type of scan and radiopharmaceutical
> Orientation of each image
> All ROIs and results of any quantitative analysis

Interpretation

In a normal ^{99m}Tc HMPAO or ^{99m}Tc ECD study, the transaxial and coronal images should show symmetric distribution of the radiotracer in both hemispheres. Because the rate of blood flow is greater in gray matter than in white matter, the greatest uptake is observed in cortical gray matter, the basal ganglia, and thalamus. *Note:* If a patient had his or her eyes open during injection of the radiotracer, significant uptake may be present in the visual cortex (occipital lobes).

Abnormal uptake patterns can be observed in various cerebrovascular diseases, epilepsy, stroke, transient ischemic attacks, acute head trauma, dementia, and other neuropsychiatric disorders. Abnormal regions may show absent, decreased, or increased uptake compared with that of adjacent areas or of corresponding areas in the contralateral hemisphere and comparison with that of the known normal appearance.

Radiation Dosimetry

The estimated absorbed doses in organs and tissues of an average subject (70 kg) from the administration of 20 mCi (740 MBq) ^{99m}Tc HMPAO or ^{99m}Tc ECD are shown in Table 3-1.[8,9]

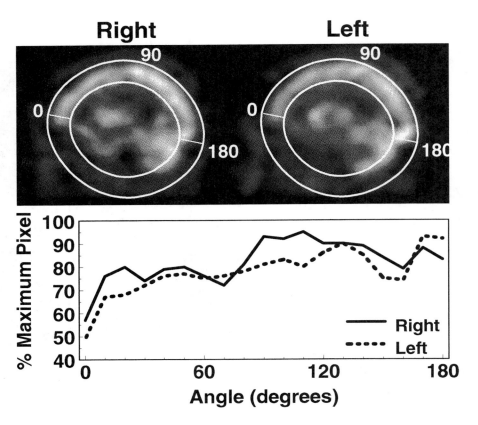

Figure 3-8. Sagittal slice with elliptical ROIs positioned for analysis of cortical activity. Comparative results of left and right counts normalized to cerebellum are shown.

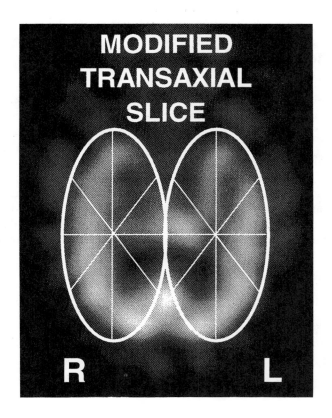

Figure 3-9. Position of elliptical ROIs over temporal lobes. The ROIs are subdivided into 8 pie segments.

Table 3-1. Absorbed Radiation Dose Estimates for a 70-kg Adult From 20 mCi (740 MBq) ^{99m}Tc HMPAO or ^{99m}Tc ECD

| | Absorbed Radiation Dose | | | |
| Tissue | 99mTc HMPAO | | 99mTc ECD | |
	rad/20 mCi	mGy/740 MBq	rad/20 mCi	mGy/740 MBq
Lacrimal glands	5.16	51.6	—	—
Gallbladder wall	3.80	38.0	1.82	18.2
Kidneys	2.60	26.0	0.54	5.40
Urinary bladder wall	0.94	9.40	5.40 (4-hr void)	54.0
Thyroid	2.00	20.0	0.26	2.60
Small bowel	0.88	8.80	0.70	7.00
Upper large intestinal wall	1.58	15.8	1.22	12.2
Lower large intestinal wall	1.08	10.8	0.96	9.62
Liver	1.08	10.8	0.39	3.92
Ovaries	0.46	4.60	0.40	4.00
Testes	0.14	1.40	0.16	1.62
Red marrow	0.26	2.60	0.18	1.78
Brain	0.52	5.20	0.40	4.00
Eyes	0.52	5.20	—	—
Bone surface	—	—	0.25	2.52
Total body	0.26	2.60	0.18	1.78

References

1. Devous MD Sr, Leroy RF, Herman RW. Single photon emission computed tomography in epilepsy. Semin Nucl Med 1990; 20: 325–341.
2. Bonte FJ, Hom J, Tintner R, Weiner MF. Single photon tomography in Alzheimer's disease and the dementias. Semin Nucl Med 1990; 20: 342–352.
3. Hellman RS, Tikofsky RS. An overview of the contribution of regional cerebral blood flow studies in cerebrovascular disease: is there a role for single photon emission computed tomography? Semin Nucl Med 1990; 20: 303–324.
4. Ballinger JR, Reid RH, Gulenchyn KY. Technetium-99m HM-PAO stereoisomers: differences in interaction with glutathione. J Nucl Med 1988; 29: 1998–2000.
5. Kung HF, Ohmomo Y, Kung MP. Current and future radiopharmaceuticals for brain imaging with single photon emission computed tomography. Semin Nucl Med 1990; 20: 290–302.
6. Friedman PJ, Davis G, Allen B. Semi-quantitative SPECT scanning in acute ischaemic stroke. Scand J Rehab Med 1993; 25: 99–105.
7. Lewis DH, Eskridge JM, Newell DW, et al. Brain SPECT and the effect of cerebral angioplasty in delayed ischemia due to vasospasm. J Nucl Med 1992; 33: 1789–1796.
8. Package insert. Ceretec: kit for the preparation of Technetium Tc-99m exametazime injection. Amersham Corp., 1995.
9. Package insert. Neurolite (Tc-99m bicisate). The Du Pont Merck Pharmaceutical Co., Nov., 1994.

Brain Imaging– Acetazolamide Challenge Study

Summary Information

Radiopharmaceutical

Adult dose: 20 mCi (740 MBq) ^{99m}Tc HMPAO or 20 mCi (740 MBq) ^{99m}Tc ECD intravenously.

Pediatric dose: Adjusted according to patient's weight (See Appendix A-3). *Notes:* Previously ^{99m}Tc HMPAO injection had to be used within 30 minutes of preparation. A more stable formulation of HMPAO (4-6 hour reconstituted shelf life) has recently been approved by the FDA.

Contraindications Acetazolamide (Diamox) is a sulfonamide derivative and may be contraindicated in patients with an allergy to sulfonamides (adverse reactions common to all sulfonamide derivatives include anaphylaxis, fever, and rash). Common short-term reactions to acetazolamide may include a tinnitus and/or a "tingling" sensation in the extremities.

In patients who have migraine headaches, acetazolamide may precipitate or exacerbate a migraine attack. Acetazolamide should be used with caution in patients with a history of recent transient ischemic attacks (within 1 week).

Dose/Scan Interval For the acetazolamide stress study, ^{99m}Tc HMPAO or ^{99m}Tc ECD is injected 20 minutes after the injection of acetazolamide. For both rest and stress studies, imaging should commence 10–15 minutes after injection of ^{99m}Tc ECD or 1 hour after injection of ^{99m}Tc HMPAO.

Views Obtained Tomographic views of the brain.

Indications

A brain scan with acetazolamide challenge is indicated in patients with suspected or known cerebrovascular disease.[1–4] Resting brain blood flow in patients with cerebrovascular disease may be focally decreased or may be normal in the absence of prior ischemic events.

However, these patients may have diminished vasodilatory reserve and an inability to increase brain blood flow at times of increased demand.

Principle

Vascular diseases such as atherosclerosis may produce blood flow abnormalities that cannot respond to a vasodilator. If the vascular disease is severe, the blood flow abnormality may be detected with a resting cerebral blood flow study. However, mild-to-moderate vascular disease may show no abnormality. After the administration of a cerebral vasodilator such as acetazolamide, normal areas show increased blood flow, whereas areas of mild-to-moderate vascular disease will remain unchanged and will appear as regions of comparatively reduced blood flow.

Patient Preparation

The patients should be kept in a quiet darkened room with their eyes closed before the ^{99m}Tc HMPAO or ^{99m}Tc ECD is administered, to decrease uptake in the visual cortex.

Pharmaceutical

Acetazolamide comes in 500-mg vials and is reconstituted in sterile water.

Adult dose: 1 g IV
Pediatric dose: 15 mg/kg body weight IV

Instrument Specifications

Gamma camera: Single-/dual- or triple-head SPECT system
Collimators: Single-head system—high-resolution fan-beam collimator
Dual-/triple-head systems—ultrahigh-resolution fan-beam collimators
Energy setting: 140 keV 15–20% energy window
Computer system: Acquisition requirements—SPECT (128 × 128 matrix)
Processing requirements—SPECT reconstruction software, optional; quantitative regional uptake program

Imaging Procedure

Stress Study

1. Inject the acetazolamide intravenously over a 5-minute period, with the patient supine. Pain at the injection site will occur if the drug is extravasated, because of its low pH. Longer infusion times are less effective.
2. Inject the ^{99m}Tc HMPAO or ^{99m}Tc ECD 20 minutes after the acetazolamide infusion is complete (time of maximum cerebral vasodilation).
3. Commence imaging about 1 hour after the ^{99m}Tc HMPAO injection or 10–15 minutes after the ^{99m}Tc ECD injection.

Rest Study (Optional—May Not Be Required If Stress Study Shows Symmetric Perfusion)

On a separate day, inject the same dose of ^{99m}Tc HMPAO or ^{99m}Tc ECD (no acetazolamide to be administered) and image at 1 hour (^{99m}Tc HMPAO) or 10–15 minutes

(^{99m}Tc ECD) after injection. *Note:* The same gamma camera should be used for the acetazolamide stress and rest studies.

Ensure that the patient's head is securely restrained in the head holder, as shown in Figure 3-1. Even small head movements during the acquisition can cause a noticeable degradation in image quality. *Note:* With fan-beam collimators, it is difficult to determine whether the brain is fully visualized in the field of view, because of distortion of the images. Hence, with the detector head close to the patient's head, move the patient up into the gantry until the shoulders just clear the edge of the detectors as shown in Figure 3-2. Perform a SPECT study using the following acquisition variables.

Single-Head System

A 128 × 128 matrix (fan-beam collimators) or a 64 × 64 matrix (parallel-hole collimators), 120 views every 3° at 20 seconds per view. Use a 360° circular orbit. For fan-beam collimators, zoom factor = 1. For parallel-hole collimators, set zoom factor = 2, with offset along the y-axis, to the lower part of the detector field of view.

Dual-/Triple-Head System

A 128 × 128 matrix with 120 views every 3° at 15 seconds per view. Use a 360° circular orbit with no zoom. If hardware permits, perform a multiorbit acquisition with 10 orbits, each with 120 views at 1.5 seconds per view.

Computer Analysis

Data Reconstruction

1. Before reconstruction, ensure that uniformity correction and center-of-rotation correction have been performed or will be performed during the reconstruction process.
2. If fan-beam collimators were used, rebin the raw data into a 64 × 64 matrix (this may be done automatically on some systems during reconstruction).
3. Planar data should be prefiltered before back-projection and reconstructed with a Ramp filter. Suggested filters are a Butterworth (order 10–15, cutoff at 0.4–0.6 Nyquist) or Weiner filter (FWHM = 7–9 mm). Reconstruct planar data into a 64 × 64 matrix. Apply attenuation correction (attenuation coefficient = 0.10–0.12 cm^{-1}).
4. For multiorbit acquisitions, if no patient motion is present, sum all 10 orbits and reconstruct as previously. Otherwise, eliminate bad orbits from summation. The multiorbit function is particularly valuable in patients who are in discomfort or are uncooperative and in children, who are most likely to move during the study. If motion is limited to 3 orbits or less, the remaining orbits may yield acceptable image quality. More extensive motion may require repeat acquisition of the study.
5. Review the sagittal slices, and check that the fronto-occipital plane is horizontal. This plane can be seen best by drawing a line on a midline sagittal slice, as shown in Figure 3-3. If the plane is not horizontal, generate a new set of oblique transaxial slices along this plane and, from these, produce new sagittal and coronal slices. Recheck the new sagittal slices to ensure correct orientation of the tomographic slices.
6. Carefully check rest and stress oblique images to ensure that both studies have been reoriented in the same plane.

Semiquantitative Analysis

Note: Software for semiquantitative analysis is not yet standardized on many nuclear medicine computer systems. A common feature of many semiquantitative analysis techniques is the use of the cerebellum as a reference activity against which activities in other regions of the brain are compared.[5,6] Comparative quantitation is possible between the rest and stress studies, because in general the cerebellum is relatively unaffected by acetazolamide. The analysis described next requires the ability to generate circumferential profiles from elliptical ROIs. This function is commonly used in cardiac analysis software to generate short-axis circumferential count profiles.

Semiquantitative analysis requires as input the oblique transaxial and sagittal data sets as described in the preceding step 5. Analysis of the temporal lobes requires oblique transaxial slices whose plane of orientation lies midway between standard transaxial and coronal orientations. These oblique slices should be oriented to cut through the long axis of the temporal lobes, as shown in Figure 3-4.

1. From the stress study, display the transaxial data, and select those slices encompassing the cerebellum. Next, place a box ROI over the region of the cerebellum in each slice. Determine and record the highest pixel count in the cerebellum.
2. Select 3 transaxial slices for analysis, showing basal, midventricle, and vertex regions of the brain (see Fig. 3-5).
3. Center and rotate 2 elliptical ROIs on a transaxial slice so that the cerebral cortex is located between the 2 ROIs (see Fig. 3-6).
4. For the region between the 2 ROIs, generate circumferential count profiles by obtaining the maximum pixel count every 6° over 360° (60 points). Decrease the 60 points to 20 by obtaining the average of every 3 points (15°). Normalize the results by dividing by the maximum count in the cerebellum. Obtain the left-to-right ratio. Typical results from this type of analysis are shown in Figure 3-6.
5. Repeat steps 3 and 4 for the other 2 transaxial slices.
6. For sagittal analysis, select right and left sagittal slices equidistant from the midline of the brain (see Fig. 3-7).
7. On the right sagittal slice, position and rotate the elliptical ROIs until the cortex is enclosed in the upper half of the 2 ellipses, as shown in Figure 3-8.
8. For the region between the 2 ROIs, generate circumferential count profiles by obtaining the maximum pixel count every 6° over 180° (30 points). Decrease the 30 points to 10 by obtaining the average of every 3 points (15°). Normalize the results by dividing by the maximum count in the cerebellum.
9. With identical ROIs, repeat this analysis on the left sagittal slice. Normalize the results by dividing by the maximum count in the cerebellum. Obtain the left-to-right ratio. Typical results from this type of analysis are shown in Figure 3-8.
10. For analysis of the temporal lobes, select the oblique transaxial data set generated at the angle shown in Figure 3-4. Position small elliptical ROIs over the right and left temporal lobes, and subdivide them as shown in Figure 3-9. Determine the maximum count in each region, normalize to cerebellum counts, and obtain the left-to-right ratio.
11. Repeat the preceding analysis with the rest images. The same ROIs should be used to permit comparison of the stress and rest studies.

Information on Film

On all computer films, ensure that the following information is recorded:

Patient's name and clinic/hospital number
Date and time of study after the injection

Acetazolamide dose and time interval between acetazolamide injection and radiopharmaceutical injection

Type of scan and radiopharmaceutical

Orientation of each image

All ROIs and results of any quantitative analysis

Interpretation

Patients with cerebrovascular disease may show abnormalities on the stress study. The rest study will indicate whether these abnormalities are fixed or reversible.

Additional Note

A patient who has normal findings on the stress study (i.e., no significant asymmetry, right-to-left differences less than 15%) does not need to have a rest study performed, as it is unlikely that a patient will have totally balanced (left = right) cerebrovascular disease.

Radiation Dosimetry

The estimated absorbed doses in organs and tissues of an average subject (70 kg) from the administration of 20 mCi (740 MBq) ^{99m}Tc HMPAO or ^{99m}Tc ECD are shown in Table 3-1.[7,8]

References

1. Knop J, Thie A, Fuchs C, Siepmann G, Zeumer H. ^{99m}Tc-HMPAO-SPECT with acetazolamide challenge to detect hemodynamic compromise in occlusive cerebrovascular disease. Stroke 1992; 23: 1733–1742.
2. Devous MD Sr, Payne JK, Lowe JL. Dual-isotope brain SPECT imaging with technetium-99m and iodine-123: clinical validation using xenon-133 SPECT. J Nucl Med 1992; 33: 1919–1924.
3. Matsuda H, Higashi S, Kinuya K, et al. SPECT evaluation of brain perfusion reserve by the acetazolamide test using Tc-99m HMPAO. Clin Nucl Med 1991; 8: 572–579.
4. Matsuda H, Tsuji S, Sumiya H, et al. Acetazolamide effect on vascular response in areas with diaschisis as measured by Tc-99m HMPAO brain SPECT. Clin Nucl Med 1992; 17: 581–586.
5. Friedman PJ, Davis G, Allen B. Semi-quantitative SPECT scanning in acute ischaemic stroke. Scand J Rehabil Med 1993; 25: 99–105.
6. Lewis DH, Eskridge JM, Newell DW, et al. Brain SPECT and the effect of cerebral angioplasty in delayed ischemia due to vasospasm. J Nucl Med 1992; 33: 1789–1796.
7. Package Insert. Ceretec: kit for the preparation of Technetium Tc-99m exametazime injection. Amersham Corp., 1990.
8. Package Insert. Neurolite (Tc-99m bicisate). The Du Pont Merck Pharmaceutical Co., Nov., 1994.

Cerebrospinal Fluid Imaging–Cisternography

Summary Information

Radiopharmaceutical

Adult dose: 500 µCi (18.5 MBq) of ^{111}In diethylenetriaminepentacetic acid (DTPA) injected intrathecally by lumbar puncture. The injection should be performed aseptically by a trained physician or nurse, with the assistance of a technologist.

Pediatric dose: Adjusted according to patient's weight (see Appendix A-3).

Injection Procedure

1. The lumbar puncture should be performed by a physician or nurse experienced in lumbar puncture injections.
2. An unopened, unused vial of ^{111}In DTPA should be used. Calculate the volume of ^{111}In DTPA to be administered to the patient (volumetric dose calculation).
3. The vial contents must never be diluted, and the only needle puncture of the vial should be that of the physician or nurse proceeding with the injection.
4. The following supplies are needed:
    1-ml syringe for ^{111}In DTPA dose
    Sterile gloves (have all sizes available)
    2 lumbar puncture trays
    Spinal needles—various lengths and gauges
    Alcohol wipes
    A table and wastebasket close to the physician
5. The required volume of ^{111}In DTPA should be withdrawn from the vial using aseptic technique.
6. After injection of the ^{111}In DTPA, the physician or nurse should rinse the syringe 2–3 times with cerebrospinal fluid (CSF) before removing the needle.

Contraindications Increased intracranial pressure. A relative contraindication is recent lumbar puncture.

Dose/Scan Interval Imaging commences about 2 hours after injection.

Views Obtained The following views should be obtained:
Posterior head and spine, including injection site on the 2-hour view
Anterior head
Right and left lateral views of the head
Occasionally, a vertex view or transmission scan through the head may be helpful

Indications

Radionuclide cisternography is used to monitor the flow of CSF through the subarachnoid space and is one of the most reliable techniques for assessing CSF hemodynamics. Clinical indications for cisternography include conditions that can block or alter the flow of CSF (e.g., meningitis, hemorrhage, tumors). Radionuclide cisternography is particularly useful in the diagnosis of CSF rhinorrhea and normal-pressure hydrocephalus.[1-3] Patients with normal-pressure hydrocephalus demonstrate the clinical triad of dementia, ataxia, and urinary incontinence. Early diagnosis of this condition may lead to surgical correction.

Principle

After the injection of ^{111}In DTPA into the lumbar subarachnoid space (generally between the 3rd and 4th lumbar vertebrae), the flow of ^{111}In DTPA through the subarachnoid space can be monitored. Altered CSF flow characterizes the diagnosis of communicating and noncommunicating hydrocephalus and may result in CSF leaks.[2,4] Minor leaks of CSF into the nasal cavity can be detected by counting the radioactivity accumulated in cotton swabs placed in the nasal passages.[4]

Patient Preparation

1. After injection of the ^{111}In DTPA into the subarachnoid space, the patient should remain supine for 2 hours to prevent headache or other side effects that are due to the temporary imbalance of the CSF.
2. If CSF rhinorrhea is suspected, small cotton swabs (pledgets), such as those shown in Figure 3-10, should be placed in the nasal sinuses either before or within 2 hours after the injection of the ^{111}In DTPA. A total of 6 pledgets should be inserted into the nasal sinuses (3 per side). The pledgets should be placed in the following locations (Fig. 3-11):
   Right and left sphenoethmoidal recess (sphenoid)
   Right and left superior meatus (cribriform)
   Right and left middle meatus

Instrument Specifications

Gamma camera:	Any large field-of-view system can be used
Collimators:	Medium energy collimator

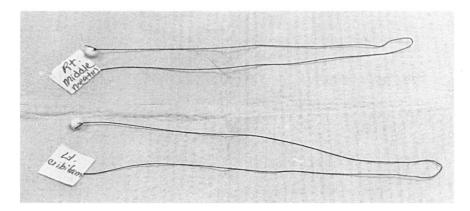

Figure 3-10. Cotton swabs (pledgets) used to detect small CSF leaks.

Energy setting: 20% energy windows around the 172-keV and 247-keV peaks of ^{111}In

Zoom factor: About 1.5 for a 40-cm field-of-view system

Analog formatter: 8 × 10 film, 70-mm (9 on 1) format

Computer system: Acquisition requirements—static (256 × 256 matrix)
Processing requirements—none

Imaging Procedure

1. At 2 hours after the injection, position the patient supine on the imaging table, with the gamma camera placed posteriorly over the head and neck.
2. Acquire a posterior view of the head and neck on the analog formatter and on the computer (256 × 256 matrix) for 50–100 kct. Note the acquisition time, and acquire a view of the injection site (if not already included in the previous image) for the same time.
3. Acquire an anterior view of the head and neck for 50–100 kct on the computer and analog formatter. Note the time of the anterior head view, and acquire the right and left lateral views for this time.
4. The posterior, anterior, and lateral views should be acquired again at 6 and 24 hours after the injection. Additional sets of images may be required at 48 and 72 hours. For these later views, the acquisition time, counts, and intensity setting of the analog formatter should be noted and adjusted to allow for decay and clearance.
5. In some patients, a vertex view may be required. This is easiest to perform if the patient is placed supine on a SPECT table top, with his or her head in the headrest and the detector facing horizontally.
6. A ^{99m}Tc or ^{57}Co transmission scan can be helpful to delineate the cranium, especially in patients with increased ventricular size.

Computer Analysis

None.

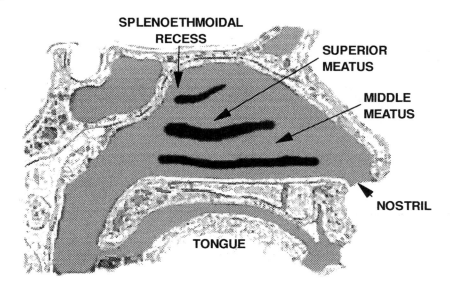

Figure 3-11. Sagittal view through the nasal sinuses showing the regions for placement of pledgets.

Laboratory Analysis

If a CSF nasal leak is present, activity will leak into the nasal passages and be absorbed onto the pledgets. Because the pledgets may be contaminated with nasal mucus or may dry out after removal, the difference between the dry and wet weight of the pledget is only a crude indication of the amount of CSF absorbed by the pledget. The fluid-retaining capacity of the pledgets can be estimated by weighing 10 dry pledgets and noting their average weight. Next, soak the pledgets in water and then remove them and weigh them again. Determine the average weight of the wet pledgets. The difference (in grams) represents the maximum fluid capacity of a pledget. Convert this to its equivalent volume of fluid (1 g water = 1 ml water). Small pledgets retain only 0.1–0.2 ml of CSF, and larger ones have a larger fluid capacity (0.5 ml) and provide a more accurate estimate of CSF leakage.

1. At about 6 hours after the injection, the nasal pledgets should be removed, and each one should be placed in a separate tube.
2. At the time the pledgets are removed, draw 3–5 ml of blood into a heparinized vial.
3. Centrifuge the blood sample, and extract the plasma. Place 1 ml of plasma in a counting tube.
4. Count an empty tube (background), each pledget, and the 1-ml plasma sample in a well counter.
5. Ensure that the well counter is set to count over the energy range 140–550 keV at 5 minutes per sample.
6. Correct the pledget activity for background and divide by the fluid capacity of the pledget to give counts per milliliter.
7. Adjust plasma counts (background corrected) to give counts per milliliter. Compare with counts per milliliter in the pledgets. Pledget activity should be less than 1.3–1.5 times the plasma activity of normal subjects.[4]
8. If a small leak is present, increased activity may be seen only in the sphenoid or cribriform pledgets, depending on the location of the leak.

Information on Film

On analog and computer film, ensure that the following information is recorded:

> Patient name and clinic/hospital number
> Date and time of each image after injection
> Type of scan and radiopharmaceutical
> Orientation of each image (e.g., ant, post)

Also, record on a worksheet the time of blood samples and pledget removal and the analysis of pledget activity.

Interpretation

Normal Flow

Activity migrates upward and reaches the cisterna magna within 2–3 hours. The activity passes forward along the base of the brain and then ascends symmetrically in front of and along the side of both cerebral hemispheres to reach the superior sagittal sinus after 24 hours. [111]In DTPA is normally reabsorbed by the arachnoid villi and enters the blood stream to be excreted by the kidneys. Reabsorption occurs slowly over several days. These times may be considerably shorter in children and longer in elderly patients.

Table 3-2. Absorbed Radiation Dose Estimates in a 70-kg Adult From Intrathecal Administration of 0.5 mCi (18.5 MBq) [111]In DTPA

Tissue	Absorbed Radiation Dose	
	rad/0.5 mCi	mGy/18.5 MBq
Kidneys	0.22	2.20
Spinal cord	2.00	20.0
Ovaries	0.06	0.60
Testes	0.05	0.49
Brain	0.40	4.00
Bladder wall (2-hr void)	0.21	2.10
Total body	0.04	0.40

Abnormal Flow

Abnormal flow patterns can include transient or prolonged entry of the tracer into the ventricles, delay in activity reaching the superior sagittal sinus, asymmetric flow patterns, and blockage of flow at any level. Occasionally, filling or trapping of tracer within cysts or surgical defects is seen. In patients with CSF leakage, activity may be seen in the nasal cavity on the lateral view.

Pledget Activity

The activity on the pledgets should be symmetric and not greater than plasma activity. Pledget activity should be compared with plasma activity, because ^{111}In DTPA may enter the blood stream either by reabsorption through the arachnoid villi or through extravasation of activity at the injection site. With a CSF leak, pledget activity per unit volume should be greater than 1.3–1.5 times the plasma activity per unit volume.[4]

Radiation Dosimetry

The estimated absorbed doses in organs and tissues of an average subject (70 kg) from an intrathecal injection of 0.5 mCi (18.5 MBq) [111]In DTPA are shown in Table 3-2.[5]

References

1. Lantz EJ, Forbes GS, Brown ML, Laws ER Jr. Radiology of cerebrospinal fluid rhinorrhea. Am J Roentgenol 1980; 135: 1023–1030.
2. McKusick KA. The diagnosis of traumatic cerebrospinal fluid rhinorrhea (editorial). J Nucl Med 1977; 18: 1234–1235.
3. Enzmann DR, Norman D, Price DC, Newton TH. Metrizamide and radionuclide cisternography in communicating hydrocephalus. Radiology 1979; 130: 681–686.
4. McKusick KA, Malmud LS, Kordela PA, Wagner HN Jr. Radionuclide cisternography: normal values for nasal secretion of intrathecally injected ^{111}In-DTPA. J Nucl Med 1973; 14: 933–934.
5. Harbert JC, Pollina R. Absorbed dose estimates for radionuclides. Clin Nucl Med 1984; 9: 210–221.

Cerebrospinal Fluid Imaging–Ventriculography

Summary Information

Radiopharmaceutical

Adult dose: 500 μCi (18.5 MBq) of ^{111}In DTPA injected directly into the lateral ventricle or external shunt reservoir. The injection will be performed by a trained physician and may require the assistance of a technologist.

Pediatric dose: Adjusted according to patient's weight (see Appendix A-3).

Injection Procedure

1. The ventricular injection should be performed in the operating room by an experienced physician or surgeon.
2. An unopened, unused vial of ^{111}In DTPA should be used. Calculate the volume of ^{111}In DTPA to be administered to the patient (volumetric dose calculation).
3. The vial contents must never be diluted, and the only needle puncture of the vial should be that of the physician or surgeon proceeding with the injection.
4. For a ventricular injection, the following supplies are needed:

   1-ml syringe for ^{111}In DTPA dose
   Sterile gloves (have all sizes available)
   2 lumbar puncture trays
   Spinal needles—various lengths and gauges
   Alcohol wipes
   A table and wastebasket close to the physician
5. The required volume of ^{111}In DTPA should be withdrawn from the vial using aseptic technique.
6. The physician or surgeon inserts the ventricular needle directly into the ventricle or into an external shunt reservoir, if present. This is done in the operating room or in the case of an external shunt reservoir, in the patient's room under sterile conditions. The technologist should assist in drawing the correct dose of ^{111}In DTPA and may have to be dressed in a sterile gown.

Continues

107

Summary Information *(Continued)*

7. After injection of the ^{111}In DTPA, the physician should rinse the syringe 2–3 times with CSF before removing the needle.

Contraindications   Relative contraindication—increased intracranial pressure.

Dose/Scan Interval

Ventricular injection: Imaging commences about 1 hour after the injection.

Shunt reservoir injection: Imaging commences immediately after the injection.

Views Obtained   Anterior and posterior views of the head

Anterior views of the chest and abdomen

Indications

Radionuclide ventriculography is used to monitor the pattern of CSF flow in patients who have had a ventriculostomy or a ventriculoperitoneal shunt (shunting of the CSF into the circulatory system or abdominal cavity is used to treat some types of hydrocephalus).[1]

Principle

[111]In DTPA is injected into the lateral ventricle or an external shunt reservoir. By monitoring the flow of ^{111}In DTPA, it is possible to determine the patency of the shunt or the location of the obstruction.[1,2]

Patient Preparation

A sterile environment is required for injection of the ^{111}In DTPA, either in an operating room (ventricular injection) or at the bedside (external shunt injection).

Instrument Specifications

Gamma camera: Any large field-of-view system can be used

Collimators: Medium-energy collimator

Energy setting: 20% energy window around the 172-keV and 247-keV peaks of [111]In

Analog formatter: 8 × 10 film, 70-mm (9 on 1) format

Computer system: Acquisition requirements—static (256 × 256 matrix), dynamic (64 × 64 matrix)

Processing requirements (optional)—ROI analysis, curve generation

Imaging Procedure

Ventricular Injection

1. At 1 hour after the injection, position the patient supine on the imaging table, and acquire anterior, lateral, and posterior images of the head on the analog formatter and on the computer (256 × 256 matrix) for 50–100 kct per view. Note the time per view.

2. Acquire anterior views of the chest and abdomen for the same time as in step 1 above.
3. Repeat steps 1 and 2 at 6 and 24 hours after the injection using the same time per view. Additional images may be required at 48 and 72 hours. Note that for shunts into the peritoneal cavity, additional views may be required to visualize the shunt.

Shunt Injection

1. After injection of the ^{111}In DTPA, the shunt reservoir should be pumped manually to aid in flushing activity into the chest and abdomen.
2. With the patient supine on the imaging table, acquire an anterior view of the injection site and shunt tubing immediately after the injection on analog formatter and on computer (256 × 256 matrix) for 50–100 kct. Note the time per view.
3. Repeat step 2 at 5, 10, and 20 minutes after the injection.
4. If there is delayed clearance of activity from the injection site, repeat step 2 at 2 and 6 hours after the injection using the same time per view as in step 2. Note that for shunts into the peritoneal cavity, additional views may be required to visualize the shunt.

Note: An alternative to injecting into the shunt reservoir is to inject directly into the shunt tubing, followed by dynamic acquisition on analog formatter (9 images at 3 minutes per image) and on computer (64 × 64 word mode matrix, 30 images at 1 minute per image). An ROI should be drawn around the injected activity, and time-activity curves should be generated to quantitate movement of activity from the injection site.

Computer Analysis

None.

Information on Film

On analog and computer film, ensure that the following information is recorded:

> Patient name and clinic/hospital number
> Date and time of each image after the injection
> Type of scan and radiopharmaceutical
> Orientation of each image (e.g., ant, post)

Interpretation

For ventricular injection, most of the activity is still in the ventricles at 1 hour after the injection, but the 1-hour image provides a baseline for comparison with later images and also helps in determining whether the dose was administered correctly. The 6- and 24-hour scans should show the passage of ^{111}In DTPA in the shunt tubing between the head and the chest or abdomen. Some renal or urinary activity may also be evident, indicating patency of the shunt. Ventricles should be empty—or nearly empty—of activity at 24 hours. If very little flow is seen with substantial activity remaining in the ventricles, 48- and 72-hour images may be appropriate for further evaluation.

Radiation Dosimetry

The estimated absorbed doses in organs and tissues of an average subject (70 kg) from an intrathecal injection of 0.5 mCi (18.5 MBq) [111]In DTPA are shown in Table 3-2.[3]

References

1. James AE Jr, DeBlanc HJ Jr, DeLand FH, Mathews ES. Refinements in cerebrospinal fluid diversionary shunt evaluation by cisternography. Am J Roentgenol Radium Ther Nucl Med 1972; 115: 766–773.
2. Sty JR, D'Souza BJ, Daniels D. Nuclear anatomy of diversionary central nervous system shunts in children. Clin Nucl Med 1978; 3: 271–275.
3. Harbert JC, Pollina R. Absorbed dose estimates for radionuclides. Clin Nucl Med 1984; 9: 210–221.

^{201}Tl Scan for Recurrent Brain Tumor

Summary Information

Radiopharmaceutical

Adult dose:	4 mCi (148 MBq) ^{201}Tl thallous chloride administered IV.
Pediatric dose:	Adjusted according to patient's weight (see Appendix A-3).

Contraindications None.

Dose/Scan Interval Commence imaging 20–30 minutes after the injection.[1]

Views Obtained Tomographic views of the brain.

Indications

^{201}Tl thallous chloride brain imaging is indicated in the differentiation of recurrent tumor from radiation necrosis in patients who have received treatment for primary malignant intracranial tumors.

Principle

Many studies have shown the uptake of thallium by primary brain tumors.[2–6] Unlike contrast enhancement in computed tomography (CT) or magnetic resonance imaging (MRI), which are dependent solely on breakdown of the blood-brain barrier, thallium uptake is related to tumor cell viability and growth rates[7,8] and is not present in normal brain cells, edematous tissue, or necrotic areas.[3] The degree of uptake in tumors appears to be correlated with tumor grade. The most malignant tumors have the greatest uptake, whereas low-grade tumors may not be visualized.[2–4] Hence, although thallium may be of limited use in the diagnosis and/or staging of primary brain tumors, it is useful in differentiating recurrent high-grade tumors from edematous or necrotic tissue after therapy.[9]

Patient Preparation

None required.

Instrument Specifications

Gamma camera:	Single-/dual-/triple-head SPECT system
Collimators:	Single-head system—high-resolution fan-beam collimator
	Dual-/triple-head systems—ultrahigh-resolution fan-beam collimators

Energy setting: 69–80 keV and 167 keV, 20% energy windows for [201]Tl

Computer system: Acquisition requirements—SPECT (128 × 128 matrix)

Processing requirements—SPECT reconstruction software, ROI analysis

Imaging Procedure

After injection, the patient should be placed supine on the imaging table. Ensure that the patient's head is securely restrained in the head holder (see Fig. 3-1). Position the patient so that the detectors can clear the shoulders (see Fig. 3-2). Perform a SPECT study using the following acquisition variables.

Single-Head System

A 128 × 128 matrix (fan-beam collimators) or a 64 × 64 matrix (parallel-hole collimators), 120 views every 3° at 20 seconds per view. Use a 360° circular orbit. For fan-beam collimators, zoom factor = 1. For parallel-hole collimators, set zoom factor = 2, with offset along the y-axis, to the lower part of the detector field of view.

Dual-/Triple-Head System

A 128 × 128 matrix with 120 views every 3° at 15 seconds per view. Use fan-beam collimator and a 360° circular orbit with no zoom.

Computer Analysis

Data Reconstruction

1. Before reconstruction, ensure that uniformity correction and center-of-rotation correction have been performed or will be performed during the reconstruction process.
2. If fan-beam collimators were used, rebin the raw data into a 64 × 64 matrix (this may be done automatically on some systems during reconstruction).
3. Planar data should be prefiltered and then reconstructed with a Ramp filter. Suitable pre-filters are a Butterworth (order 10–20) or Hann (or Hanning) with a cutoff at 0.5–0.8 cycles/cm. This corresponds to a cutoff at approximately 0.5 Nyquist for a 128 matrix. Reconstruct the planar data into a 64 × 64 matrix. Apply attenuation correction using an attenuation coefficient = 0.14 cm^{-1}.[10]

Thallium Uptake Index

To quantitate the degree of uptake of ^{201}Tl in a lesion, select the transaxial slice that demonstrates the highest tumor uptake. Draw a 50% isocontour ROI around the tumor uptake. Determine average counts per pixel. Mirror the ROI about the y-axis, and determine the average counts per pixel in the normal contralateral region of the brain (Fig. 3-12). The thallium uptake index (TUI) is defined as the ratio of average count per pixel in tumor to average count per pixel in normal background tissue.[4] Low-grade lesions have a TUI of 1–2 (mean ± SD = 1.27 ± 0.40), and high-grade lesions have a TUI greater than 2 (mean ± SD = 2.40 ± 0.61).[4]

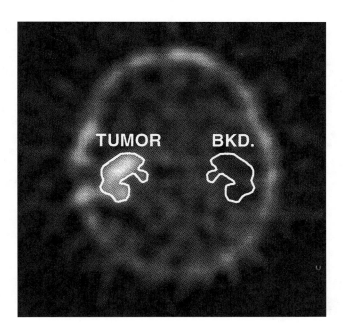

Figure 3-12. Transaxial slice showing ^{201}Tl uptake in a tumor. An isocontour (50%) ROI has been drawn around the tumor and mirrored to the contralateral side as a background ROI.

Information on Film

On all computer films, ensure that the following information is recorded.:

> Patient's name and clinic/hospital number
> Date and time of study after the injection
> Type of scan and radiopharmaceutical
> Orientation of each image
> All ROIs and results from measurement of the TUI

Interpretation

In a normal study, mild-to-moderate uptake should be seen in the scalp and in the orbital region. Occasionally, faint uptake may be seen in the choroid plexus. Areas of increased uptake are seen in patients with recurrent tumor, with the degree of uptake depending on the size and malignancy of the tumor. Uptake has also been reported in patients with hemorrhagic infarctions.[2] There is also evidence for some uptake of ^{201}Tl in patients with angiomas, epidural hematomas, or intracranial hemorrhages.[2]

Radiation Dosimetry

The estimated absorbed doses in organs and tissues of an average subject (70 kg) from the administration of 4 mCi (148 MBq) ^{201}Tl are shown in Table 3-3.[11]

Table 3-3. Absorbed Radiation Dose Estimates in a 70-kg Adult From 4 mCi (148 MBq) ^{201}Tl

Tissue	Absorbed Radiation Dose	
	rad/4 mCi	mGy/148 MBq
Heart wall	2.00	20.0
Liver	2.20	22.0
Kidneys	4.80	48.0
Testes	2.00	20.0
Ovaries	1.88	18.8
Thyroid	2.60	26.0
Stomach wall	1.68	16.8
Small intestine	1.52	15.2
Upper large intestinal wall	1.00	10.0
Lower large intestinal wall	0.84	8.40
Total body	0.82	8.20

References

1. Sehweil A, McKillop JH, Ziada G, et al. The optimum time for tumour imaging with thallium-201. Eur J Nucl Med 1988; 13: 527–529.
2. Dierckx RA, Martin JJ, Dobbeleir A, et al. Sensitivity and specificity of thallium-201 single-photon emission tomography in the functional detection and differential diagnosis of brain tumors. Eur J Nucl Med 1994; 21: 621–633.
3. Gruber ML, Hochberg FH. Systematic evaluation of primary brain tumors. J Nucl Med 1990; 31: 969–971.
4. Kim BT, Black KL, Marciano D, et al. Thallium-201 SPECT imaging of brain tumors: methods and results. J Nucl Med 1990; 31: 965–969.
5. Black KL, Hawkins RA, Kim KT, et al. Use of thallium-201 SPECT to quantitate malignancy grade of gliomas. J Neurosurg 1989; 71: 342–346.
6. Kaplan WD, Takvorian T, Morris JH, et al. Thallium-201 brain tumor imaging: a comparative study with pathologic correlation. J Nucl Med 1987; 28: 47–52.
7. Elligsen JD, Thompson JE, Frey HE, Kruuv J. Correlation of (Na+–K+)-ATPase activity with growth of normal and transformed cells. Exp Cell Res 1974; 87: 233–240.
8. Kasarov LB, Friedman H. Enhanced Na+–K+-activated adenosine triphosphatase activity in transforming fibroblasts. Cancer Res 1974; 34: 1862–1865.
9. Carvalho PA, Schwartz RB, Alexander E, et al. Initial experience with the use of sequential Tl-201/Tc-99m-HMPAO SPECT in the detection of recurrent malignant gliomas after I-125 brachytherapy (abstract). J Nucl Med 1990; 31: 826.
10. Wallis JW, Miller TR, Koppel P. Attenuation correction in cardiac SPECT without a transmission measurement. J Nucl Med 1995; 36: 506–512.
11. Harbert JC, Pollina R. Absorbed dose estimates from radionuclides. Clin Nucl Med 1984; 9: 210–221.

Confirmation of Brain Death

Summary Information

Radiopharmaceutical

Adult dose: 20 mCi (740 MBq) ^{99m}Tc HMPAO usually injected via a central or peripheral venous catheter.

Pediatric dose: Based on body surface area (see Appendix A-3).

Notes: Previously ^{99m}Tc HMPAO injection had to be used within 30 minutes after preparation. A more stable formulation of HMPAO (4-6 hour reconstituted shelf life) has recently been approved by the FDA. Although ^{99m}Tc ECD (bicisate) has properties similar to those of ^{99m}Tc HMPAO, no studies have yet been performed to demonstrate its usefulness in determining brain death.

Contraindications None.

Dose/Scan Interval

Flow study: Imaging commences immediately after the injection.

Static views/SPECT: Imaging commences 5–10 minutes after the injection.

Views Obtained Anterior flow study followed by planar (anterior, posterior, left and right lateral views) or tomographic views of the brain.

Indications

The President's Commission, in the Uniform Determination of Death Act, defined brain death as deep unresponsive coma, no brain stem function, and no respiratory reflex (defined by apnea despite arterial PCO_2 greater than 60 mm Hg). Recent studies have recommended that cerebral blood flow be the method of choice to confirm brain death when clinical criteria are equivocal, when a complete neurologic examination cannot be performed, or in patients younger than 1 year.[1] Several authors have recommended SPECT imaging with ^{99m}Tc HMPAO as the method of choice for confirmation of brain death, because the method allows better evaluation of the perfusion status of the brain stem.[2,3] ^{99m}Tc HMPAO is a perfusion agent, but it can also be used to determine the viability of internal organs, such as the heart, lungs, kidneys, and liver. This information is of value if organ transplantation is a possibility.[3]

Principle

^{99m}Tc HMPAO is a lipophilic agent capable of penetrating the intact blood–brain barrier. In vivo, it displays high instability, reacting within seconds after intravenous injection. On crossing the blood–brain barrier, it loses its lipophilic characteristics and becomes trapped inside the brain.[4] The regional uptake and retention are generally related to the regional perfusion.[5] The absence of uptake in the cerebral cortex and cerebellum is consistent with brain death.

Patient Preparation

None required.

Instrument Specifications

Gamma camera:	Small field-of-view mobile system (bedside determination of brain death)
	Single-/dual-/triple-head SPECT system (laboratory determination of brain death)
Collimators:	Low-energy all-purpose or high-resolution collimator for flow and planar views
	Fan-beam or high-resolution collimators for SPECT study
Energy setting:	140-keV 15–20% energy window
Analog formatter:	8 × 10 film, 70-mm (9-on-1) format
Computer system:	Acquisition requirements—dynamic (64 × 64 matrix), static (256 × 256 matrix), SPECT (128 × 128 matrix)
	Processing requirements—SPECT reconstruction software

Imaging Procedure

Immediate Flow Study

1. With the patient supine on the imaging table or bed, place the detector anteriorly over the head and neck.
2. Give a bolus injection of ^{99m}Tc HMPAO into a central or peripheral catheter, and flush the line with 30–50 ml of saline.
3. When activity begins to appear in the field of view, acquire a dynamic study on an analog formatter (9 frames at 3 seconds per frame) and/or on computer (a 64 × 64 word mode matrix, 30 frames at 1 second per frame).

Static Views

After injection, wait 5–10 minutes and acquire an anterior view for 200 kct on an analog formatter and on computer (256 × 256 matrix). Acquire the right lateral, left lateral, and posterior views in a similar manner.

SPECT Study

Ensure that the patient's head is adequately secured in the head holder (see Fig. 3-1). To ensure that the brain is fully visualized in the field of view, move the patient up into the gantry until the shoulders just clear the edge of the detectors (see Fig. 3-2). A SPECT study may be commenced 10 minutes after the injection using the following acquisition variables.

1. Single-head system: 128 × 128 matrix (fan-beam collimators) or 64 × 64 matrix (parallel-hole collimators), 120 views every 3° at 15 seconds per view. Use a 360° circular orbit. For fan-beam collimators, zoom factor = 1. For parallel-hole collimators, set zoom factor = 2, with offset along the y-axis, to the lower part of the detector field of view.
2. Dual-/triple-head system: 128 × 128 matrix (fan-beam collimators) with 120 views every 3° at 10 seconds per view. Use a 360° circular orbit with no zoom.

Computer Analysis

Flow Study/Planar views

No analysis required.

SPECT Study

1. Before reconstruction, ensure that uniformity correction and center-of-rotation correction have been performed or will be performed during the reconstruction process.
2. If fan-beam collimators were used, rebin the raw data into a 64 × 64 matrix (this may be done automatically on some systems during reconstruction).
3. Planar data should be prefiltered with a Butterworth or Hanning filter (the exact filter is not critical, because the purpose is to determine the presence or absence of cerebral uptake of the radiotracer). Reconstruct the planar data into a 64 × 64 matrix.

Information on Film

On all analog and computer films, ensure that the following information is recorded:

> Patient's name and clinic/hospital number
> Date and time of study after the injection
> Type of scan and radiopharmaceutical
> Orientation of each image

Interpretation

It is important that the ^{99m}Tc HMPAO preparation has passed quality control. Free ^{99m}Tc pertechnetate in the preparation could result in uptake in the brain, and give a misleading result.

Flow Study

Absence of flow above the base of the skull is consistent with brain death.

Planar Views

In brain death, the planar views should show complete absence of perfusion in both hemispheres.

SPECT Study

In a normal ^{99m}Tc HMPAO, the transaxial images should show symmetric distribution of the radiotracer in both hemispheres. Because the rate of blood flow is higher in gray matter than in white matter, the greatest uptake is observed in the cortical gray matter, the basal ganglia, and the thalamus.

In patients with brain death, a rim of scalp activity may be seen because of blood flow through the external carotid artery circulation; however, no uptake should be visible in the cerebral cortex or cerebellum. Occasionally, uptake may be seen in the cerebellum. Patients without uptake in the cerebral hemispheres, but with persistent flow in the cerebellum or brain stem, cannot be considered brain dead, although the prognosis is poor, and death usually occurs within a short time.[6]

Radiation Dosimetry

The estimated absorbed doses in organs and tissues of an average subject (70 kg) from the administration of 20 mCi (740 MBq) ^{99m}Tc HMPAO are shown in Table 3-1.[7]

References

1. Galaske RG, Schober O, Heyes R. ^{99m}Tc-HM-PAO and ^{123}I-amphetamine cerebral scintigraphy: a new, non invasive method in determination of brain death in children. Eur J Nucl Med 1988; 14: 446–452.
2. Adelstein W. Confirmation of brain death using ^{99m}Tc HM-PAO. J Neurosci Nurs 1994; 26: 118–120.
3. Wieler H, Marohl K, Kaiser KP, et al. Tc-99m HMPAO cerebral scintigraphy. A reliable, noninvasive method for determination of brain death. Clin Nucl Med 1993; 18: 104–109.
4. Ballinger JR, Reid RH, Gulenchyn KY. Technetium-99m HM-PAO stereoisomers: differences in interaction with glutathione. J Nucl Med 1988; 29: 1998–2000.
5. Kung HF, Ohmomo Y, Kung MP. Current and future radiopharmaceuticals for brain imaging with single photon emission computed tomography. Semin Nucl Med 1990; 20: 290–302.
6. Valle G, Ciritella P, Bonetti MG, et al. Considerations of brain death on a SPECT cerebral perfusion study. Clin Nucl Med 1993; 18: 953–954.
7. Package insert. Ceretec: kit for the preparation of Technetium Tc-99m exametazime injection. Amersham Corp., 1990.

4

Cardiovascular System

Michael K. O'Connor
Todd D. Miller
Timothy F. Christian
Raymond J. Gibbons

Cardiac Left-to-Right Shunt

Summary Information

Radiopharmaceutical

Adult dose: 20 mCi (740 MBq) ^{99m}Tc-DTPA.

Pediatric dose: Minimal dose is 3 mCi (111 MBq) ^{99m}Tc-DTPA; maximal dose is 20 mCi (740 MBq) of ^{99m}Tc-DTPA.[1] Dose should be adjusted according to body surface area (see Appendix A-3). *Note:* All injected doses should be in a volume of 0.2 ml or less.

Contraindications Severe tricuspid regurgitation or severe pulmonary hypertension.

Dose/Scan Interval Computer should be started 1–2 seconds before injection.

Views Obtained Anterior view to include the heart and lungs.

Indications

A cardiac shunt study can be used to assess the magnitude of a left-to-right shunt caused by an atrial or ventricular septal defect or by patent ductus arteriosus. This assessment can be useful in the management of cyanotic newborn infants and in the preoperative and postoperative evaluation of patients who have undergone corrective procedures.

Principle

After an IV bolus injection of a radioisotope, a sharp peak of activity is seen in the lungs, followed by a trough and a smaller recirculation peak as activity circulates through the systemic system and returns again to the lungs. In patients with left-to-right shunts, some activity is diverted back to the right side of the heart and reappears in the lungs before the arrival of the recirculation peak. From a time activity curve of lung activity, a quantitative measurement of the degree of shunting can be obtained by performing curve fitting to the first-pass and recirculation peaks.[1–6] ^{99m}Tc-DTPA (diethylenetriamine pentaacetic acid) is the preferred radiopharmaceutical, because rapid renal clearance permits repeat studies over a short interval.

Patient Preparation

In pediatric studies, it is important that the child be relaxed at the time of injection. Crying or a Valsalva maneuver can result in a fragmented injection bolus and a poor-quality study.

Instrument Specifications

Gamma camera: Any large field-of-view system can be used, provided it has adequate count rate capability (20% count loss greater than 70 kcps).

Collimator: Low-energy all-purpose or high-sensitivity collimator.

Energy setting: 140 keV, 15–20% energy window.

Analog formatter: Not applicable.

Computer system: Acquisition requirements—dynamic (64 × 64 matrix) at 2–4 frames per second.

Processing requirements—image manipulation, region of interest analysis, curve generation, curve fitting (gamma variate fit).

Imaging Procedure

1. The patient should be positioned supine on the imaging table, with the gamma camera positioned anteriorly over the chest.
2. The ^{99m}Tc-DTPA should be injected in the right antecubital vein. If possible, the injection should be given in the right external jugular vein, because a better quality study is obtained.[7]
3. For children less than 10 years old, a 20–21 gauge IV catheter/needle set should be used. For older children and adults, an 18–19 gauge IV catheter/needle set should be used. Connect a 60-ml syringe to a 40-inch extension set, and attach the other end of the extension set to the IV catheter/needle set as shown in Figure 4-1. Both should be prefilled with saline.

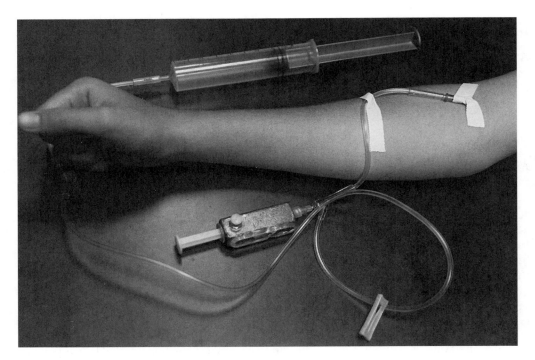

Figure 4-1. Arrangement of the IV catheter/needle set, 40° extension set, and 60-ml syringe for a first-pass study.

4. Gently flush the extension set with 5–10 ml of saline to ensure good positioning and flow through the injection site.

5. Before injection, ensure that the patient is comfortable and relaxed. Inject the ^{99m}Tc-DTPA into the side port closest to the IV catheter/needle set (see Fig. 4-1). *Note:* Ensure that the needle of the injection syringe is inserted fully into the side port past the dead space at the top of the side port. Remove the empty syringe.

6. Start acquisition on the computer. After 1–2 seconds, rapidly inject 60 ml of saline (for children less than 10 years of age, inject only 20–30 ml).

7. For adults and children greater than 10 years old, data should be acquired on the computer in a 64 × 64 word mode matrix at 0.5 seconds per frame for 50 seconds. For children less than 10 years old, data should be acquired with a zoom of 1.5–2.0 and at 0.25 seconds per frame for 30 seconds to compensate for their shorter circulation time.[8]

Computer Analysis

1. From the acquired 100–120 images, sum groups of 10 images to give 10–12 new output images. Save the output.

2. In region of interest (ROI) analysis, select the summed image that best shows the superior vena cava and right ventricle. Draw an ROI over the upper portion of the superior vena cava, as shown in Figure 4-2.

3. Select an image that best shows lung activity. Draw an ROI over the right lung, ensuring that the ROI is free of contamination from activity in the superior vena cava, right and left atria and ventricles, and the aorta (Fig. 4-3).

4. Use the raw data to generate time-activity curves from these ROIs. Check the superior vena cava curve for bolus fragmentation or delayed bolus clearance. A poor-quality bolus may invalidate the study.

5. Perform a gamma variate fit to the main first-pass peak. The limits of the fit should be from 10% of maximum activity on the upslope to 70% of maximum activity on the downslope.[1] Subtract the gamma variate fit curve from the lung curve to obtain the subtraction curve (Fig. 4-4A).

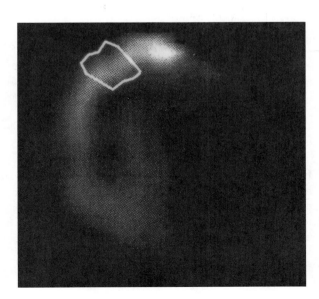

Figure 4-2. Image of bolus in superior vena cava (SVC) and right ventricle with ROI over SVC.

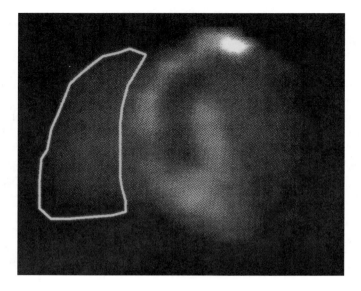

Figure 4-3. Image of bolus in lungs and right ventricle with ROI over right lung.

6. If a shunt is present, it will be manifested as a discontinuity in the downslope of the lung curve. The corresponding portion of the subtraction curve should be fitted with a second gamma variate fit.

7. If difficulty is encountered in performing the second fit, a gamma variate fit can be performed on the recirculation portion of the subtraction curve (Fig. 4-4B) and subtracted from it to yield only the shunt component of the curve. A third gamma variate fit can now be performed on this shunt component.[5]

8. Determine the integral under the first (P) and third (S) gamma variate fit curves (Fig. 4-4C). The pulmonary/systemic flow ratio (Qp/Qs) is defined as P/(P-S).

9. Obtain a hard copy of the summed images, ROIs, and superior vena cava and lung curves, as well as each phase of the curve fitting process.

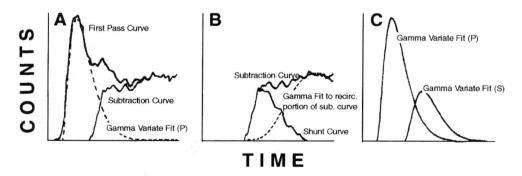

Figure 4-4. (**A**) First-pass curve with gamma variate fit (dotted line). Subtraction of gamma fit from first-pass curve gives subtraction curve. (**B**) Gamma variate fit to recirculation portion of subtraction curve. This fit is again subtracted from the subtraction curve to yield the shunt curve, which is then fitted with a third gamma variate fit. (**C**) Pulmonary/systemic flow ratio calculated as ratio of areas under first (P) and third (S) gamma variate curves = P/(P-S). (Adapted from Houser et al.,[5] with permission.)

Information on Film

On each computer film, ensure that the following information is recorded:

1. Patient name and clinic/hospital number
2. Date, type of scan, and radiopharmaceutical used
3. Appropriate labels for ROIs and curves
4. Integral of curves P and S and Qp/Qs ratio

Interpretation

In normal subjects, the Qp/Qs ratio is less than 1.2.[1] The method is reliable over the range Qp/Qs = 1.2 to 3.0. Above 3.0, the method is inaccurate because of the difficulty in correctly fitting the downslope of the initial pulmonary transit.[3] The lungs are often poorly visualized, particularly for large shunts, with some radioactivity persisting in the lungs between the first pass and recirculation.

Additional Notes

None.

Radiation Dosimetry

The estimated absorbed doses in organs and tissues of an average subject (70 kg) from an IV injection of 20 mCi (740 MBq) ^{99m}Tc-DTPA are shown in Table 4-1.[9]

Table 4-1. Absorbed Radiation Dose Estimates in a 70-kg Adult After Intravenous Administration of 20 mCi (740 MBq) ^{99m}Tc-DTPA

| | Absorbed Radiation Doses—^{99m}Tc-DTPA | |
Tissue	rad/20 mCi	mGy/740 MBq
Kidneys	1.8	18.0
Bladder wall		
2-hr void	2.3	23.0
4.8-hr void	5.4	54.0
Testes		
2-hr void	0.15	1.5
4.8-hr void	0.21	2.1
Ovaries		
2-hr void	0.22	2.2
4.8-hr void	0.31	3.1
Total body	0.12	1.2

References

1. Maltz DL, Treves S. Quantitative radionuclide angiocardiography: determination of Qp:Qs in children. Circulation 1973; 47: 1049–1056.
2. Anderson PA, Jones RH, Sabiston DC Jr. Quantitation of left-to-right cardiac shunts with radionuclide angiography. Circulation 1974; 49: 512–516.
3. Askenazi J, Ahnberg DS, Korngold E, et al. Quantitative radionuclide angiocardiography: detection and quantitation of left-to-right shunts. Am J Cardiol 1976; 37: 382–387.
4. Ham HR, Dobbeleir A, Viart P, Piepsz A, Lenaers A. Radionuclide quantitation of left-to-right cardiac shunts using deconvolution analysis: concise communication. J Nucl Med 1981; 22: 688–692.
5. Houser TS, MacIntyre WJ, Cook SA, et al. Recirculation subtraction for analysis of left-to-right cardiac shunts: concise communication. J Nucl Med 1981; 22: 1033–1038.
6. Madsen MT, Argenyi E, Preslar J, Grover-McKay M, Kirchner PT. An improved method for the quantification of left-to-right cardiac shunts. J Nucl Med 1991; 32: 1808–1812.
7. Parker JA, Treves S. Radionuclide detection, localization and quantitation of intracardiac shunts and shunts between the great arteries. In: "Principles of Cardiovascular Nuclear Medicine," eds Holman BL, Sonnenblick EH, Lesch M. Grune & Stratton, 1978, pp 189–218.
8. Silver HK, Kempe CH, Bruyn HB. "Handbook of Pediatrics." Lange Medical Publications, Los Altos, CA, 1973, p 212.
9. Kit for the Preparation of Technetium Tc-99m Mertiatide, Product #096. Mallinckrodt Medical Inc., St. Louis. Revised Nov. 1992.

Resting Radionuclide Angiographic Study

Summary Information

Radiopharmaceutical
Adult dose: 30 mCi (1,110 MBq) ^{99m}Tc-labeled red blood cells (RBCs).
Pediatric dose: Adjusted according to the patient's weight (see Appendix A-3).

Contraindications Optimum image quality in radionuclide angiography (RNA) requires that the patient be in normal sinus rhythm so that successive cardiac cycles can be accurately summed. In patients with severe arrhythmia, the study may be suboptimal. If more than 20% of the beats are premature ventricular contractions, antiarrhythmic therapy and/or alternative techniques should be considered.

Dose/Scan Interval Imaging can commence immediately after the injection.

Views Obtained Studies of the heart should be obtained in the anterior, left lateral, and left anterior oblique positions. A fourth study may be acquired in the left anterior oblique (LAO) position using the alternate gating method described later.

Indications

Gated RNA can be used to measure left ventricular ejection fraction (LVEF)[1] and to evaluate left ventricular regional wall motion. The cardiac applications of resting RNA include the evaluation of patients with stable angina (risk stratification), dyspnea (differentiate cardiac from pulmonary cause), acute infarction (evaluate for prognosis) and left-sided heart failure (differentiate systolic from diastolic dysfunction).[2,3] Other applications include the monitoring of patients with valvular heart disease (aortic and mitral regurgitation) or cardiomyopathy.[3,4] It can also be used to monitor the cardiotoxic effects of chemotherapeutic agents such as doxorubicin.[5]

Principle

RNA requires that the blood be labeled with a suitable tracer such as ^{99m}Tc-tagged RBCs. The technique is based on imaging the left ventricle for a large number of beats and summing the image data from each beat to produce a composite beat with adequate count statistics for analysis. RNA requires the simultaneous acquisition of the patient's electrocardiogram (ECG) and images of the left ventricle. Starting with an R-wave trigger, the image data are loaded sequentially into 20–30 frames spanning a single cardiac cycle. The next R wave resets the system so that image data from the next cardiac cycle are loaded into the same 20–30 frames. This summing process continues until sufficient counts are present in each frame to permit analysis of this 20–30 frame composite cardiac cycle. Chamber size and wall motion may be assessed qualitatively by replaying the images in a closed-loop display, and LVEF may be calculated from a time–activity curve generated using a left ventricular ROI. In addition to LVEF, an estimate of left ventricular volume can be obtained from the resting RNA study with a blood sample.[6,7]

The standard RNA technique assumes all heart beats are of equal duration. In practice, it is necessary to place upper and lower limits on the acceptable R-R interval to eliminate ectopic beats. Despite this, some of the latter frames of the RNA study often have fewer counts than anticipated, making it difficult to interpret the later portions of the time–activity curve. The alternate gating LAO study is designed to overcome this problem by acquiring 2 cardiac cycles into 56 frames rather than 1 cycle into 20 frames. This permits accurate analysis of the filling phase (from end-systole to end-diastole) from the first of the 2 cardiac cycles.[8] To perform alternate gating, a "divide-by-two" circuit must be placed in line between the ECG leads and the ECG gate so that only every second pulse is counted, thereby simulating a heart rate half the true rate.[9]

Patient Preparation

Preparation of the ^{99m}Tc-labeled RBCs (modified in vivo labeling technique):

1. Place 4 ml of heparinized saline in a 6-ml syringe.
2. Place 30 mCi (1,110 MBq) ^{99m}Tc sodium pertechnetate in a volume of 1 ml into a 12-ml syringe.
3. Attach the 6-ml syringe and the 12-ml syringe to a 3-way stopcock.
4. Reconstitute a vial of sodium pyrophosphate (PYP). Optimal labeling requires at minimum a dose of 5 mg Sn-PYP per 70 kg of body weight or 10 µg Sn (II)/kg.[10] Inject the required amount of Sn-PYP into the patient with a 21-gauge butterfly infusion set positioned in an arm vein. Wait 15 minutes.
5. Connect the syringes and stopcock to the butterfly infusion set (Fig. 4-5). Draw 6–10 ml of blood into the 12-ml syringe.
6. Draw 2 ml of heparinized saline through the stopcock into the 12-ml syringe. Push the rest of the heparinized saline through the butterfly infusion set.
7. Mix the blood, and let it stand for 10 minutes, then reinject it into the patient.

Before commencing the study, position 3 electrodes in the right and left midclavicular area and below the heart, as shown in Figure 4-6. Before the electrodes are placed, the skin should be prepared as follows:[11]

1. Shave any superficial hair over the area of electrode placement.
2. With an alcohol-saturated gauze pad, clean the area to remove any oils.
3. Lightly abrade the skin with 200-grit emery paper.

The ECG signal from these electrodes provides a gating signal to the computer. If the heart rate displayed on the computer does not match that shown on the ECG system, adjust the strength of the trigger signal until concordance is obtained.

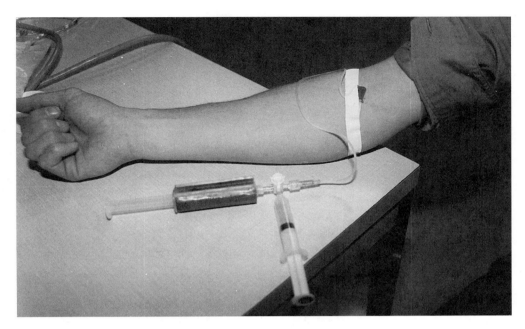

Figure 4-5. Arrangement of butterfly infusion set, stopcock, and syringes for modified in vivo RBC labeling.

Instrument Specifications

Gamma camera:	Any small or large field-of-view system may be used.
Collimator:	Low-energy all-purpose collimator.
Energy setting:	140-keV peak, 15–20% window.
Additional items:	ECG gating system and "divide by two" circuit box if alternate gating is required.
Computer system:	Acquisition requirements—gated acquisition (64 × 64 matrix), 20 frames per cardiac cycle (56 frames for alternate gating). Processing requirements—semiautomated or automated analysis software for ejection fraction and wall motion analysis of gated study.

Imaging Procedure

1. Place the patient supine on the imaging table with the feet down. Position the detector anteriorly over the chest, and using the persistence screen, check that the heart is located centrally in the field of view.
2. Set up the computer acquisition with the following variables: 64 × 64 word mode matrix, 20 frames per cycle, acquisition should terminate at 300 kct per frame. If available, use a "rubber band" framing method (rubber banding is used to eliminate drop-off in image counts at the end of the composite cardiac cycle by stretching or compressing each cardiac cycle to match the time per frame used by the system). On the patient's R-wave histogram, set a ±25% window around the primary heart rate. Check that the heart rate is stable. Acquire the anterior RNA study.

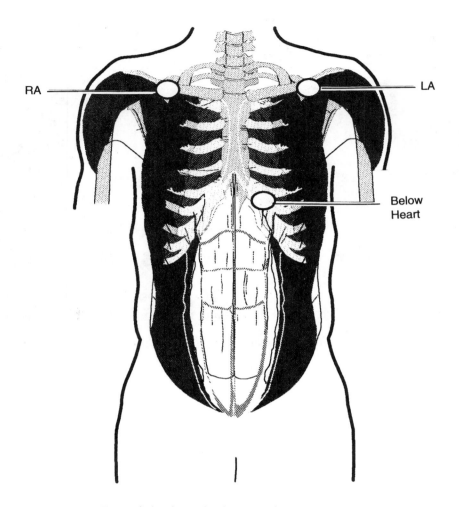

RA

LA

Below
Heart

Figure 4-6. Electrode placement for rest RNA study.

3. Rotate the detector to the left lateral position, and move the patient's left arm above the head to permit the detector to be positioned close to the chest wall. Acquire the left lateral study as described in step 2. Review the image for visualization of the inferobasal segment of the left ventricle. Adjust the camera position, and reacquire the image if necessary.

4. Reposition the detector to the LAO position, and acquire the study as described in step 2. *Note:* The optimal LAO angle for separation of the left and right ventricles varies from patient to patient. Visually inspect the images on the persistence screen to determine the optimal angle. The interventricular septum should appear as a nearly vertical dark band on the image. A caudal tilt of 10°–20° (Fig. 4-7) should be used to obtain optimal separation of the atria and ventricles.

5. If an alternate gating acquisition is requested, leave the detector in the LAO position. The alternate trigger box eliminates every other trigger pulse, decreasing the heart rate displayed on the computer to half its true value.

6. Set up the acquisition with the following variables: 64 × 64 word mode matrix, 56 frames per cycle (2 cycles), framing method should be set to constant time per frame, acquisition

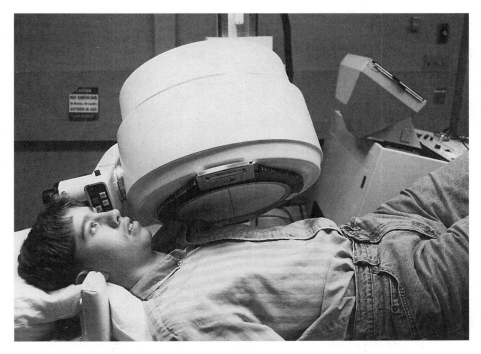

Figure 4-7. Detector positioned for the LAO view. Note use of caudal tilt for better separation of atria and ventricles.

should terminate after 10 minutes. On the patient's R-wave histogram, set a ±50% window around the primary heart rate.

7. After completion of these studies, draw a 10-ml sample of blood into a glass vial. Place the vial on top of the collimator, as shown in Figure 4-8, and count for 2 minutes.

Computer Analysis

Analysis is performed on standard and 56-frame LAO studies. Select the standard LAO study. Analysis software on the computer generally requires that a seed ROI be placed over the left ventricle. A combination of a second-derivative edge-detection routine and a fixed count threshold is commonly used to determine the left ventricular boundary. In most cases, the fixed count threshold should be adjusted so that most of the left ventricular boundary is determined by the second-derivative edge-detection routine. Irrespective of the edge-detection algorithm, visually check during the analysis that the left ventricular ROI boundaries are consistent with the outline of the left ventricle. If they are not consistent, adjust the edge-detection variables until an acceptable boundary is obtained. The background ROI should be determined from the end-systole frame and should be displaced 2–3 pixels to the right of the left ventricle (Fig. 4-9). Repeat this process with the 56-frame LAO study. At minimum, the analysis software should display the time-activity curve, global or regional left ventricular wall motion analysis, and phase and amplitude images of the heart.

Measurement of left ventricular volume requires the following information from the LAO study and the 10-ml blood sample:

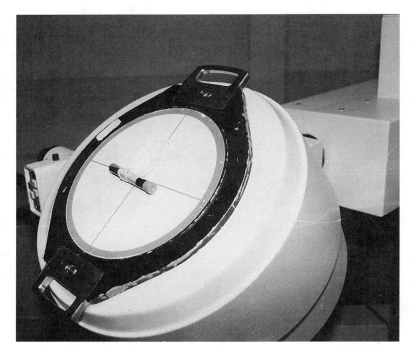

Figure 4-8. Setup for acquisition of 10-ml blood sample on gamma camera.

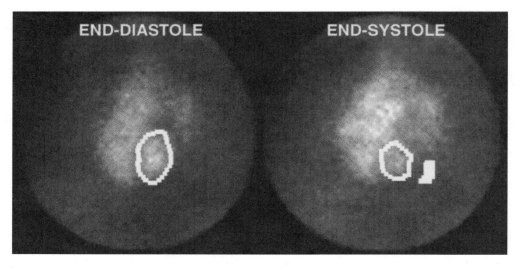

Figure 4-9. End-diastolic and end-systolic frames showing acceptable boundaries for the left ventricle and correct placement of the background ROI.

1. Left ventricular end-diastole counts (ct) (EDC)
2. Left ventricular end-systole counts (ct) (ESC)
3. Total number of cardiac cycles acquired in the study (TC)
4. Duration of each frame in the composite cardiac cycle (sec) (DUR)
5. Two-minute counts in the 10-ml blood sample (ct) (BLD)

Analysis requires that the end-diastole and end-systole counts be normalized (n) to counts per second, as follows:

$$nEDC = \frac{EDC}{TC \times DUR} \ ct/sec$$

$$nESC = \frac{ESC}{TC \times DUR} \ ct/sec$$

The blood sample must be normalized to counts per second per milliliter as follows:

$$nBLD = \frac{BLD}{2 \times 60 \times 10} \ ct/sec/ml$$

Note: If there is a significant delay (greater than 20 minutes) between the patient study and counting of the blood sample, then a decay-correction factor should be applied to the blood counts. Use the following nomograms to calculate the end-diastole and end-systole volumes:[7]

$$End\text{-}diastole\ blood\ volume = \frac{nEDC}{nBLD} \times 66.3 + 2.2 \ ml$$

$$End\text{-}systole\ blood\ volume = \frac{nESC}{nBLD} \times 67.8 + 0.77 \ ml$$

The time–activity curve from the 56-frame study permits analysis of left ventricular filling/emptying rates. The start of the fast and slow phases of ventricular filling and the start of the atrial filling phase can be identified by using Figure 4-10 as a guide. Filling/emptying rates can be determined from the derivative of the time–activity curve (perform curve differentiation).

Information on Film

The content of hard copies of the results of the RNA analysis will vary depending on the computer system but should include the time–activity curve and LVEF value, information on the patient's R-R histogram, end-diastole/end-systole ROIs for wall motion assessment, and phase/amplitude analysis images. If computed, left ventricular volumes and left ventricular filling/emptying rates should also be obtained.

Interpretation

In normal subjects, the LVEF should be about 60% (range, 50–80%).[12] There should be no area of abnormal wall motion (hypokinesis or dyskinesis). Abnormalities in cardiac function may be manifested as a decrease in LVEF and/or the presence of abnormalities in global and regional wall motion. For normal subjects, peak filling rates should be between

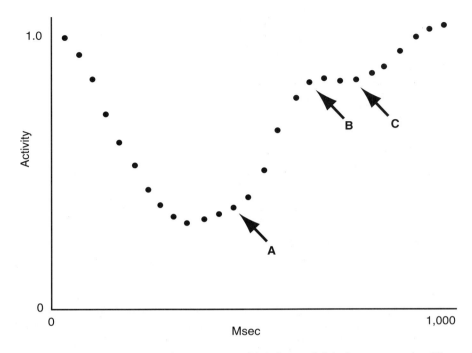

Figure 4-10. Time–activity curve showing start of (**A**) fast and (**B**) slow ventricular filling phases and (**C**) start of atrial filling phase. (Adapted from Sinak and Clements,[8] with permission.)

Table 4-2. Absorbed Radiation Dose Estimates in a 70-kg Adult After Intravenous Administration of 30 mCi (1,110 MBq) ^{99m}Tc-labeled Red Blood Cells[a]

	Absorbed Radiation Doses	
Tissue	rad/30 mCi	mGy/1,110 MBq
Heart wall	1.62	16.2
Bladder wall	1.53	15.3
Spleen	1.23	12.3
Lungs	1.23	12.3
Blood	1.05	10.5
Liver	0.78	7.8
Kidneys	0.75	7.5
Red marrow	0.57	5.7
Thyroid	0.54	5.4
Ovaries	0.51	5.1
Testes	0.21	2.1
Total body	0.45	4.5

[a]Assumes a 2.4-hr voiding schedule.

2.4 and 3.6 end-diastolic volume (EDV) per second, and the time-to-peak-filling rate should be 135–212 msec.[8]

Radiation Dosimetry

The estimated absorbed doses in organs and tissues of an average subject (70 kg) from an IV injection of 30 mCi (1,110 MBq) ^{99m}Tc-labeled RBCs are shown in Table 4-2.[13]

References

1. Borer JS, Bacharach SL, Green MV, et al. Real-time radionuclide cineangiography in the noninvasive evaluation of global and regional left ventricular function at rest and during exercise in patients with coronary-artery disease. N Engl J Med 1977; 296: 839–844.
2. Rocco TP, Dilsizian V, Fischman AJ, Strauss HW. Evaluation of ventricular function in patients with coronary artery disease. J Nucl Med 1989; 30: 1149–1165.
3. Gibbons RJ. Nuclear cardiology. In "Cardiology: Fundamentals and Practice," vol. 1, 2nd Edition, eds Giuliani ER, Fuster V, Gersh BJ, McGoon MD, McGoon DC. Mosby Year Book, St. Louis, 1991, pp 459–491.
4. Dilsizian V, Rocco TP, Bonow RO, et al. Cardiac blood-pool imaging. II: Applications in noncoronary heart disease. J Nucl Med 1990; 31: 10–22.
5. Alexander J, Dainiak N, Berger HJ, et al. Serial assessment of doxorubicin cardiotoxicity with quantitative radionuclide angiocardiography. N Engl J Med 1979; 300: 278–283.
6. Dehmer GJ, Lewis SE, Hillis LD, et al. Nongeometric determination of left ventricular volumes from equilibrium blood pool scans. Am J Cardiol 1980; 45: 293–300.
7. Clements IP, Brown ML, Smith HC. Radionuclide measurement of left ventricular volume. Mayo Clin Proc 1981; 56: 733–739.
8. Sinak LJ, Clements IP. Influence of age and sex on left ventricular filling at rest in subjects without clinical cardiac disease. Am J Cardiol 1989; 64: 646–650.
9. Clements IP, Nelson MA, O'Connor MK, et al. Diastolic measurements from alternate R-wave gating of radionuclide angiograms. Am Heart J 1988; 116: 113–117.
10. Hamilton RG, Alderson PO. A comparative evaluation of techniques for rapid and efficient in vivo labeling of red cells with [^{99m}Tc] pertechnetate. J Nucl Med 1977; 18: 1010–1013.
11. Froelicher VF, Myers J, Follansbee WP, Labovitz AJ. Exercise testing methodology. In "Exercise and the Heart," Mosby, St. Louis, 1993.
12. Hanley PC, Zinsmeister AR, Clements IP, et al. Gender-related differences in cardiac response to supine exercise assessed by radionuclide angiography. J Am Coll Cardiol 1989; 13: 624–629.
13. Atkins HL, Thomas SR, Buddemeyer U, Chervu LR. MIRD dose estimate report No. 14: radiation absorbed dose from technetium-99m-labeled red blood cells. J Nucl Med 1990; 31: 378–380.

Resting Radionuclide Angiography–Ejection Fraction Only

Summary Information

Radiopharmaceutical

    Adult dose: 20 mCi (740 MBq) ^{99m}Tc-labeled RBCs.

    Pediatric dose: Adjusted according to the patient's weight (see Appendix A-3).

Contraindications   Optimal image quality in RNA requires that the patient be in normal sinus rhythm so that successive cardiac cycles can be accurately summed. In patients with severe arrhythmia, the study may be suboptimal.

Dose/Scan Interval   Imaging can commence immediately after the injection.

Views Obtained   Images of the heart should be obtained in the left anterior oblique position.

Indications

This procedure is designed to provide an inexpensive measurement of LVEF. This is useful in monitoring patients with coronary artery disease,[1,2] valvular heart disease (aortic and mitral regurgitation), or cardiomyopathy.[2,3] It can also be used to monitor the cardiotoxic effects of chemotherapeutic agents such as doxorubicin.[4]

Principle

RNA requires that the blood be labeled with a suitable tracer such as ^{99m}Tc-tagged RBCs. The technique is based on imaging the left ventricle for a large number of beats and summing the image data from each beat to produce a composite beat with adequate count statistics for analysis. RNA requires the simultaneous acquisition of the patient's electrocardiogram and images of the left ventricle. Starting with an R-wave trigger, the image data are loaded sequentially into 20–30 frames spanning a single cardiac cycle. The next R wave resets the system so that image data from the next cardiac cycle are loaded into the same 20–30 frames. This summing process continues until sufficient counts are present in each frame to permit analysis of this 20–30 frame-composite cardiac cycle.

The ejection fraction can be calculated from the time–activity curve generated by ROIs placed over the left ventricle.

Patient Preparation

This procedure uses in vivo labeling of RBCs.

1. Reconstitute a vial of PYP. Optimal labeling requires at minimum a dose of 5 mg Sn-PYP per 70 kg of body weight or 10 µg Sn (II)/kg.[5] Inject the required amount of Sn-PYP into the patient. Wait 15 minutes.
2. Inject 20 mCi (740 MBq) ^{99m}Tc pertechnetate intravenously.

Before commencing the study, position three electrodes in the right and left midclavicular areas and below the heart, as shown in Figure 4-6. Before the electrodes are placed, the skin should be prepared as follows:

1. Shave any superficial hair over the area of electrode placement.
2. With an alcohol-saturated gauze pad, clean the area to remove any oils.
3. Lightly abrade the skin with 200-grit emery paper.[6]

The ECG signal from these electrodes provides a gating signal to the computer. If the heart rate displayed on the computer does not match that shown on the ECG system, adjust the strength of the trigger signal until concordance is obtained.

Instrument Specifications

Gamma camera:	Any small or large field-of-view system may be used.
Collimator:	Low-energy all-purpose collimator.
Energy setting:	140-keV peak, 15–20% window.
Additional items:	ECG gating system.
Computer system:	Acquisition requirements—gated acquisition (64 × 64 matrix), 20 frames per cycle.
	Processing requirements—semiautomated or automated analysis software for measurement of ejection fraction.

Imaging Procedure

1. Place the patient supine on the imaging table with the feet down. Position the detector in the LAO position, and move the patient's left arm above the head to permit the detector to be positioned close to the chest wall. *Note:* The optimal LAO angle for separation of the left and right ventricles varies from patient to patient. Visually inspect the images on the persistence screen to determine the optimal angle. Also, a caudal tilt of 10°–20° should be used to obtain optimal separation of the atria and ventricles, as shown in Figure 4-7.
2. Set up the computer acquisition with the following variables: 64 × 64 word mode matrix, 20 frames per cycle, acquisition should terminate at 250 kct per frame. If available, use a rubber band framing method (rubber banding is used to eliminate drop-off in image counts at the end of the composite cardiac cycle by stretching or compressing each cardiac cycle to match the time per frame used by the system). On the patient's R-wave histogram, set a ±25% window around the primary heart rate. Check that the heart rate is stable. Acquire the LAO RNA study.

Computer Analysis

Analysis software on the computer generally requires that a seed ROI be placed over the left ventricle. A combination of a second-derivative edge-detection routine and a fixed count threshold is commonly used to determine the left ventricular boundary. In most cases, the fixed count threshold should be adjusted so that most of the left ventricular boundary is determined by the second-derivative edge-detection routine. Irrespective of the edge-detection algorithm, visually check during the analysis that the left ventricular ROI boundaries are consistent with the outline of the left ventricle. If they are not consistent, adjust the edge-detection variables until an acceptable boundary is obtained. The background ROI should be determined from the end-systole frame and should be displaced 2–3 pixels to the right of the left ventricle (see Fig. 4-9). For this procedure, all that is required from the analysis is the LVEF.

Information on Film

No output of the analysis to a hard copy is required for this study. The physician will dictate a report indicating the LVEF.

Interpretation

In normal subjects, the LVEF should be in the range of 50–80%.[7]

Radiation Dosimetry

The estimated absorbed doses in organs and tissues of an average subject (70 kg) from an IV injection of 20 mCi (740 MBq) ^{99m}Tc-labeled RBCs are shown in Table 4-3.[8]

Table 4-3. Absorbed Radiation Dose Estimates for a 70-kg Adult After Intravenous Injection of 20 mCi (740 MBq) ^{99m}Tc-Labeled Red Blood Cells[a]

Tissue	Absorbed Radiation Doses	
	rad/20 mCi	mGy/740 MBq
Heart wall	1.14	11.4
Bladder wall	0.76	7.6
Spleen	0.86	8.6
Lungs	0.86	8.6
Blood	0.74	7.4
Liver	0.56	5.6
Kidneys	0.54	5.4
Red marrow	0.40	4.0
Thyroid	0.38	3.8
Ovaries	0.36	3.6
Testes	0.15	1.5
Total body	0.32	3.2

[a]Assumes a 2.4-hr voiding schedule.

References

1. Rocco TP, Dilsizian V, Fischman AJ, Strauss HW. Evaluation of ventricular function in patients with coronary artery disease. J Nucl Med 1989; 30: 1149–1165.

2. Gibbons RJ. Nuclear cardiology. In "Cardiology: Fundamentals and Practice", vol. 1, 2nd Edition, eds Giuliani ER, Fuster V, Gersh BJ, McGoon MD, McGoon DC. Mosby Year Book, St. Louis, 1991, pp 459–491.

3. Dilsizian V, Rocco TP, Bonow RO, et al. Cardiac blood-pool imaging. II: Applications in noncoronary heart disease. J Nucl Med 1990; 31: 10–22.

4. Alexander J, Dainiak N, Berger HJ, et al. Serial assessment of doxorubicin cardiotoxicity with quantitative radionuclide angiocardiography. N Engl J Med 1979; 300: 278–283.

5. Hamilton RG, Alderson PO. A comparative evaluation of techniques for rapid and efficient in vivo labeling of red cells with [^{99m}Tc] pertechnetate. J Nucl Med 1977; 18: 1010–1013.

6. Froelicher VF, Myers J, Follansbee WP, Labovitz AJ. Exercise testing methodology. In "Exercise and the Heart." Mosby, St. Louis, 1993.

7. Hanley PC, Zinsmeister AR, Clements IP, et al. Gender-related differences in cardiac response to supine exercise assessed by radionuclide angiography. J Am Coll Cardiol. 1989; 13: 624–629.

8. Atkins HL, Thomas SR, Buddemeyer U, Chervu LR. MIRD dose estimate report No. 14: radiation absorbed dose from technetium-99m-labeled red blood cells. J Nucl Med 1990; 31: 378–380.

Exercise Radionuclide Angiography

Note: All stress testing should be performed only if a qualified physician is in the immediate area and available to monitor any problems that may arise during or following the exercise procedure.

Summary Information

Radiopharmaceutical

Adult dose: Approximately 30 mCi (1,110 MBq) ^{99m}Tc-labeled RBCs. See the administered dose tables (see Tables 4-6 and 4-7) for the appropriate height- and weight-adjusted doses for males and females.

Pediatric dose: Adjusted according to the patient's weight (see Appendix A-3).

Contraindications Optimal image quality in RNA requires that the patient be in normal sinus rhythm so that successive cardiac cycles can be accurately summed. In patients with severe arrhythmia, the study may be suboptimal.

Dose/Scan Interval Imaging can commence immediately after the injection.

Views Obtained Images of the heart should be obtained in the anterior, left lateral, and LAO positions during the rest study and in the LAO position during exercise.

Indications

Gated RNA is one of the most accurate techniques available for measuring LVEF.[1] Exercise RNA has been used widely in examining patients with known or suspected coronary artery disease.[2,3] It can also be used for assessing prognosis in patients with stable coronary artery disease, in postinfarction patients, and in postrevascularization patients.[4–6]

Principle

RNA requires that the blood be labeled with a suitable tracer such as ^{99m}Tc-tagged RBCs. The technique is based on imaging the left ventricle for a large number of beats and summing the image data from each beat to produce a composite beat with adequate count statistics for analysis. RNA requires the simultaneous acquisition of the patient's ECG and images of the left ventricle. Starting with an R-wave trigger, the image data are sequentially loaded into 20–30 frames spanning a single cardiac cycle. The next R wave resets the system so that image data from the next cardiac cycle are loaded into the same 20–30 frames. This summing process continues until sufficient counts are present in each frame to permit analysis of this 20–30 frame-composite cardiac cycle. Chamber size and wall motion may be assessed qualitatively by replaying the images in a closed-loop display, and the LVEF may be calculated from the time–activity curve that is generated.

Exercise is performed during RNA, because in many patients with coronary artery disease or other limitations of cardiac function, these limitations may be manifested only when the heart is stressed. For diagnostic and prognostic purposes, the best criterion is a decreased exercise LVEF.

Patient Preparation

The patient should not eat more than a light meal 1–2 hours before the study. Whenever appropriate, the patient should discontinue the use of nitrates 12 hours before the study and the use of calcium channel and beta-blockers 24 hours before the study.

Preparation of the ^{99m}Tc-labeled RBCs (modified in vivo labeling technique):

1. Place 4 ml of heparinized saline in a 6-ml syringe.
2. Place the appropriate dose of ^{99m}Tc sodium pertechnetate (Tables 4-6 and 4-7) into a volume of 1 ml in a 12-ml syringe.
3. Attach the 6- and 12-ml syringes to a 3-way stopcock.
4. Reconstitute a vial of sodium PYP. Optimal labeling requires at minimum a dose of 5 mg Sn-PYP per 70 kg of body weight or 10 µg Sn (II)/kg.[7] Inject the required amount of Sn-PYP into the patient with a 21-gauge butterfly infusion set positioned in an arm vein. Wait 15 minutes.
5. Connect the syringes and the stopcock to the butterfly infusion set (see Fig. 4-5). Draw 6–10 ml of blood into the 12-ml syringe.
6. Draw 2 ml of heparinized saline through the stopcock into the 12-ml syringe. Push the remainder of the heparinized saline through the butterfly infusion set.
7. Mix the blood, and let it stand for 10 minutes, then reinject it into the patient.

Before commencing the study, attach electrodes for ECG recording. Twelve electrodes should be positioned on the body, as shown in Figure 4-11 (these permit a full-stress ECG to be recorded with the exercise RNA study). Before the electrodes are placed, prepare the skin as follows:[8]

1. The patient should be supine.
2. Shave any superficial hair over the area of electrode placement.
3. With an alcohol-saturated gauze pad, clean the area to remove any oils.
4. Lightly abrade the skin with 200-grit emery paper.
5. Use the diagram in Figure 4-11 as a guide to place the 12 electrodes.
6. Attach the leads, and check that all the connections are secure and that good-quality ECG tracings are obtained.

Instrument Specifications

Gamma camera: A small field-of-view (20–30 cm) system is preferred, because a large field-of-view system may hinder leg movement during exercise.

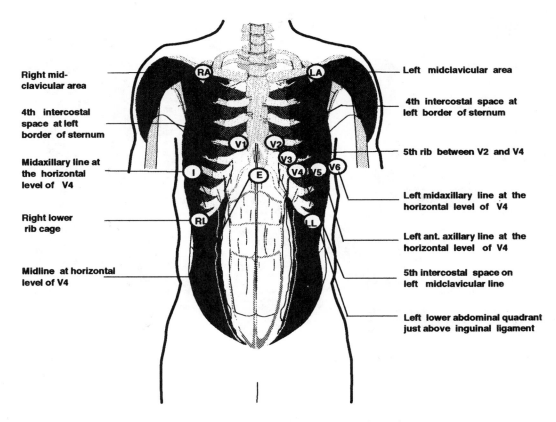

Right mid-
clavicular area

4th intercostal
space at left
border of sternum

Midaxillary line at
the horizontal
level of V4

Right lower
rib cage

Midline at horizontal
level of V4

Left midclavicular area

4th intercostal space at
left border of sternum

5th rib between V2 and V4

Left midaxillary line at the
horizontal level of V4

Left ant. axillary line at the
horizontal level of V4

5th intercostal space on
left midclavicular line

Left lower abdominal quadrant
just above inguinal ligament

Figure 4-11. Placement of 12-lead ECG electrodes.

Collimator:	Low-energy, all-purpose collimator.
Energy setting:	140-keV peak, 15–20% window.
Additional items:	ECG gating system and "divide-by-two" circuit box if alternate gating is required.
Computer system:	Acquisition requirements—gated acquisition (64 × 64 matrix), 20 frames per cardiac cycle (56 frames for alternate gating).
	Processing requirements—semiautomated or automated analysis software for LVEF and wall motion analysis of gated study.

Imaging Procedure

1. Position the patient supine on the ergometer table with the feet down. Connect all the ECG leads, and verify that the ECG tracings are acceptable.
2. Place a blood pressure cuff on the patient's arm. The patient's systolic and diastolic blood pressures should be measured and recorded during each stage of the study.
3. Position the detector anteriorly over the chest, and using the persistence screen, check that the heart is located centrally in the field of view. Check that the patient is positioned correctly for exercise as shown in Figure 4-12 (i.e., the legs are clear of the detector, and the hand grips are in the appropriate position).

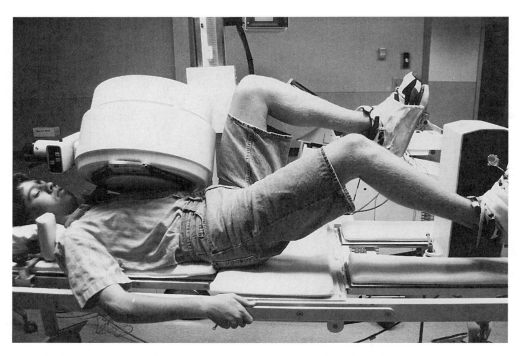

Figure 4-12. Patient in position on ergometer table for exercise. Note clearance between legs and detector head.

4. Set up the computer acquisition with the following variables: 64 × 64 word mode matrix, 20 frames per cycle, acquisition should terminate at 300 kct per frame. If available, use a rubber band framing method (rubber banding is used to eliminate drop-off in image counts at the end of the composite cardiac cycle by stretching or compressing each cardiac cycle to match the time per frame used by the system). On the patient's R-wave histogram, set a ±25% window around the primary heart rate. Check that the heart rate is stable. Acquire the anterior RNA study.

5. Rotate the detector to the left lateral position, and move the patient's left arm above the head to permit the detector to be positioned close to the chest wall. Acquire the left lateral study as described in step 4.

6. Reposition the detector to the LAO position, and with the patient's feet down, acquire the study as described in step 4. *Note:* The optimal LAO angle for separation of the left and right ventricles varies from patient to patient. Visually inspect the images on the persistence screen to determine the optimal angle. Also, a caudal tilt of 10°–20° should be used to obtain optimal separation of the atria and ventricles (Fig. 4-7).

7. If a 56-frame LAO study is requested for analysis of left ventricular filling or emptying rates (or both), acquire the study at this point, before exercise (see details of the acquisition and processing in Procedure 4-3, "Resting Radionuclide Angiography").

8. After completion of the rest views, set up the computer for a maximum of 7 acquisitions. Each acquisition should be acquired with the following variables: 64 × 64 word mode matrix, 16 frames per cycle, acquisition should terminate at 2 minutes. Rubber banding should be used if available. On the patient's R-wave histogram, do not set any upper or

lower limits on the heart rate (if a window is required by the system, set it to the widest possible limit around the primary heart rate).

9. Securely strap the patient's feet into the pedals of the ergometer. With the detector still in the LAO position, acquire a resting LAO study for 2 minutes, with the patient's feet up on the pedals.

10. The patient should now begin to exercise. The standard exercise protocol consists of 7 possible stages: 300, 600, 900, 1,200, 1,500, and 1,800 kg-m/min, followed by one stage immediately after exercise (300 kg-m/min is approximately 50 watts). *Note:* This protocol occasionally needs to be modified to meet the exercise ability of the patient.

11. Starting at 300 kg-m/min, the patient should be instructed to exercise at a predetermined number of revolutions per minute (typically 50–60) for 3 minutes. After 55 seconds, start the 2-minute RNA acquisition.

12. In some cases (e.g., evaluation of the postinfarction patients), a submaximal exercise protocol is used. In these patients, the exercise protocol consists of only two stages: 200 and 400 kg-m/min.

13. After 3 minutes of exercise, increase the workload on the ergometer by 300 kg-m/min, and repeat the preceding process. It is important to note any significant arrhythmias.

14. Continue step 13 until the patient can no longer maintain the exercise level (because of fatigue, chest pain, etc.). *Note:* Most patients will not be able to complete the protocol.

15. After exercise, the patient should stop pedaling, but the feet should remain up on the pedals. Wait 55 seconds, and acquire a further 2-minute acquisition (immediate postexercise LAO study).

16. After completion of the study, obtain a 10-ml blood sample in a glass vial. Place the vial on top of the collimator, and count for 2 minutes, as shown in Figure 4-8.

Computer Analysis

Analysis is performed on all rest and stress LAO studies. For the analysis of each study, the RNA analysis software on the computer generally requires that a seed ROI be placed over the left ventricle. A combination of a second-derivative edge-detection routine and a fixed count threshold is commonly used to determine the left ventricular boundary. In most cases, the fixed count threshold should be adjusted so that most of the left ventricular boundary is determined with the second-derivative edge-detection routine. Irrespective of the edge-detection algorithm, visually check during the analysis that the left ventricular ROI boundaries are consistent with the outline of the left ventricle. If they are not consistent, adjust the edge-detection variables until an acceptable boundary is obtained. The background ROI should be determined from the end-systole frame and should be displaced 2–3 pixels to the right of the left ventricle (see Fig. 4-9). The analysis software should, at minimum, output the LVEF curve, global or regional left ventricular wall motion analysis, and phase and amplitude images of the heart. Save the final LVEF curve. Repeat this process for each LAO study. Label the LVEF curves appropriately, e.g., E300 for 300 kg-m/min exercise level.

Measurement of left ventricular volumes requires the following information from each LAO study and the 10-ml blood sample:

1. Left ventricular end-diastolic counts (ct) (EDC)
2. Left ventricular end-systolic counts (ct) (ESC)
3. Total number of cardiac cycles acquired in the study (TC)

4. Duration of each frame in the composite cardiac cycle (seconds) (DUR)
5. Two-minute counts in a 10-ml blood sample (ct) (BLD)

Analysis requires that the end-diastole and end-systole counts be normalized (n) to counts per second, as follows:

$$nEDC = \frac{EDC}{TC \times DUR} \text{ ct/sec}$$

$$nESC = \frac{ESC}{TC \times DUR} \text{ ct/sec}$$

The blood sample must be normalized (n) to counts per second per milliliter as follows:

$$nBLD = \frac{BLD}{2 \times 60 \times 10} \text{ ct/sec per ml}$$

Note: If there is a significant delay (greater than 20 minutes) between the patient study and counting of the blood sample, then a decay-correction factor should be applied to the blood counts. Use the following nomograms to calculate the end-diastole and end-systole volumes:[9]

$$\text{End-diastole blood volume} = \frac{nEDC}{nBLD} \times 66.3 + 2.2 \text{ ml}$$

$$\text{End-systole blood volume} = \frac{nESC}{nBLD} \times 67.8 + 0.77 \text{ ml}$$

In addition, the following patient information is useful in the interpretation of the data:

1. Age, height, weight, and whether sedentary or active
2. Systolic/diastolic blood pressures for each LAO study

Table 4-4 illustrates a standard report from an exercise RNA study.

Information on Film

No image hard copy is generated. Results of the preceding analysis are tabulated and printed.

Interpretation

Normal Subjects

In normal subjects, the change in LVEF with exercise is determined partly by the resting LVEF. In normal subjects with high resting LVEF, the LVEF may not change with exercise.[10] The normal LVEF response to exercise is also different between men and women, as shown in Figure 4-13.[11,12]

Coronary Artery Disease/Prognosis

In the detection of coronary artery disease and in the estimation of prognosis, the LVEF at peak exercise is considered the most important variable.[13] Table 4-5 shows the sensitivity

Table 4-4. Sample Output From 7-Stage Exercise RNA Study in a Patient With Cardiomyopathy Who Exercised to Fatigue[a]

Work (kg-m/min)	Rest	300	600	900	1,200	1,500	1,800	Postexercise
Duration (min)	0.0	3.0	3.0	3.0	3.0	3.0	—	
HR (beats/min)	61	95	117	140	147	172		
SBP (mm Hg)	130	150	160	195	200	215		
DBP (mm Hg)	80	90	100	80	80	80		
LVEF (%)	44	48	51	48	49	44		
CI (L/min per m²)	4.7	8.1	10.0	11.0	11.0	13.0		
LVEDVI	181	180	174	179	157	185		
LVESVI	103	94	87	95	81	106		
SBP/LVESVI	1.25	1.58	1.82	2.04	2.46	2.01		

Abbreviations: CI, cardiac index; HR, heart rate; LVEDVI, LVESI, left ventricular and diastolic/systolic volume index; LVEF left ventricular ejection fraction; SBP/DBP, systolic/diastolic systolic blood pressure.
[a]Age: 31, Height: 176 cm, Weight: 70 kg, B.S.A.: 1.86 m². Procedure: Exercise, peak exercise.
Pressure-rate double product: 36,980.
Metabolic equivalents (METS): 13.5.

and normalcy rate of LVEF at peak exercise for the diagnosis of coronary artery disease.[14] In assessing prognosis, the reported results indicate that the LVEF at peak exercise and peak heart rate provide 80–90% of the prognostic power.[15] Figure 4-14 shows the probability of survival at 5 years relative to LVEF at peak exercise.[16]

Prediction of Disease Severity

The ability to identify severe disease depends primarily on four variables, which are in order (1) magnitude of ST-segment depression, (2) LVEF at peak exercise, (3) peak double product (peak heart rate × systolic blood pressure), and (4) patient sex. Probability graphs that predict disease in men and women have been generated from these four variables.[17]

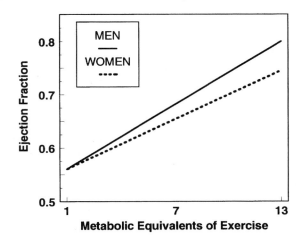

Figure 4-13. Gender difference in the LVEF response to supine exercise. (Adapted from Hanley et al.,[11] with permission.)

Table 4-5. Sensitivity and Normalcy Rate of Ejection Fraction at Peak Exercise for Diagnosis of Coronary Artery Disease

Ejection Fraction at Peak Heart Rate	Sensitivity %	Normalcy Rate %
0.50	55	98
0.55	66	93
0.57	72	90
0.60	77	82
0.63	84	72
0.65	86	67

(Adapted from Gibbons,[14] with permission.)

Radiation Dosimetry

The estimated absorbed doses in organs and tissues of an average subject (70 kg) from an IV injection of 30 mCi (1,110 MBq) ^{99m}Tc-labeled RBCs are shown in Table 4-2.[18]

Administered Dose Tables

Tables 4-6 and 4-7 are based on the 1983 Metropolitan Weight and Height Tables and are designed to give consistent count statistics for patients of different height and weight.[19,20] The height and weight measurements are based on subjects wearing indoor clothes but no shoes. To determine the appropriate dose, check the left-hand column for the patient's height and, in the corresponding horizontal column, identify the square with the patient's weight (in pounds). The appropriate administered dose (in mCi and MBq) is given at the top of the weight column.

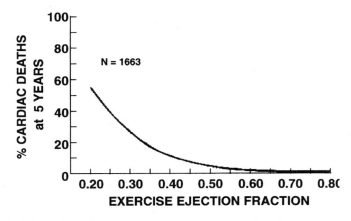

Figure 4-14. Probability of survival at 5 years relative to ejection fraction at peak exercise, for patients with stable angina. (Data from Jones et al.[16])

Table 4-6. Administered Dose Tables for Males

Height	25 mCi 925 MBq	26 mCi 962 MBq	27 mCi 999MBq	28 mCi 1036 MBq	29 mCi 1073 MBq	30 mCi 1110 MBq	31 mCi 1147 MBq	32 mCi 1184 MBq	33 mCi 1221 MBq	34 mCi 1258 MBq	35 mCi 1295 MBq	36 mCi 1332 MBq	37 mCi 1369 MBq	38 mCi 1406 MBq	39 mCi 1443 MBq	40 mCi 1480 MBq
5' 1"	90–100	101–110	111–120	121–130	131–140	141–150	151–160	161–170	171–180	181–190	191–200	201–210	211–220	221–230	231–240	241–250
5' 2"	93–103	104–113	114–123	124–133	134–143	144–153	154–163	164–173	174–183	184–193	194–203	204–213	214–223	224–233	234–243	244–253
5' 3"	96–106	107–116	117–126	127–136	137–146	147–156	157–166	167–176	177–186	187–196	197–206	207–216	217–226	227–236	237–246	247–256
5' 4"	100–110	111–120	121–130	131–140	141–150	151–160	161–170	171–180	181–190	191–200	201–210	211–220	221–230	231–240	241–250	251–260
5' 5"	104–114	115–124	125–134	135–144	145–154	155–164	165–174	175–184	185–194	195–204	205–214	215–224	225–234	235–244	245–254	255–264
5' 6"	108–118	119–128	129–138	139–148	149–158	159–168	169–178	179–188	189–198	199–208	209–218	219–228	229–238	239–248	249–258	259–268
5' 7"	112–122	123–132	133–142	143–152	153–162	163–172	173–182	183–192	193–202	203–212	213–222	223–232	233–242	243–252	253–262	263–272
5' 8"	116–126	127–136	137–146	147–156	157–166	167–176	177–186	187–196	197–206	207–216	217–226	227–236	237–246	247–256	257–266	267–276
5' 9"	120–130	131–140	141–150	151–160	161–170	171–180	181–190	191–200	201–210	211–220	221–230	231–240	241–250	251–260	261–270	271–280
5' 10"	124–134	135–144	145–154	155–164	165–174	175–184	185–194	195–204	205–214	215–224	225–234	235–244	245–254	255–264	265–274	275–284
5' 11"	128–138	139–148	149–158	159–168	169–178	179–188	189–198	199–208	209–218	219–228	229–238	239–248	249–258	259–268	269–278	279–288
6' 0"	132–142	143–152	153–162	163–172	173–182	183–192	193–202	203–212	213–222	223–232	233–242	243–252	253–262	263–272	273–282	283–292
6' 1"	137–147	148–157	158–167	168–177	178–187	188–197	198–207	208–217	218–227	228–237	238–247	248–257	258–267	268–277	278–287	288–297
6' 2"	142–152	153–162	163–172	173–182	183–192	193–202	203–212	213–222	223–232	233–242	243–252	253–262	263–272	273–282	283–292	293–302
6' 3"	147–157	158–167	168–177	178–187	188–197	198–207	208–217	218–227	228–237	238–247	248–257	258–267	268–277	278–287	288–297	298–307

Table 4-7. Administered Dose Tables for Females

Height	25 mCi 925 MBq	26 mCi 962 MBq	27 mCi 999MBq	28 mCi 1036 MBq	29 mCi 1073 MBq	30 mCi 1110 MBq	31 mCi 1147 MBq	32 mCi 1184 MBq	33 mCi 1221 MBq	34 mCi 1258 MBq	35 mCi 1295 MBq	36 mCi 1332 MBq	37 mCi 1369 MBq	38 mCi 1406 MBq	39 mCi 1443 MBq	40 mCi 1480 MBq
4' 9"	71–81	82–91	92–101	102–111	112–121	122–131	132–141	142–151	152–161	162–171	172–181	182–191	192–201	202–211	212–221	222–231
4' 10"	74–84	85–94	95–104	105–114	115–124	125–134	135–144	145–154	155–164	165–174	175–184	185–194	195–204	205–214	215–224	225–234
4' 11"	77–87	88–97	98–107	108–117	118–127	128–137	138–147	148–157	158–167	168–177	178–187	188–197	198–207	208–217	218–227	228–237
5' 0"	80–90	91–100	101–110	111–120	121–130	131–140	141–150	151–160	161–170	171–180	181–190	191–200	201–210	211–220	221–230	231–240
5' 1"	83–93	94–103	104–113	114–123	124–133	134–143	144–153	154–163	164–173	174–183	184–193	194–203	204–213	214–223	224–233	234–243
5' 2"	87–97	98–107	108–117	118–127	128–137	138–147	148–157	158–167	168–177	178–187	188–197	198–207	208–217	218–227	228–237	238–247
5' 3"	91–101	102–111	112–121	122–131	132–141	142–151	152–161	162–171	172–181	182–191	192–201	202–211	212–221	222–231	232–241	242–251
5' 4"	95–105	106–115	116–125	126–135	136–145	146–155	156–165	166–175	176–185	186–195	196–205	206–215	216–225	226–235	236–245	246–255
5' 5"	99–109	110–119	120–129	130–139	140–149	150–159	160–169	170–179	180–189	190–199	200–209	210–219	220–229	230–239	240–249	250–259
5' 6"	103–113	114–123	124–133	134–143	144–153	154–163	164–173	174–183	184–193	194–203	204–213	214–223	224–233	234–243	244–253	254–263
5' 7"	107–117	118–127	128–137	138–147	148–157	158–167	168–177	178–187	188–197	198–207	208–217	218–227	228–237	238–247	248–257	258–267
5' 8"	110–120	121–130	131–140	141–150	151–160	161–170	171–180	181–190	191–200	201–210	211–220	221–230	231–240	241–250	251–260	261–270
5' 9"	113–123	124–133	134–143	144–153	154–163	164–173	174–183	184–193	194–203	204–213	214–223	224–233	234–243	244–253	254–263	264–273
5' 10"	116–126	127–136	137–146	147–156	157–166	167–176	177–186	187–196	197–206	207–216	217–226	227–236	237–246	247–256	257–266	267–276
5' 11"	119–129	130–139	140–149	150–159	160–169	170–179	180–189	190–199	200–209	210–219	220–229	230–239	240–249	250–259	260–269	270–279

References

1. Borer JS, Bacharach SL, Green MV, et al. Real-time radionuclide ventriculography in the non-invasive evaluation of global and regional left ventricular function at rest and during exercise in patients with coronary-artery disease. N Engl J Med 1977; 296: 839–844.

2. Jones RH, McEwan P, Newman GE, et al. Accuracy of diagnosis of coronary artery disease by radionuclide management of left ventricular function during rest and exercise. Circulation 1981; 64: 586–601.

3. Gibbons RJ. Nuclear cardiology. In "Cardiology: Fundamentals and Practice," vol. 1, 2nd Edition, eds Giuliani ER, Fuster V, Gersh BJ, McGoon MD, McGoon DC. Mosby Year Book, St. Louis, 1991, pp 459–491.

4. Iqbal A, Gibbons RJ, Zinsmeister AR, Mock MB, Ballard DJ. Prognostic value of exercise radionuclide angiography in a population-based cohort of patients with known or suspected coronary artery disease. Am J Cardiol 1994; 74: 119–124.

5. Lavie CJ, Gibbons RJ, Zinsmeister AR, Gersh BJ. Interpreting results of exercise studies after acute myocardial infarction altered by thrombolytic therapy, coronary angioplasty or bypass. Am J Cardiol 1991; 67: 116–120.

6. Jones RH, Floyd RD, Austin EH, Sabiston DC Jr. The role of radionuclide angiography in the preoperative prediction of pain relief and prolonged survival following coronary artery bypass grafting. Ann Surg 1983; 197: 743–754.

7. Hamilton RG, Alderson PO. A comparative evaluation of techniques for rapid and efficient in vivo labeling of red cells with [^{99m}Tc] pertechnetate. J Nucl Med 1977; 18: 1010–1013.

8. Froelicher VF, Myers J, Follansbee WP, Labovitz AJ. "Exercise and the Heart." Mosby, St. Louis, 1993.

9. Clements IP, Brown ML, Smith HC. Radionuclide measurement of left ventricular volume. Mayo Clin Proc 1981; 56: 733–739.

10. Port S, McEwan P, Cobb FR, Jones RH. Influence of resting left ventricular function on the left ventricular response to exercise in patients with coronary artery disease. Circulation 1981; 63: 856–863.

11. Hanley PC, Zinsmeister AR, Clements IP, et al. Gender-related differences in cardiac response to supine exercise assessed by radionuclide angiography. J Am Coll Cardiol 1989; 13: 624–629.

12. Higginbotham MB, Morris KG, Coleman RE, Cobb FR. Sex-related differences in normal cardiac response to upright exercise. Circulation 1984; 70: 357–366.

13. Gibbons RJ, Lee KL, Pryor D, et al. The use of radionuclide angiography in the diagnosis of coronary artery disease—a logistic regression analysis. Circulation 1983; 68: 740–746.

14. Gibbons RJ. Rest and exercise radionuclide angiography for diagnosis in chronic ischemic heart disease. Circulation 1991; 84 (Suppl. 3): 193–199.

15. Lee KL, Pryor DB, Pieper KS, et al. Prognostic value of radionuclide angiography in medically treated patients with coronary artery disease. A comparison with clinical and catheterization variables. Circulation 1990; 82: 1705–1717.

16. Jones RH, Johnson SH, Bigelow C, et al. Exercise radionuclide angiography predicts cardiac death in patients with coronary artery disease. Circulation 1991; 84 (Suppl. 3): 152–158.

17. Gibbons RJ, Fyke FE III, Clements IP, et al. Noninvasive identification of severe coronary artery disease using exercise radionuclide angiography. J Am Coll Cardiol 1988; 11: 28–34.

18. Atkins HL, Thomas SR, Buddemeyer U, Chervu LR. MIRD dose estimate report No. 14: radiation absorbed dose from technetium-99m-labeled red blood cells. J Nucl Med 1990; 31: 378–380.

19. Glynn RB, Narveson LG, Hung JC, Gibbons RJ. Adjustment to radionuclide angiogram dose based upon patient's physical parameters. J Nucl Med Technol 1994; 22: 17–20.

20. Glynn RB, Hung JC, Mahoney DW, Wollan PC. Simplification of radionuclide angiogram dosage adjustment chart using linear equations (abstract). J Nucl Med Technol 1994; 22: 105–106.

Dobutamine Radionuclide Angiography

Note: Pharmacologic stress should be performed only if a cardiologist is in the immediate area and available to monitor any problem that may arise during or following the stress procedure.

Summary Information

Radiopharmaceutical

Adult dose: Approximately 30 mCi (1,110 MBq) ^{99m}Tc-labeled RBCs. See Tables 4-6 and 4-7 for the appropriate height- and weight-adjusted doses for males and females.

Pediatric dose: Adjusted according to the patient's weight (see Appendix A-3).

Contraindications Optimum image quality in RNA requires that the patient be in normal sinus rhythm so that successive cardiac cycles can be summed accurately. In patients with severe arrhythmia, the study may be suboptimal. Contraindications for dobutamine stress are current use of beta-blockers, hypertrophic cardiomyopathy, uncontrolled hypertension (blood pressure greater than 200/110 mm Hg) and ventricular arrhythmias.[1,2] During and after dobutamine infusion, about 75% of patients experience some side effects. Palpitations and chest pain occur in about 30% of patients, and other side effects (arrhythmias, nausea, headache, tremor, ECG changes) occur in less than 5%.[2] Most of these effects are transient, because dobutamine has a biologic half-life of only 2 minutes.[3] Occasionally, esmolol may be administered to neutralize the side effects.

Dose/Scan Interval Imaging can commence immediately after injection of the radiolabeled RBCs.

Views Obtained Images of the heart should be obtained in the anterior, left lateral, and LAO positions during the rest study and in the LAO position during the dobutamine stress study.

Indications

Although exercise RNA has been used widely in the examination of patients with known or suspected coronary artery disease,[4,5] many patients are unable or unwilling to exercise effectively. In such patients, the use of a pharmacologic agent such as dobutamine to stress the heart may be the most appropriate choice.

Principle

RNA requires that the blood be labeled with a suitable tracer such as ^{99m}Tc-tagged RBCs. The technique is based on imaging the left ventricle for a large number of beats and summing the image data from each beat to produce a composite beat with adequate count statistics for analysis. RNA requires the simultaneous acquisition of the patient's ECG and images of the left ventricle. Chamber size and wall motion may be assessed qualitatively by replaying the images in a closed-loop display, and LVEF may be calculated from the time–activity curve that is generated.

Dobutamine is a synthetic sympathetic amine that causes an increase in the rate pressure product, stroke volume, and cardiac output, with a resultant increase in heart rate and myocardial contractility.[3,6] Dobutamine has a biologic half-life in plasma of about 2 minutes. RNA can be performed during dobutamine infusion, similar to an exercise RNA study. With stepped increases in the infused dose of dobutamine, changes in LVEF and myocardial contractility can be determined from the RNA study.

Patient Preparation

Patients should fast for at least 3 hours before the administration of dobutamine, because potential side effects of this drug include nausea and vomiting.

Electrocardiogram Recording

Before commencing the study, position the electrodes for recording the ECG. Twelve electrodes should be positioned on the body, as shown in Figure 4-11 (these permit a full-stress ECG to be recorded with the dobutamine stress RNA study). Before the electrodes are placed, prepare the skin as follows:[7]

1. The patient should be supine.
2. Shave any superficial hair over the area of electrode placement.
3. With an alcohol-saturated gauze pad, clean the area to remove any oils.
4. Lightly abrade the skin with 200-grit emery paper.
5. Use the diagram in Figure 4-11 as a guide to place the 12 electrodes.
6. Attach the leads, and check that all the connections are secure and that good-quality ECG tracings are obtained.

Preparation of the ^{99m}Tc-Labeled Red Blood Cells

1. Place 4 ml of heparinized saline in a 6-ml syringe.
2. Place the appropriate dose of ^{99m}Tc pertechnetate (Tables 4-6 and 4-7), in a volume of 1 ml into a 12-ml syringe.
3. Place a 20-gauge IV catheter/needle set into an antecubital vein. Reconstitute a vial of sodium PYP. Optimal labeling requires, at minimum, a dose of 5 mg Sn-PYP per 70 kg body weight or 10 µg Sn (II)/kg.[8] Inject PYP into patient through the IV catheter/needle set.

4. Attach the distal end of a T-piece infusion set to the IV catheter/needle set. One port on a 3-way stopcock should be attached to the T-piece extension set. Connect the 6- and 12-ml syringes to the other ports on the stopcock.
5. Wait 15 minutes, then draw 6–10 ml of blood into the 12-ml syringe.
6. Draw 2 ml of heparinized saline through the stopcock into the 12-ml syringe. Push the rest of the heparinized saline through the T-piece infusion set.
7. Mix the blood, and let it stand for 10 minutes, then reinject it into the patient.

Dobutamine Infusion Preparation

The dobutamine infusion should be prepared as follows:

1. Place the contents of a vial (20 ml) of dobutamine into a 250-ml saline bag (final concentration is about 1 mg/ml).
2. Connect the saline bag to an infusion pump administration set. Prime the administration set with saline, and install it in the infusion pump, as shown in Figure 4-15.
3. Attach a 50–70 inch solution set to a 250-ml saline bag. After the blood has been radiolabeled as described, remove the 6- and 12-ml syringes, and attach the end of the solution set to one port on the 3-way stopcock. Attach the infusion pump administration set to the other port on the 3-way stopcock.
4. Figure 4-16 shows the arrangement of the IV catheter/needle set, T-piece set, stopcock, and infusion sets.
5. Calculate the appropriate pump settings in milliliters per hour for the patient's weight that correspond to infusion rates of 10, 20, 30, and 40 µg/kg per minute.

Instrument Specifications

Gamma camera:	Any small or large field-of-view system can be used.
Collimator:	Low-energy, all-purpose collimator.
Energy setting:	140-keV peak, 20% window.
Additional items:	ECG gating system.

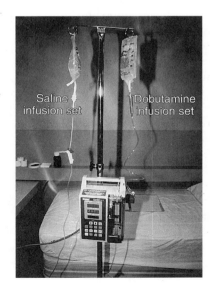

Figure 4-15. A 250-ml saline bag containing dobutamine (right side) with administration set for infusion pump. Standard 250-ml saline bag and extension set (left side) connect directly to stopcock.

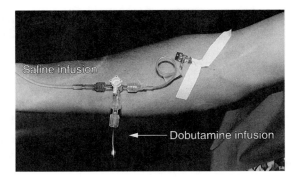

Figure 4-16. Arrangement of 20-gauge IV catheter/needle set, T-piece, stopcock, and infusion sets for dobutamine administration.

Computer system: Acquisition requirements—gated acquisition (64 × 64 matrix), 20 frames per cardiac cycle.

Processing requirements—semiautomated or automated analysis software for ejection fraction and wall motion analysis of gated study.

Imaging Procedure

1. Position the patient supine on the imaging table. Connect all the ECG leads, and verify that ECG tracings are acceptable.
2. Place a blood pressure cuff on the patient's arm. Measure and record the patient's systolic and diastolic blood pressures during each stage of the study.
3. Position the detector anteriorly over the chest, and using the persistence screen, check that the heart is located centrally in the field of view.
4. Set up the computer acquisition with the following variables: 64 × 64 word mode matrix, 20 frames per cycle, acquisition should terminate at 300 kct per frame. If available, use a rubber band framing method (rubber banding is used to eliminate drop-off in image counts at the end of the composite cardiac cycle by stretching or compressing each cardiac cycle to match the time per frame used by the system). On the patient's R-wave histogram, set a ±25% window around the primary heart rate. Check that the heart rate is stable. Acquire the anterior RNA study.
5. Rotate the detector to the left lateral position, and move the patient's left arm above the head to permit the detector to be positioned close to the chest wall. Acquire the left lateral study, as described in step 4.
6. Reposition the detector to the LAO position, and acquire the study, as described in step 4. *Note:* The optimum LAO angle for separation of the left and right ventricles varies from patient to patient. Visually inspect the images on the persistence screen to determine the optimal angle. Also, a caudal tilt of 10°–20° should be used to obtain optimal separation of the atria and ventricles, as shown in Figure 4-7.
7. Occasionally, the referring physician will request a 56-frame LAO study for analysis of left ventricular filling/emptying rates. If so, this study should be acquired at this point, before dobutamine infusion (see details of acquisition and processing in Procedure 4-3, "Resting Radionuclide Angiography").
8. After completion of the rest views, set up the computer for a maximum of 5 acquisitions. Each acquisition should be acquired with the following variables: 64 × 64 word mode matrix, 16 frames per cycle, and acquisition should terminate at 2 minutes. Rubber banding

should be used if available. On the patient's R-wave histogram, do not set any upper or lower limits on heart rate (if a window is required by the system, set it to the widest possible limit around the primary heart rate).

9. Dobutamine infusion should now be started at a rate of 10 µg/kg per minute for 3 minutes. After 55 seconds, start the 2-minute RNA acquisition.
10. After 3 minutes, increase the infusion rate to 20 µg/kg per minute and repeat step 9.
11. Repeat step 10 with infusion rates of 30 and 40 µg/kg per minute.
12. Infusion rate may be increased to a maximum of 50 µg/kg per minute if the patient fails to have an adequate increase in heart rate. *Note:* Dosage end points are as follows:
    a. 85% of predicted maximal value for age
    b. 70% of predicted maximal value for age in postmyocardial infarction patients
    c. Marked hypertensive/hypotensive response
    d. Ischemic symptoms
13. The patient's ECG should be monitored during the dobutamine infusion, and blood pressure should be measured every minute. Any significant arrhythmia should be noted, as dobutamine occasionally induces significant ectopy.
14. If severe side effects occur, the cardiologist may request that the infusion be stopped. If necessary, esmolol (a rapidly acting beta-blocker) can be used to neutralize the side effects of dobutamine.
15. After cessation of dobutamine infusion, the patient's condition should be monitored for 5 minutes.
16. If no side effects persist, monitoring may be stopped, and the ECG leads and electrodes removed.
17. After completion of the study, obtain a 10-ml sample of blood in a glass vial. Place the vial on top of the collimator, and count for 2 minutes, as shown in Figure 4-8.
18. After the blood sample has been drawn, remove the IV catheter/needle set and associated tubing, and discard them in the radioactive waste bin.

Computer Analysis

Analysis is performed on all rest and stress LAO studies. For the analysis of each study, the RNA analysis software on the computer generally requires that a seed ROI be placed over the left ventricle. A combination of a second-derivative edge-detection routine and a fixed count threshold is commonly used to determine the left ventricular boundary. In most cases, the fixed count threshold should be adjusted so that most of the left ventricular boundary is determined by the second-derivative edge-detection routine. Irrespective of the edge-detection algorithm, visually check during the analysis that the left ventricular ROI boundaries are consistent with the outline of the left ventricle. If they are not consistent, adjust the edge-detection variables until an acceptable boundary is obtained. The background ROI should be determined from the end-systole frame and should be displaced 2-3 pixels to the right of the left ventricle (Fig. 4-9). The analysis software should, at minimum, output the time–activity curve, global or regional left ventricular wall motion analysis, and phase and amplitude images of the heart. Save the final time–activity curve. Repeat this process for each LAO study. Label the time–activity curves appropriately, e.g., D10 for a 10-µg/kg per minute dobutamine infusion level.

Measurement of left ventricular volumes requires the following information from each LAO study and the 10-ml blood sample:

1. Left ventricular end-diastolic counts (ct) (EDC)
2. Left ventricular end-systolic counts (ct) (ESC)
3. Total number of cardiac cycles acquired in the study (TC)
4. Duration of each frame in the composite cardiac cycle (sec) (DUR)
5. Two-minute counts in the 10-ml blood sample (ct) (BLD)

Analysis requires that the end-diastole and end-systole counts be normalized (n) to counts/second, as follows:

$$nEDC = \frac{EDC}{TC \times DUR} \ ct/sec$$

$$nESC = \frac{ESC}{TC \times DUR} \ ct/sec$$

The blood sample must be normalized (n) to counts per second per milliliter as follows:

$$nBLD = \frac{BLD}{2 \times 60 \times 10} \ ct/sec \ per \ ml$$

Note: If there is a significant delay (greater than 20 minutes) between the patient study and counting of the blood sample, then a decay-correction factor should be applied to the blood counts. Use the following nomograms to calculate the end-diastole and end-systole volumes:[9]

$$\text{End-diastole blood volume} = \frac{nEDC}{nBLD} \times 66.3 + 2.2 \ ml$$

$$\text{End-systole blood volume} = \frac{nESC}{nBLD} \times 67.8 + 0.77 \ ml$$

In addition, the following patient information is recorded:

1. Age, height, weight, and whether sedentary or active
2. Systolic/diastolic blood pressures for each LAO study

A standard report is produced for the dobutamine RNA study, similar to that for exercise RNA (see Table 4-4). In addition to LVEF and blood volume, the patient's heart rate and blood pressure are recorded for each level of dobutamine infusion.

Information on Film

No image hard copy is generated. Results of the preceding analysis are tabulated and printed.

Interpretation

The results obtained with dobutamine generally parallel those obtained with exercise. Some studies have shown that exercise testing and dobutamine testing have comparable sensitivity and accuracy, although differences in the type of abnormal response occur.[10] In particular, with dobutamine, some patients may demonstrate wall motion abnormalities without an abnormal ejection fraction response.[10]

Radiation Dosimetry

The estimated absorbed doses to organs and tissues of an average subject (70 kg) from an IV injection of 30 mCi (1,110 MBq) ^{99m}Tc-labeled RBCs are shown in Table 4-2.[11] The exact dose to be administered is determined from Tables 4-6 and 4-7, which are based on the 1983 Metropolitan Weight and Height Tables and are designed to give consistent count statistics for patients of different height and weight.[12,13] The height and weight measurements are based on subjects wearing indoor clothes but no shoes. To determine the appropriate dose, check the left-hand column for the patient's height and, in the corresponding horizontal column, identify the square with the patient's weight (in pounds). The appropriate administered dose (in millicuries and megabecquerels) is given at the top of the weight column.

References

1. Package insert. Dobutrex solution (dobutamine hydrochloride injection). Eli Lilli & Co., Indianapolis, IN. Revised Dec. 22, 1992.
2. Hays JT, Mahmarian JJ, Cochran AJ, Verani MS. Dobutamine thallium-201 tomography for evaluating patients with suspected coronary artery disease unable to undergo exercise or vasodilatory pharmacologic stress testing. J Am Coll Cardiol 1993; 21: 1583–1590.
3. Verani MS. Dobutamine myocardial perfusion imaging. J Nucl Med 1994; 35: 737–739.
4. Jones RH, McEwan P, Newman GE, et al. Accuracy of diagnosis of coronary artery disease by radionuclide management of left ventricular function during rest and exercise. Circulation 1981; 64: 586–601.
5. Gibbons RJ. Nuclear cardiology. In "Cardiology: Fundamentals and Practice," vol. 1, 2nd Edition, eds Giuliani ER, Fuster V, Gersh BJ, McGoon MD, McGoon DC. Mosby Year Book, St. Louis, 1991, pp 459–491.
6. Krivokapich J, Huang SC, Schelbert HR. Assessment of the effects of dobutamine on myocardial blood flow and oxidative metabolism in normal human subjects using nitrogen-13 ammonia and carbon-11 acetate. Am J Cardiol 1993; 71: 1351–1356.
7. Froelicher VF, Myers J, Follansbee WP, Labovitz AJ. "Exercise and the Heart." Mosby Year Book, St. Louis, 1993, pp 10–31.
8. Hamilton RG, Alderson PO. A comparative evaluation of techniques for rapid and efficient in vivo labeling of red cells with [^{99m}Tc] pertechnetate. J Nucl Med 1977; 18: 1010–1013.
9. Clements IP, Brown ML, Smith HC. Radionuclide measurement of left ventricular volume. Mayo Clin Proc 1981; 56: 733–739.
10. Freeman ML, Palac R, Mason J, et al. A comparison of dobutamine infusion and supine bicycle exercise for radionuclide cardiac stress testing. Clin Nucl Med 1984; 9: 251–255.
11. Atkins HL, Thomas SR, Buddemeyer U, Chervu LR. MIRD dose estimate report No. 14: radiation absorbed dose from technetium-99m-labeled red blood cells. J Nucl Med 1990; 31: 378–380.
12. Glynn RB, Narveson LG, Hung JC, Gibbons RJ. Adjustment to radionuclide angiogram dose based upon patient's physical parameters. J Nucl Med Technol 1994; 22: 17–20.
13. Glynn RB, Hung JC, Mahoney DW, Wollan PC. Simplification of radionuclide angiogram dosage adjustment chart using linear equations (abstract). J Nucl Med Technol 1994; 22: 105–106.

Aortic/Mitral Regurgitant Index

Summary Information

Radiopharmaceutical

Adult dose: 20–30 mCi (740–1,110 MBq) ^{99m}Tc-labeled RBCs.

Pediatric dose: Adjusted according to the patient's weight (see Appendix A-3).

Contraindications   The regurgitant fraction is obtained from analysis of a gated RNA study. Hence, it requires that the patient be in normal sinus rhythm so that successive cardiac cycles can be accurately summed. In patients with severe arrhythmia, the study may be suboptimal.

Dose/Scan Interval   Imaging can commence immediately after injection.

Views Obtained   Images of the heart should be obtained with the patient in the LAO position with a 30° caudal tilt.

Indications

This procedure is an adjunct to a rest or exercise RNA study. It provides a rough index of the severity of valvular regurgitation in patients with aortic or mitral valve regurgitation (or both).

Principle

From an RNA study, it is possible to determine the relative right and left ventricular stroke volumes. In normal patients, these volumes should be about equal. However, in patients with left-sided valvular insufficiency, the stroke volume of the left ventricle should increase in proportion to the degree of insufficiency.[1] Hence, determination of the left ventricle-to-right ventricle stroke volume ratio (SVR) provides a quantitative estimate of the degree of valvular incompetence. This technique has been validated in animal studies[2] and in clinical studies with contrast angiography.[3,4] These studies have shown that a simple index, the regurgitant fraction (RF), provides an excellent method of quantitating relative left ventricular volume overload:

$$RF = (LV - RV)/LV \text{ or}$$
$$RF = 1 - 1/SVR$$

where LV and RV are the left and right ventricular stroke counts, respectively.

This technique has several limitations. If both ventricles are overloaded, then only the combined effects will be determined and the individual performance of each ventricle cannot be obtained. Poor separation of atria and ventricles, in particular, overlap of the right ventricle and right atrium, and overlap with the ascending aorta decrease the sensitivity and specificity of this procedure.[5] Thus, this technique cannot accurately distinguish patients with mild valvular disease from normal subjects.

Patient Preparation

Standard patient preparation for a rest or exercise RNA study is used. Labeling of the RBCs should be performed as described in the rest or exercise RNA procedures.

Instrument Specifications

Gamma camera:	Any small or large field-of-view system can be used.
Collimator:	Low-energy 30° slant hole collimator.
Energy setting:	140-keV peak, 20% window.
Additional items:	ECG gating system.
Computer system:	Acquisition requirements—gated acquisition (64 × 64 matrix), 20 frames per cardiac cycle.
	Processing requirements—phase and amplitude analysis software, ROI and curve analysis software.

Imaging Procedure

1. The patient should be supine on the imaging table with the feet down. Place the detector in the LAO position, and move the patient's left arm above the head to permit the detector to be positioned close to the chest wall. *Note:* The optimal LAO angle for separation of the left and right ventricles varies from patient to patient. Visually inspect the images on the persistence screen to determine the optimal angle.
2. No caudal tilt is required, because this is provided by the 30° slant hole collimator. This gives optimal separation between the atria and ventricles.[6,7]
3. Set up the computer acquisition with the following variables: 64 × 64 word mode matrix, 20 frames per cycle, acquisition should terminate at 300 kct per frame. If available, use a rubber band framing method (rubber banding is used to eliminate drop-off in image counts at the end of the composite cardiac cycle by stretching or compressing each cardiac cycle to match the time per frame used by the system). On the patient's R-wave histogram, set a ±25% window around the primary heart rate. Check that the heart rate is stable. Acquire the LAO RNA study.

Computer Analysis

1. After analysis of the conventional RNA study, select the slant-hole LAO study. Filter it with a Hann filter (cutoff, 0.5 Nyquist), and perform phase and amplitude analyses. The output from this should be stored as a phase image set.
2. From the phase and amplitude display, carefully note the regions corresponding to the ventricles and atria (typically displayed in blue and yellow, respectively).

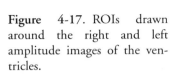 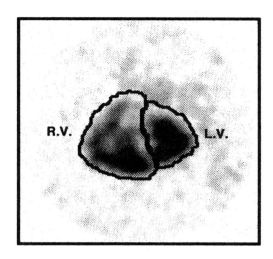

Figure 4-17. ROIs drawn around the right and left amplitude images of the ventricles.

3. Run the ROI analysis software. Display the amplitude image, and draw ROIs around the amplitude images of the right and left ventricles, as shown in Figure 4-17.
4. Select the original unfiltered slant-hole LAO study. Using curve analysis software, generate time–activity curves of counts in the right and left ventricles with the ROIs generated in step 3.
5. Record the maximum (RV_{max} and LV_{max}) and minimum counts (RV_{min} and LV_{min}) from each curve on the regurgitant fraction form shown in Figure 4-18, and calculate the RF with the following equation:

$$\% \, RF = \left(1 - \frac{RV_{max} - RV_{min}}{LV_{max} - LV_{min}}\right) \times 100$$

REGURGITANT FRACTION WORKSHEET

Patient Name : _____

Clinic No. _____   Date : _____

RT. / LT. VENTRICULAR TIME ACTIVITY CURVES	
RIGHT VENTRICLE	**LEFT VENTRICLE**
Max. Count : _____	Max. Count : _____
Min. Count : _____	Min. Count : _____
Difference : _____ (A)	Difference : _____ (B)
% Regurgitant Fraction (1 - A/B) x 100 = _____	

Figure 4-18. Worksheet for calculation of the regurgitant fraction.

Information on Film

Obtain a hard copy of the amplitude image and the ROIs for the right and left ventricles. Obtain a hard copy of the time–activity curves for both ventricles.

Interpretation

The normal value for the RF varies among laboratories, depending on the type of equipment available and the analysis performed.[8] In our laboratory, the normal range for the RF is 8% ± 6% (mean ± 1 SD).

Radiation Dosimetry

The estimated absorbed doses in organs and tissues of an average subject (70 kg) from an IV injection of 20 or 30 mCi (740 or 1,110 MBq) ^{99m}Tc-labeled RBCs are shown in Tables 4-3 and 4-2, respectively.[9]

References

1. Rigo P, Alderson PO, Robertson RM, Becker LC, Wagner HN Jr. Measurement of aortic and mitral regurgitation by gated cardiac blood pool scans. Circulation 1979; 60: 306–312.
2. Baxter RH, Becker LC, Alderson PO, et al. Quantitation of aortic valvular regurgitation in dogs by nuclear imaging. Circulation 1980; 61: 404–410.
3. Manyari DE, Nolewajka AJ, Kostuk WJ. Quantitative assessment of aortic valvular insufficiency by radionuclide angiography. Chest 1982; 81: 170–176.
4. Taylor DN, Harris DN, Condon B, et al. Radionuclide evaluation of valvular regurgitation. Br J Radiol 1982; 55: 204–207.
5. Rigo P, Chevigne M. Quantitation of valvular regurgitation using radioisotopes. Eur Heart J 1987; 8 (Suppl. C): 63–69.
6. Parker JA, Uren RF, Jones AG, et al. Radionuclide left ventriculography with the slant hole collimator. J Nucl Med 1977; 18: 848–851.
7. Gandsman EJ, North DL, Shulman RS, Bough EW. Measurement of the ventricular stroke volume ratio by gated radionuclide angiography. Radiology 1981; 138: 161–165.
8. Alderson PO. Radionuclide quantification of valvular regurgitation. J Nucl Med 1982; 23: 851–855.
9. Atkins HL, Thomas SR, Buddemeyer U, Chervu LR. MIRD dose estimate report No. 14: radiation absorbed dose from technetium-99m-labeled red blood cells. J Nucl Med 1990; 31: 378–380.

Stress Testing (Myocardial Perfusion Studies)

Note: All stress tests should be performed only if a cardiologist is in the immediate area and available to monitor any problem that may arise during or following the stress procedure.

Indications

In many patients with coronary artery disease, clinical symptoms may become evident only when the heart is stressed. Exercise and pharmacologic stress are used in conjunction with myocardial perfusion agents such as ^{201}Tl thallous chloride or ^{99m}Tc sestamibi to demonstrate abnormalities in regional myocardial blood flow.

Principle

The heart is an aerobic organ with oxygen demands that are higher than any other organ in the body (the oxygen requirements of the left ventricle are about 20 times those of any other organ in the body per gram of tissue). The most important determinant of myocardial oxygen demand is heart rate. Because oxygen extraction from the coronary circulation is almost maximal at rest, the only way for the heart to meet an increased energy demand is to increase coronary blood flow. Patients with coronary artery disease have limited capacity to increase their coronary blood flow. By increasing heart rate through exercise or by increasing blood flow through pharmacologic methods and by injecting a radiotracer such as ^{201}Tl or ^{99m}Tc sestamibi, one can demonstrate limitations in coronary blood flow as a decrease in the uptake of the radiotracer in the diseased regions of the myocardium.

Stress Testing Methods

Currently, four different methods of stress testing are used: exercise, adenosine, dipyridamole, and dobutamine. The relative contraindications, patient preparation, stress test procedure, and potential side effects of each method follow. The choice of the method appropriate for a given patient is determined by the cardiologist. Exercise testing is the method of choice in most patients; however, some patients are unable or unwilling to exercise effectively, or their performance may be affected by antianginal drugs. In such cases, the use of pharmacologic agents to stress the heart may be the most appropriate choice.

Crash Cart

A crash cart must be available and in proximity to the patient during stress testing. A recommended list of the contents for a crash cart is given in Appendix A-7.

Electrocardiogram Preparation

Before commencing the stress test, position the electrodes for ECG recording. Twelve electrodes should be positioned on the body, as shown in Figure 4-11 (these permit a full-stress ECG to be recorded with the stress test). Before the electrodes are placed, prepare the skin as follows:[1]

1. The patient should be supine.
2. Shave any superficial hair over the area of electrode placement.
3. With an alcohol-saturated gauze pad, clean the area to remove any oils.
4. Lightly abrade the skin with 200-grit emery paper.
5. Place the 12 electrodes using the diagram in Figure 4-11 as a guide.
6. Attach the leads, and check that all the connections are secure and that good-quality ECG tracings are obtained at rest.

Exercise Stress Test

Introduction

Exercise testing is preferred to pharmacologic stress testing for several reasons. It provides information about the patient's overall cardiovascular fitness, which can be helpful in patient management, and it has none of the unpleasant side effects associated with many of the pharmacologic agents. Several large surveys have shown exercise testing to be a safe procedure, with complication rates of less than 10 per 10,000 tests.[1-3]

Contraindications

Potential contraindications to exercise testing are listed in Table 4-8.

Pretest Preparation

1. The patient should not eat or smoke for at least 2–3 hours before the test.
2. Attach the ECG electrodes and leads as described.

Table 4-8. Potential Contraindications to Exercise Testing

Acute myocardial infarction
Recent change in resting ECG
Unstable angina
Serious cardiac dysrhythmias
Acute pericarditis/myocarditis
Endocarditis
Severe aortic stenosis
Acute aortic dissection
Acute pulmonary embolus or pulmonary infarction
Any acute or serious noncardiac disorder
Severe physical handicap

3. Place a blood pressure cuff on the patient's arm.
4. Place a 20-gauge IV catheter/needle set in an antecubital vein and attach a 50–70-inch-long solution set and a 250-ml saline bag to the angiographic catheter. The extension set should be preloaded with saline. Figure 4-19 shows the arrangement of IV catheter/needle set, extension set, and saline bag in a patient being prepared for a treadmill test.
5. To reduce the likelihood of leakage or separation of tubing from the catheter set during exercise, check that all the connections are secure.

Instrumentation

A programmable treadmill and ECG monitor are used.

Stress Test Procedure

1. The stress test procedure should be explained fully to the patient before exercise.
2. Demonstrate to the patient the proper procedure for getting on and off the treadmill as well as walking on it.
3. The patient may hold the handrail for the first minute of exercise but should only use finger touch thereafter to maintain balance, because tight gripping of the handrail can increase ECG muscle artifact.[1]
4. Many different exercise regimens are available; the four most commonly used ones are the Bruce, Naughton, modified Bruce, and Cornell regimens. The cardiologist determines the regimen appropriate for the patient. The details of each exercise regimen are listed in Table 4-9.
5. The patients should then begin to exercise.
6. For ^{201}Tl: Approximately 60 seconds before peak exercise, the ^{201}Tl should be injected into the side port on the solution set (Fig. 4-20). The solution set should then be flushed with saline to ensure that all the radiopharmaceutical has been injected.
7. For ^{99m}Tc sestamibi: The injection should be given approximately 90 seconds before peak exercise.
8. It is important that the patient continue to exercise for up to 60 seconds after a ^{201}Tl injection or for 90 seconds after a ^{99m}Tc sestamibi injection, while coronary blood flow is still at peak level.
9. In some patients, the stress test may be terminated before peak exercise is achieved. In such cases, the radiopharmaceutical should be injected when it becomes apparent that the patient

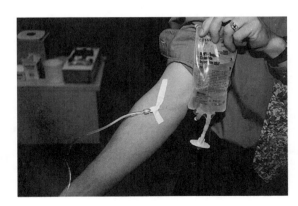

Figure 4-19. Arrangement of IV catheter/needle set, solution set, and saline bag for exercise study.

Table 4-9. Details of the Four Most Commonly Used Exercise Protocols (Treadmill)

Protocol	Stage	Speed (MPH)	Grade (%)	Duration	METs
Bruce	R&R	1.2	0.00	0:00	1.9
	1	1.7	10.00	3:00	4.6
	2	2.5	12.00	3:00	7.0
	3	3.4	14.00	3:00	10.1
	4	4.2	16.00	3:00	12.9
	5	5	18.00	3:00	15.0
	6	5.5	20.00	3:00	16.9
	7	6.0	22.00	3:00	19.1
Naughton	R&R	1.0	0	—	1.8
	1	1.0	0	2:00	1.8
	2	2.0	0	2:00	2.5
	3	2.0	3.5	2:00	3.4
	4	2.0	7	2:00	4.4
	5	2.0	10.5	2:00	5.3
	6	2.0	14	2:00	6.3
	7	2.0	17.5	2:00	7.3
Cornell	R&R	1.7	0	—	2.3
	1	1.7	0	2:00	2.3
	2	1.7	5	2:00	3.5
	3	1.7	10	2:00	4.6
	4	2.1	11	2:00	5.8
	5	2.5	12	2:00	7.0
	6	3.0	13	2:00	8.6
	7	3.4	14	2:00	10.1
	8	3.8	15	2:00	11.6
	9	4.2	16	2:00	12.9
	10	4.6	17	2:00	14.0
	11	5.0	18	2:00	15.0
Modified Bruce	R&R	1.2	0	—	1.9
	1	1.7	0	3:00	2.3
	2	1.7	5	3:00	3.5
	3	1.7	10	3:00	4.6
	4	2.5	12	3:00	7.0
	5	3.4	14	3:00	10.1
	6	4.2	16	3:00	12.9
	7	5.0	18	3:00	15.0
	8	5.5	20	3:00	16.9
	9	6.0	22	3:00	19.1

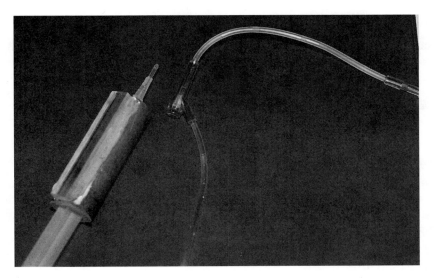

Figure 4-20. Shielded syringe with radiopharmaceutical and injection side port on solution set.

     cannot continue. Whenever possible, the patient should try to continue to exercise for another 30 seconds to 1 minute after injection.

10. Absolute indications for the termination of the exercise test are given in Table 4-10.

11. After exercise, the patient should be seated for about 6 minutes. The ECG recordings should be continued during this time.

12. If the patient's condition is stable, the catheter set and tubing should be removed and discarded in the radioactive waste bin. The ECG monitor may be disconnected from the patient and the electrodes removed. For ^{201}Tl studies, the patient should be brought immediately to the gamma camera. For ^{99m}Tc sestamibi studies, the patient may remain seated until it is time for the imaging study (about 30 minutes).

Table 4-10. Absolute Indications for Termination of Stress Test

Acute myocardial infarction or suspicion thereof
Onset of severe angina
Decrease in systolic blood pressure with increasing workload accompanied by signs or symptoms
Serious dysrhythmias
Signs of poor perfusion, including pallor, cyanosis, or cold and clammy skin
Central nervous system symptoms, including ataxia, vertigo, visual or gait problems, and confusion
Technical problems with monitoring ECG or blood pressure
ST depression greater than 2 mm without factors that would cause false-positives

Side Effects

Most exercise-related side effects cease with the termination of exercise. The cardiologist should continue to monitor the patient after exercise for any problems. Note that in many patients, abnormal ECG changes are recorded for up to 4–5 minutes after exercise. Hence, patients should be monitored carefully during this period.

Adenosine Stress Test

Introduction

Adenosine is a powerful coronary vasodilator. It is a naturally occurring nucleotide with an extremely short biologic half-life of the order of seconds.[4,5] After IV infusion of this agent, coronary blood flow increases considerably (up to 4 times that at rest) and often exceeds that achieved with maximal exercise.[6]

Contraindications

Contraindications to the use of adenosine are severe asthma, chronic obstructive pulmonary disease, unstable angina, sick sinus syndrome, 2nd- or 3rd-degree atrioventricular block, oral dipyridamole use, or hypotension (systolic pressure less than 80 mm Hg).[7]

Pretest Preparation

1. Patients should fast for at least 4 hours before adenosine testing, because potential side effects include nausea and vomiting.
2. Ingestion of all foods and beverages containing caffeine must be stopped for at least 12 hours before the study.[8] Patients taking long-acting aminophylline should discontinue its use 48–72 hours before the study. *Note:* Patients taking pentoxifylline (Trental) need not discontinue this medication.[9]
3. If the patient has chronic obstructive pulmonary disease, a pulmonary function test is required before adenosine is administered (see "Additional Notes," following).
4. Attach the ECG electrodes and leads as described.
5. Place a blood pressure cuff on the patient's arm.
6. Draw a vial (30 ml) of adenosine into a 60-ml syringe (concentration, 3 mg/ml). If the patient's weight is greater than 80 kg, draw two vials (60 ml).
7. Connect the 60-ml syringe to an infusion pump administration set. Prime the administration set with saline, and install it in the infusion pump, as shown in Figure 4-21.
8. Attach a 50–70 inch solution set to a 250-ml saline bag. The other end of the solution set should be attached to a 3-way stopcock. The distal port on the stopcock should be attached to a T-piece extension set. The middle port on the stopcock is attached to the infusion pump administration set (Fig. 4-22).
9. Place a 20-gauge IV catheter/needle set into an antecubital vein, and attach the distal end of the T-piece to the catheter set. Figure 4-22 shows the arrangement of catheter, T-piece, stopcock, and infusion sets.
10. Calculate the appropriate pump settings in milliliters per hour for the patient's weight that corresponds to infusion rates of 50, 75, 100, and 140 μg/kg per minute.

Stress Test Procedure

1. Two infusion sequences can be used for adenosine:

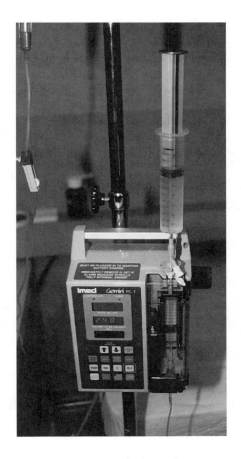

Figure 4-21. Arrangement of infusion pump, administration set, and syringe for adenosine infusion.

Standard Infusion Procedure—Adenosine is infused at a rate of 140 µg/kg per minute for 6 minutes. After 3 minutes, the radiopharmaceutical should be injected slowly over a 15–20 second period through the injection port on the T-piece set.

Graded Infusion Procedure—In high-risk patients, a graded infusion procedure may be used. The adenosine infusion should be started at 50 µg/kg per minute for the first minute, followed by stepped increases to 75, 100, and 140 µg/kg per minute for each consecutive minute. After 4 minutes of infusion, inject the radiopharmaceutical as described. Continue adenosine infusion at 140 µg/kg per minute for another 3 minutes.

Figure 4-22. Arrangement of 20-gauge IV catheter/needle set, T-piece, stopcock, and infusion sets for adenosine administration.

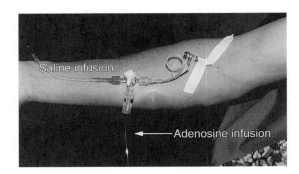

2. The patient's ECG should be monitored during the adenosine infusion, and blood pressure should be measured every minute.
3. If severe side effects occur, the cardiologist may request that the infusion be stopped or the infusion rate be reduced. Aminophylline should be available in all cases and may be required to reverse the side effects in some patients.
4. If possible, adenosine infusion should be continued for at least 1 minute after injection of the radiopharmaceutical.
5. After cessation of adenosine infusion, the patient's condition should be monitored for 5 minutes.
6. If no side effects persist, monitoring may be stopped, and the ECG leads and electrodes removed.
7. Remove the catheter set and tubing, and discard them in the radioactive waste bin. For ^{201}Tl studies, the patient should be brought immediately to the gamma camera. For ^{99m}Tc sestamibi studies, the patient may remain seated until it is time for the imaging study (about 30 minutes).

Additional Notes

Patients with chronic obstructive pulmonary disease may experience breathing difficulties with adenosine, particularly those with reversible airways disease (asthma). The following criteria are used in our laboratory to determine patient suitability for adenosine infusion. These criteria are determined from measurement of forced expired volume in the first second (FEV_1).

> FEV_1 = 30–39% of predicted for age, height, and weight AND bronchodilator response less than 15%.
> FEV_1 = 40–100% of predicted for age, height, and weight AND bronchodilator response less than 30%.
> Methocholine challenge test less than 30% decrease in resting FEV_1.

Table 4-11. Incidence of Adenosine-Induced Side Effects Reported in 5,500 Patients

Side Effect	Incidence, %
Mild hypotension and tachycardia	Usual
Flushing/warmth	35–40
Chest pain	35–40
Dyspnea	35
Nausea/abdominal pain	15–20
Dizziness or headache	15
Throat/neck/jaw discomfort	10–15
Ischemia (ST change)	<10
1st- or 2nd-degree atrioventricular block	<5
Arrhythmias	<5

(Adapted from Blust et al.,[10] with permission.)

If a patient does not meet these criteria, dobutamine should be considered as an alternative. If the patient has not undergone pulmonary function testing before arriving in the nuclear medicine department, the measurement of FEV_1 can be performed with a pulmonary function kit.

Side Effects

The side effects of adenosine and their relative incidence are listed in Table 4-11. About 50–60% of patients experience some side effects. Flushing and chest pain are the most frequent, occurring in about 40% of patients.[10] Severe complications (such as severe bronchospasm, ischemia, induced hypotension, or conduction abnormalities) generally abate promptly with the termination of the adenosine infusion.[11]

Dipyridamole Stress Test

Introduction

Dipyridamole is a pyrimidopyrimidine compound that has both antithrombotic and vasodilating properties.[12] Dipyridamole acts by inhibiting the reuptake of adenosine by myocardial cells, thereby increasing the local myocardial levels of this nucleotide, which has strong coronary vasodilatory properties (see preceding section). Because dipyridamole acts indirectly via adenosine, the peak effect of an IV infusion of dipyridamole on coronary blood flow is not seen for 7–8 minutes after the start of the infusion.[13] The effects produced by dipyridamole last for 30–60 minutes and are prolonged in hepatic failure.[12]

Contraindications

Contraindications to the use of dipyridamole are severe asthma, chronic obstructive pulmonary disease, unstable angina, sick sinus syndrome, 2nd- or 3rd-degree atrioventricular block, hypotension (systolic pressure less than 80 mm Hg), allergy to dipyridamole or aminophylline, or current use of aminophylline.[7,14]

Pretest Preparation

1. The patient should fast for at least 4 hours before the dipyridamole test, because potential side effects include nausea and vomiting.
2. Ingestion of all foods and beverages containing caffeine must be stopped for at least 12 hours before the study.[8] Patients taking long-acting aminophylline should discontinue its use 48–72 hours before the study. *Note:* Patients taking pentoxifylline (Trental) need not discontinue this medication.[9]
3. Attach the ECG electrodes and leads as described.
4. Place a blood pressure cuff on the patient's arm.
5. Dipyridamole is administered at a dose of 0.56 mg/kg body weight to a maximum dose of 60 mg. Based on the patient's weight, calculate the dose of dipyridamole (in milligrams) to be administered.
6. Dipyridamole generally is supplied in 10-ml vials at a concentration of 5 mg/ml.
7. Draw the required dose of dipyridamole into a 60-ml syringe and dilute up to 50 ml with saline.

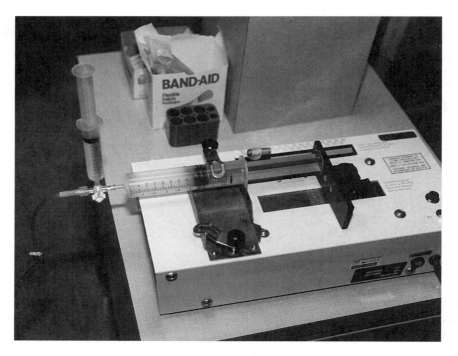

Figure 4-23. Arrangement of Harvard pump, 60-ml syringe, stopcock, 12-ml syringe, and extension set for dipyridamole infusion.

8. Install the 60-ml syringe in a Harvard infusion pump, and check that the pump is set to infuse at a rate of 10 ml/min.
9. Attach a 3-way stopcock to the 60-ml syringe. Attach a 12-ml syringe filled with saline and a 40-inch extension set with a syringe cannula to the other ports on the stopcock, as shown in Figure 4-23. Prime the extension set with the dipyridamole solution.
10. Attach a 50–70-inch solution set to a 250-ml saline bag. Place a 20-gauge IV catheter/needle set into an antecubital vein, and attach the other end of the 50–70-inch solution set to the catheter.

Stress Test Procedure

1. Insert the syringe cannula into the side port on the 50–70-inch solution set (Fig. 4-24), and turn on the Harvard infusion pump.

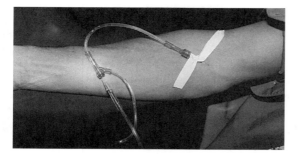

Figure 4-24. Intravenous catheter/needle set with 70-inch extension set to saline bag and side port connection to dipyridamole infusion pump.

2. Dipyridamole should be infused for 4–5 minutes. When the dipyridamole syringe is empty, turn the stopcock and flush the tubing with the 12-ml saline syringe.

3. The patient's ECG should be monitored during the dipyridamole infusion, and the blood pressure should be measured every minute.

4. After completion of dipyridamole infusion, remove the syringe cannula and extension set from the solution set.

5. Four minutes later, inject the radiopharmaceutical through the side port on the solution set. Flush the solution set with saline to ensure that all the radiopharmaceutical has been injected.

6. If severe side effects occur, the cardiologist may administer aminophylline to reverse the effects of the dipyridamole. If possible, aminophylline should not be given until 3 minutes after the radiopharmaceutical has been injected.

7. If aminophylline is required, it should be administered slowly through the side port of the solution set at a dose of 75–100 mg. If symptoms persist, the dose may be increased as high as 300 mg.

8. After cessation of dipyridamole infusion, the patient's condition should be monitored for 5 minutes.

9. If no side effects persist, monitoring may be stopped and the ECG leads and electrodes removed.

10. a. For ^{201}Tl studies, the patient should be brought immediately to the gamma camera. The IV catheter/needle and extension sets should be left in place until after the single photon emission computed tomography (SPECT) acquisition in case of delayed side effects.

    b. For ^{99m}Tc studies, the IV catheter/needle and extension sets should be left in place until imaging commences (about 30 minutes).

11. After removal, the catheter and extension sets should be discarded in the radioactive waste bin.

Note: In patients with severe side effects, monitoring should be continued for 3–5 minutes after administration of aminophylline. This is necessary because aminophylline has a shorter biologic half-life than dipyridamole and the side effects of dipyridamole may recur as the counteracting effects of aminophylline diminish.

Side Effects

The side effects of IV dipyridamole and their relative incidence are listed in Table 4-12.[15] About 25% of the patients experience some side effects. If severe complications occur (such as severe bronchospasm, ischemia, induced hypotension, or conduction abnormalities), administer aminophylline as described. This indirectly blocks the action of dipyridamole by blocking the action of adenosine.

Table 4-12. Incidence of Dipyridamole-Induced Side Effects Observed in 4,000 Patients

Side Effect	Incidence (%)
Chest pain/angina pectoris	20–25
Dizziness or headache	10–15
ECG abnormalities	5–10
Flushing or warmth	<5
Nausea or abdominal pain	<5
Shortness of breath/wheezing	<5

Dobutamine Stress Test

Introduction

Dobutamine is a synthetic sympathetic amine that is widely used in stress echocardiography. It causes an increase in the rate pressure product, stroke volume, and cardiac output, with a resultant increase in myocardial oxygen consumption.[16] The resulting increase in coronary blood flow is approximately twice the level at rest.[17] Dobutamine has a biologic half-life in plasma of about 2 minutes.[16] Dobutamine should be used in patients who have bronchospastic disease in whom dipyridamole or adenosine is contraindicated. Other potential candidates for dobutamine are patients who take oral dipyridamole or who have ingested caffeine or xanthine in the preceding 12 hours.

Contraindications

Contraindications to dobutamine are current use of beta-blockers, hypertrophic cardiomyopathy, uncontrolled hypertension (blood pressure greater than 200/110 mm Hg), and ventricular arrhythmias.[18,19]

Pretest Preparation

1. Patients should fast for at least 3 hours before the dobutamine is administered, because potential side effects include nausea and vomiting.
2. Attach the ECG electrodes and leads as described.
3. Place a blood pressure cuff on the patient's arm.
4. Place the contents of a vial (20 ml) of dobutamine into a 250-ml saline bag (final concentration about 1 mg/ml).
5. Connect the saline bag to an infusion pump administration set. Prime the administration set with saline, and install it in the infusion pump, as shown in Figure 4-15.
6. Attach a 50–70 inch solution set to a 250-ml saline bag. The other end of the solution set should be attached to a 3-way stopcock. The distal port on the stopcock should be attached to a T-piece extension set. The middle port on the stopcock is attached to the infusion pump administration set.
7. Place a 20-gauge IV catheter/needle set into an antecubital vein, and attach the distal end of the T-piece set to the catheter. Figure 4-16 shows the arrangement of the catheter, T-piece, stopcock, and infusion sets.
9. Calculate the appropriate pump settings in milliliters per hour for the patient's weight that correspond to infusion rates of 10, 20, 30, and 40 µg/kg per minute.

Stress Test Procedure

1. Dobutamine is administered in a graded dose. Start the infusion at a rate of 10 µg/kg per minute for 3 minutes, followed by stepped increases to 20, 30, and 40 µg/kg per minute for each consecutive 3-minute interval.

   Note 1: The infusion rate may be increased to a maximum of 50 µg/kg per minute if an adequate increase in heart rate fails to develop.
   Note 2: In patients whose condition is unstable, the dose increment may be reduced to 5 µg/kg per minute.

2. The patient's heart rate and ECG should be monitored during the dobutamine infusion, and the blood pressure should be measured every minute.

3. When a satisfactory increase in heart rate has been achieved, inject the radiopharmaceutical through the side port on the T-piece set. Dobutamine infusion should be continued for another 2 minutes. *Note:* Dosage end points are as follows:

   a. 85% of predicted maximum value for age
   b. 70% of predicted maximum value for age in postmyocardial infarction patients
   c. Marked hypertensive/hypotensive response
   d. Ischemic symptoms

4. DO NOT inject the radiopharmaceutical if the heart rate does not increase by 15 beats per minute over the baseline heart rate.

5. If severe side effects occur, the cardiologist may request that the infusion be stopped. If necessary, esmolol (a rapidly acting beta-blocker) can be used to neutralize the side effects of dobutamine.

6. After cessation of dobutamine infusion, the patient's condition should be monitored for 5 minutes.

7. If no side effects persist, monitoring may be stopped and the ECG leads and electrodes removed.

8. Remove the catheter set and tubing, and discard them in the radioactive waste bin. For ^{201}Tl studies, the patient should be brought immediately to the gamma camera. For ^{99m}Tc sestamibi studies, the patient may remain seated until it is time for the imaging study (about 30 minutes).

Side Effects

About 75% of patients experience some side effects. Palpitations and chest pain occur in about 30% of them. Other side effects (arrhythmias, nausea, headache, tremor, ECG changes) occur in less than 5% of patients.[19] Most of these effects are transient. Occasionally, esmolol may be administered to neutralize the side effects of dobutamine.

References

1. Exercise standards. A statement for health professionals from the American Heart Association. Circulation 1990; 82: 2286–2322.

2. Rochmis P, Blackburn H. Exercise tests. A survey of procedures, safety, and litigation experience in approximately 170,000 tests. JAMA 1971; 217: 1061–1066.

3. Gibbons L, Blair SN, Kohl HW, Cooper K. The safety of maximal exercise testing. Circulation 1989; 80: 846–852.

4. Berne RM. Cardiac nucleotides in hypoxia: possible role in regulation of coronary blood flow. Am J Physiol 1963; 204: 317–322.

5. Belardinelli L, Linden J, Berne RM. The cardiac effects of adenosine. Prog Cardiovasc Dis 1989; 32: 73–97.

6. Froelicher VF, Myers J, Follanbee WP, Labovitz AJ. Stress radionuclide myocardial perfusion imaging. In "Exercise and the Heart." Mosby Year Book, St. Louis, 1993, pp 252–293.

7. Verani MS. Pharmacological stress with adenosine for myocardial perfusion imaging. Semin Nucl Med 1991; 21: 266–272.

8. Jacobson AF, Cerqueira MD, Raisys V, Shattuc S. Serum caffeine levels following twenty-four hour abstention from caffeine prior to myocardial perfusion imaging with dipyridamole or adenosine (abstract). J Nucl Med 1992; 33: 866.

9. Brown KA, Slinker BK. Pentoxifylline (Trental) does not inhibit dipyridamole-induced coronary hyperemia: implications for dipyridamole-thallium-201 myocardial imaging. J Nucl Med 1990; 31: 1020–1024.
10. Blust JS, Boyce TM, Moore WH. Pharmacologic cardiac intervention: comparison of adenosine, dipyridamole, and dobutamine. J Nucl Med Tech 1992; 20: 53–59.
11. Iskandrian AS. Single-photon emission computed tomographic thallium imaging with adenosine, dipyridamole, and exercise. Am Heart J 1991; 122: 279–284.
12. Botvinick EH, Dae MW. Dipyridamole perfusion scintigraphy. Semin Nucl Med 1991; 21: 242–265.
13. Nielsen-Kudsk F, Pedersen AK. Pharmacokinetics of dipyridamole. Acta Pharmacol Toxicol 1979; 44: 391–399.
14. Gibbons RJ. Nuclear cardiology. In "Cardiology: Fundamentals and Practice," vol. 1, 2nd Edition, eds Giuliani ER, Fuster V, Gersh BJ, McGoon MD, McGoon DC. Mosby Year Book, St. Louis, 1991, pp 459–491.
15. Package insert. IV Persantine. The Du Pont Merck Pharmaceutical Co., Billerica, MA. Revised July 1993.
16. Verani MS. Dobutamine myocardial perfusion imaging. J Nucl Med 1994; 35: 737–739.
17. Krivokapich J, Huang SC, Schelbert HR. Assessment of the effects of dobutamine on myocardial blood flow and oxidative metabolism in normal human subjects using nitrogen-13 ammonia and carbon-11 acetate. Am J Cardiol 1993; 71: 1351–1356.
18. Package insert. Dobutrex solution (dobutamine hydrochloride injection). Eli Lilli & Co., Indianapolis, IN. Revised Dec. 22, 1992.
19. Hays JT, Mahmarian JJ, Cochran AJ, Verani MS. Dobutamine thallium-201 tomography for evaluating patients with suspected coronary artery disease unable to undergo exercise or vasodilator pharmacologic stress testing. J Am Coll Cardiol 1993; 21: 1583–1590.

^{201}Tl Myocardial Perfusion Study

Summary Information

Radiopharmaceutical

Adult dose: Stress study—3 mCi (111 MBq) thallous chloride ^{201}Tl administered intravenously during stress test.

1 mCi (37 MBq) ^{201}Tl administered intravenously before the delayed study.

Rest study—4 mCi (148 MBq) ^{201}Tl administered intravenously before the rest study.

Pediatric dose: See pediatric dose chart in Appendix A-3.

Contraindications

Rest ^{201}Tl study: None.

Stress ^{201}Tl study: See previous section entitled "Stress Test Procedure" for appropriate contraindications for exercise and pharmacologic stress. It is recommended that whenever possible, ^{99m}Tc sestamibi be used in place of ^{201}Tl for patients who exceed the weight limits specified next (one exception to this recommendation is ^{201}Tl for the assessment of myocardial viability):

Men—weight limit = 100 kg
Women—weight limit = 80 kg

Dose/Scan Interval

Rest study: SPECT imaging can commence 5 minutes after the injection.

Stress study: Anterior view of the chest and heart should be acquired at 10 minutes after the injection. SPECT acquisition should begin within 15 minutes after the injection but should not be performed earlier than 10 minutes because of the possibility of myocardial creep after exercise.[1] *Note:* In patients who have achieved stage 3 or higher on the Bruce protocol (see Table 4-9), imaging should not start earlier than 15 minutes after the injection and the respiratory rate should be less than 20 respirations per minute at the start of imaging to reduce the likelihood of upward creep.

Views Obtained

Anterior planar view of the chest and heart, followed by a 180° SPECT study (45° right anterior oblique to 45° left posterior oblique).

Indications

Stress (exercise or pharmacologic) ^{201}Tl studies have a high sensitivity and specificity for the diagnosis of coronary artery disease.[2,3] They can also aid in the stratification of the severity of disease and in the assessment of prognosis.[4,5] Also, ^{201}Tl studies have been used to assess myocardial viability in patients with known coronary artery disease[6] and to evaluate patients after revascularization.[7] Resting ^{201}Tl studies have been used to detect the presence and extent of myocardial damage in the early (6–24 hours) period after acute myocardial infarction[8] and to determine myocardial viability in patients with coronary artery disease and severely depressed left ventricular function.[9]

Principle

Thallium is an analog of potassium and has a high rate of extraction by the myocardium over a wide range of metabolic and physiologic conditions. It is distributed in the myocardium in proportion to regional blood flow and myocardial cell viability.[10] During stress, myocardial thallium uptake peaks within 1 minute after injection.[11] Its uptake in the heart ranges from about 1% of the injected dose at rest[12] to about 4% with maximal exercise.[13] Regions of the heart that are infarcted or underperfused at the time of injection extract less ^{201}Tl than normal myocardium and appear as areas of decreased activity on the ^{201}Tl scans. After initial ^{201}Tl uptake by the myocardium, activity decreases with time as ^{201}Tl washes out of the myocardium into the blood pool. Simultaneously, there is wash-in of activity as the heart continues to extract some of the ^{201}Tl from the circulating blood.[14] The washout and wash-in of ^{201}Tl from normal and ischemic regions of the heart, respectively, are manifested by the reversibility of defects seen on ^{201}Tl scans and provide information on the viability of the abnormal myocardial tissue.[15]

Patient Preparation

Rest ^{201}Tl study:	None.
Stress ^{201}Tl study:	See previous section on preparation for stress test. For all studies, ensure that all metal objects in the region of the chest (metal buttons, coins, etc.) are removed before imaging commences.

Instrument Specifications

Gamma camera:	Single, dual-head (90° orientation) or triple-head SPECT system.
Collimator:	Low-energy all-purpose collimator.
Energy setting:	68–80 keV, 30% window.
	167 keV, 20% window.
Additional items:	An armrest should be attached to the end of the SPECT table (Fig. 4-25).
Computer system:	Acquisition requirements—static acquisition (256 × 256 matrix), tomographic acquisition (64 × 64 matrix, 30°–60° views).
	Processing requirements—tomographic reconstruction software, permitting oblique reorientation of transaxial data. Quantitative analysis requires additional software to generate short-axis circumferential profiles or bull's-eye images.

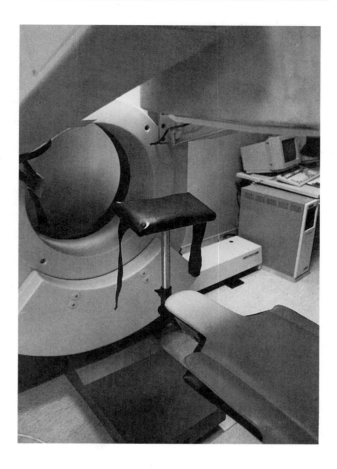

Figure 4-25. Armrest attached to end of SPECT table. Patient's arms are secured to it by means of Velcro straps.

Imaging Procedure

Stress Thallium Study

1. Before the patient arrives for the test, set up a static acquisition on the gamma camera/computer system with the following variables: 256×256 word mode matrix for 1,000 kct or 5 minutes (whichever comes first).
2. After completion of the stress test, position the patient supine on the imaging table. Rotate the gantry so that the detector is positioned anteriorly over the chest.
3. Acquire the anterior chest view.
4. After completion of the chest view, the patient's arms should be positioned above the head and strapped to the arm holder (Fig. 4-26).
5. Cushions or a pillow should be placed under the patient's feet, as shown in Figure 4-27, to make them more comfortable and to reduce the likelihood of patient motion.
6. Adjust the table height and gantry radius of rotation to minimize patient-to-collimator separation over the range 45° right anterior oblique to 45° left posterior oblique, and rotate the gantry to the 45° right anterior oblique position.
7. The following are the recommended acquisition variables for the tomographic study:

   Single-head system: 180° circular orbit, 30–32 views at 40 seconds per view, approximately every 6° for step and shoot or continuous step and shoot rotations; 60–64 views at 20 seconds per view, approximately every 3° for continuous rotations, 64×64 word mode matrix.

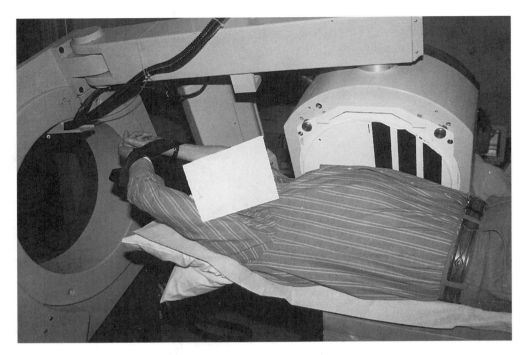

Figure 4-26. Patient setup for ^{201}Tl studies. Arms should be secured to armrest by means of the Velcro straps.

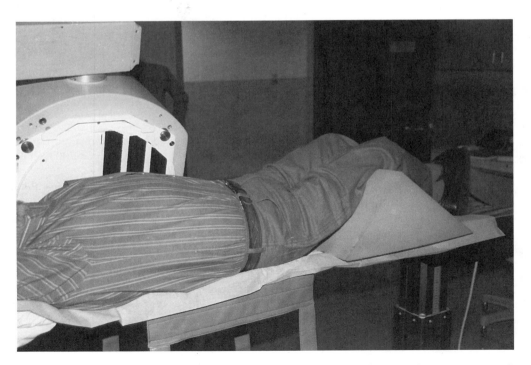

Figure 4-27. For SPECT studies, cushions may be placed under the feet to reduce pressure on the lower back and increase patient comfort.

Dual-head system: 90° circular orbit per detector, 15–16 views per detector at 40–60 seconds per view, approximately every 6° for step and shoot or continuous step and shoot rotations; 30–32 views at 20–30 seconds per view, approximately every 3° for continuous rotations; 64 × 64 word mode matrix.

Triple-head system: 120° circular orbit per detector, giving a total orbit of 360°; 20 views per detector at 30–40 sec/view, approximately every 6° for step and shoot or continuous step and shoot rotations; 40 views per detector at 10–15 seconds per view, approximately every 3° for continuous rotations; 64 × 64 word mode matrix. *Note:* If possible, reconstruct only 180° of the 360° data (45° right anterior oblique to 45° left posterior oblique).

Note: A circular orbit is preferred because a noncircular orbit may introduce artifacts.[16]

8. On completion of acquisition, replay the raw tomographic data, and check image quality (inspect data for patient motion and myocardial creep).
9. After completion of the stress study, instruct the patient to return 4 hours later. The patient may eat a light lunch with small amount of fluid intake; a heavy meal may alter the redistribution of ^{201}Tl in the body.[17] Patients should not exercise between the rest and stress images. *Note:* Patients with diabetes can continue their normal routine.
10. At 4 hours after injection, the patient should be reinjected with 1 mCi (37 MBq) [201]Tl. Steps 1–8 should be repeated, with the exception of the anterior chest view, which is not acquired on the redistribution study.

Rest Thallium Study

1. After the IV injection of 4 mCi (148 MBq) ^{201}Tl, the patient should be positioned supine on the imaging table (see Fig. 4-27) with the arms positioned above the head and strapped to the arm holder (see Fig. 4-26).
2. Acquire the rest ^{201}Tl study as per steps 5–8 above.

Computer Analysis

No analysis is required for the anterior chest image. For the tomographic images, perform uniformity and center-of-rotation corrections to the planar data. If possible, prefilter the planar data before back-projection. The optimum filter varies depending on how the filter algorithms have been implemented on the system. The most commonly used filter for ^{201}Tl studies is a Hann filter (sometimes called Hanning filter). For a standard 40-cm field-of-view system with a pixel size of 6–7 mm/pixel for a 64 × 64 matrix, the Nyquist frequency is approximately 0.75 cycles/cm. For this type of system, the cutoff value for the Hann filter should be in the range 0.4–0.6 cycles/cm (0.5–0.7 Nyquist or 0.25–0.35 cycles/pixel).

The prefiltered data should then be reconstructed using a simple Ramp filter and a zoom of 2. One-pixel-thick transaxial slices should be generated and oblique reformatting performed to generate conventional long- and short-axis slices of the heart. For stress studies, record the horizontal and vertical angular rotation of the heart so that both stress and rest studies can be reconstructed in a similar manner.

Additional Notes

1. With exercise studies, upward creep of the myocardium during SPECT acquisition appears to be associated with patients who have exercised to exhaustion. If the patient's breathing is

still labored at 15 minutes after exercise (greater than 20 respirations per minute), imaging should be delayed until their respiratory rate is at baseline.[15]

2. Patients with veins difficult for IV placement of catheters should be given 4 mCi (148 MBq) of ^{201}Tl during exercise. No reinjection of ^{201}Tl before the delayed imaging should be performed.

3. Some patients may be unable to raise their arms above their head. If possible, ask them to raise only their left arm, with the right arm by their side. If this is not possible, acquire the SPECT study from 90° right lateral to 90° left lateral. The patient's arms should then be by the side and positioned posteriorly so that they are out of the field of view.

4. Artifacts produced by attenuation of photons by the breasts or the diaphragm may cause apparent perfusion defects. Suspected artifacts caused by the breast may be detected by a careful review of the anterior chest view and the rotating planar images.

Information on Film

Obtain hard copies of the stress and rest images displayed side by side. Images should be displayed using the orientation shown in Figure 4-28.[18]

Interpretation

Regions of decreased perfusion or absence of perfusion on a resting study usually represent acute or old myocardial infarction. Areas of decreased perfusion or absence of

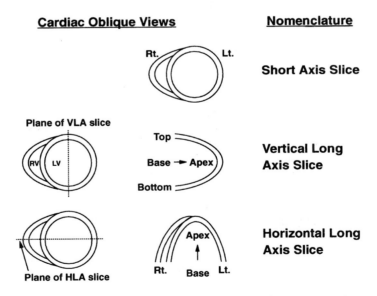

Figure 4-28. Correct orientation of short- and long-axis slices of the heart, for both display and hard copy purposes.

perfusion on the stress images, which partly or completely fill in on the redistribution images, may be due to transient ischemia. A constant deficit is usually due to myocardial infarction. The normal right ventricle is frequently visualized on the stress images.

Visualization of the right ventricle on resting images is a sign of right ventricular hypertrophy. An increase in the size of the septum relative to the posterolateral wall is seen in asymmetric septal hypertrophy. Uniform widening of all the walls and increased tracer uptake are characteristic of concentric left ventricular hypertrophy. Increased lung uptake is a manifestation of left ventricular dysfunction during exercise and generally indicates severe exercise-induced ischemia and/or resting left ventricular dysfunction.[19]

Exercise thallium scintigraphy has a high sensitivity (about 90%) and specificity (about 75%) in the detection of coronary artery disease.[20] Equally important is its ability to stratify disease severity and assess prognosis.[4,5] Figure 4-29 shows the ability of ^{201}Tl to predict the probability of a future cardiac event in patients without previous myocardial infarction.[21]

Radiation Dosimetry

The estimated absorbed doses in organs and tissues of an average subject (70 kg) from an IV injection of 4 mCi (148 MBq) ^{201}Tl are shown in Table 4-13.[12]

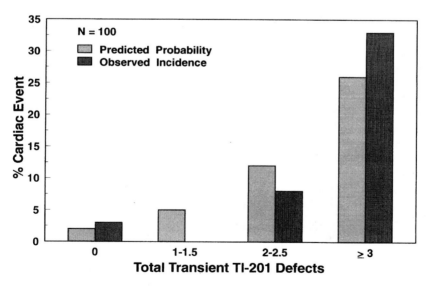

Figure 4-29. Probability of a future cardiac event and observed incidence of events as a function of the number of transient ^{201}Tl defects in 100 patients without prior myocardial infarction. (Adapted from Brown et al.,[21] with permission.)

Table 4-13. Absorbed Radiation Dose Estimates in a 70-kg Adult After Intravenous Administration of 4 mCi (148 MBq) ^{201}Tl Thallous Chloride

Tissue	Absorbed Radiation Dose	
	rad/4 mCi	mGy/148 MBq
Heart	2.67	26.7
Small bowel	2.0	20.0
Upper large intestine	1.33	13.3
Lower large intestine	1.07	10.7
Kidney	6.40	64.0
Liver	2.93	29.3
Stomach wall	2.27	22.7
Testes	2.67	26.7
Ovaries	2.53	25.3
Thyroid	3.47	34.7
Total body	1.07	10.7

References

1. Friedman J, Van Train K, Maddahi J, et al. "Upward creep" of the heart: a frequent source of false-positive reversible defects during thallium-201 stress-redistribution SPECT. J Nucl Med 1989; 30: 1718–1722.
2. Kotler TS, Diamond GA. Exercise thallium-201 scintigraphy in the diagnosis and prognosis of coronary artery disease. Ann Intern Med 1990; 113: 684–702.
3. Beller GA. Pharmacologic stress imaging. JAMA 1991; 265: 633–638.
4. Gibbons RJ. The use of radionuclide techniques for identification of severe coronary disease. Curr Probl Cardiol 1990; 15: 301–352.
5. Brown KA. Prognostic value of thallium-201 myocardial perfusion imaging. A diagnostic tool come of age. Circulation 1991; 83: 363–381.
6. Bonow RO, Dilsizian V, Cuocolo A, Bacharach SL. Identification of viable myocardium in patients with chronic coronary artery disease and left ventricular dysfunction. Comparison of thallium scintigraphy with reinjection and PET imaging with 18F-fluorodeoxyglucose. Circulation 1991; 83: 26–37.
7. DePuey EG. Radionuclide methods to evaluate percutaneous transluminal coronary angioplasty. Semin Nucl Med 1991; 21: 102–115.
8. Wackers FJ, Sokole EB, Samson G, et al. Value and limitations of thallium-201 scintigraphy in the acute phase of myocardial infarction. N Engl J Med 1976; 295: 1–5.
9. Ragosta M, Beller GA, Watson DD, Kaul S, Gimple LW. Quantitative planar rest-redistribution ^{201}Tl imaging in detection of myocardial viability and prediction of improvement in left ventricular function after coronary bypass surgery in patients with severely depressed left ventricular function. Circulation 1993; 87: 1630–1641.
10. Nielsen AP, Morris KG, Murdock R, Bruno FP, Cobb FR. Linear relationship between the distribution of thallium-201 and blood flow in ischemic and nonischemic myocardium during exercise. Circulation 1980; 61: 797–801.

11. Okada RD. Myocardial kinetics of thallium-201 after stress in normal and perfusion-reduced canine myocardium. Am J Cardiol 1985; 56: 969–973.

12. Atkins HL, Budinger TF, Lebowitz E, et al. Thallium-201 for medical use. Part 3: Human distribution and physical imaging properties. J Nucl Med 1977; 18: 133–140.

13. Krahwinkel W, Herzog H, Feinendegen LE. Pharmacokinetics of thallium-201 in normal individuals after routine myocardial scintigraphy. J Nucl Med 1988; 29: 1582–1586.

14. Grunwald AM, Watson DD, Holzgrefe HH Jr, Irving JF, Beller GA. Myocardial thallium-201 kinetics in normal and ischemic myocardium. Circulation 1981; 64: 610–618.

15. Bonow RO, Dilsizian V. Thallium-201 for assessment of myocardial viability. Semin Nucl Med 1991; 21: 230–241.

16. Maniawski PJ, Morgan HT, Wackers FJ. Orbit-related variation in spatial resolution as a source of artifactual defects in thallium-201 SPECT. J Nucl Med 1991; 32: 871–875.

17. Nelson CW, Wilson RA, Angello DA, Palac RT. Effect of thallium-201 blood levels on reversible myocardial defects. J Nucl Med 1989; 30: 1172–1175.

18. ACC/AHA/SNM policy statement. Standardization of cardiac tomographic imaging. J Nucl Med 1992; 33: 1434–1435.

19. Homma S, Kaul S, Boucher CA. Correlates of lung/heart ratio of thallium-201 in coronary artery disease. J Nucl Med 1987; 28: 1531–1535.

20. Froelicher VF, Myers J, Follansbee WP, Labowitz AJ. Stress radionuclide myocardial perfusion imaging. In "Exercise and the Heart." Mosby Year Book, St. Louis, 1993, pp 252–293.

21. Brown KA, Boucher CA, Okada RD, et al. Prognostic value of exercise thallium-201 imaging in patients presenting for evaluation of chest pain. J Am Coll Cardiol 1983; 1: 994–1001.

^{99m}Tc Sestamibi Myocardial Perfusion Study

Summary Information

Radiopharmaceutical

Adult dose: See Dose/Scan Interval.

Stress study—10–30 mCi (370–1,110 MBq) ^{99m}Tc sestamibi (methoxyisobutyl isonitrile) administered intravenously during the stress test.

Rest study—10–30 mCi (370–1,110 MBq) ^{99m}Tc sestamibi administered intravenously before the rest study.

Pediatric dose: Adjusted according to the patient's weight (see Appendix A-3).

Contraindications

Stress study: See previous section entitled "Stress Test Procedure" for appropriate contraindications for exercise and pharmacologic stress.

Rest study: None.

Dose/Scan Interval For stress studies, SPECT imaging should be performed 30–60 minutes after injection. For rest studies, SPECT imaging should be performed 30-60 minutes after injection, but it may be performed as long as 6 hours after injection. A wide range of possible imaging protocols exist for ^{99m}Tc sestamibi.[1] The 2-day protocol provides optimal image quality, but the 1-day protocol is more convenient for both patients and physicians.

Two-Day Imaging Protocol Day 1—Stress study in afternoon, with 30 mCi (1,110 MBq) of ^{99m}Tc sestamibi.

Day 2—Rest study in morning, with 30 mCi (1,110 MBq) of ^{99m}Tc sestamibi.

Note: The order of rest and stress can be reversed, or the stress study can be performed in the morning, if it is inconvenient to stress the patient in the afternoon.

Continues

Summary Information *(Continued)*

One-Day Imaging Protocol   Rest study in the morning, with 10 mCi (370 MBq) of ^{99m}Tc sestamibi.

Stress study in the afternoon, with 30 mCi (1,110 MBq) of ^{99m}Tc sestamibi.

Views Obtained   Obtain a 180° SPECT study from 45° right anterior oblique to 45° left posterior oblique.

Indications

Indications for myocardial perfusion imaging with ^{99m}Tc sestamibi are generally the same as those for ^{201}Tl, with two important exceptions. Because of minimal redistribution after injection in patients with severely decreased resting flow, ^{99m}Tc sestamibi has some limitations in the assessment of myocardial viability.[2,3]

However, this same feature permits ^{99m}Tc sestamibi to be used to assess myocardial salvage resulting from therapeutic intervention in acute infarction[4,5] and to assess myocardial blood flow during periods of spontaneous chest pain.[6]

Principle

^{99m}Tc sestamibi is a cation, like thallium; however, it has a lower fractional extraction than thallium (0.57 versus 0.80), particularly at high flow rates.[7] Nevertheless, its distribution in the myocardium is proportional to blood flow in a manner parallel to that observed with ^{201}Tl.[8] Uptake in the heart at rest is approximately 1.2% of the injected dose, increasing to 1.5% with maximal exercise.[9] Sestamibi has a high cell retention efficiency, and as a result, the washout of sestamibi is very slow (half-life greater than 6 hours), with minimal redistribution within the myocardium.[10] ^{99m}Tc sestamibi is cleared from the blood by the hepatobiliary system, resulting in high uptake in the liver and gallbladder. Radioactivity in the liver decreases rapidly, allowing imaging to commence 30–60 minutes after injection.

Patient Preparation

      Rest study: None.
     Stress study: See previous section on preparation for stress test.
Note: For all studies, ensure that all metal objects in the region of the chest (metal buttons, coins, etc.) are removed before imaging begins.

Instrument Specifications

    Gamma camera: Single, dual-head (90° orientation), or triple-head SPECT system.
        Collimator: Low-energy all-purpose or low-energy high-resolution collimator.
   Energy setting: 140 keV, 20% window.

Additional items: An armrest, such as that shown in Figure 4-25, should be attached to the end of the SPECT table.

                                 Lead shield (composed of two layers of flexible lead rubber, with a total lead equivalency of 1 mm Pb) attached to the collimator face with Velcro strips (Fig. 4-30).

Computer system: Acquisition requirements—tomographic acquisition (64×64 matrix, 30–60 views).

                                 Processing requirements—tomographic reconstruction software, permitting oblique reorientation of transaxial data. Quantitative analysis requires additional software to generate short-axis circumferential profiles or bull's-eye images.

Imaging Procedure

1. Before the patient is positioned on the table, attach the flexible lead shield (see Fig. 4-30) to the collimator face so that it covers the lower half of the field of view. This is designed to reduce interference from activity in the small bowel and gallbladder.

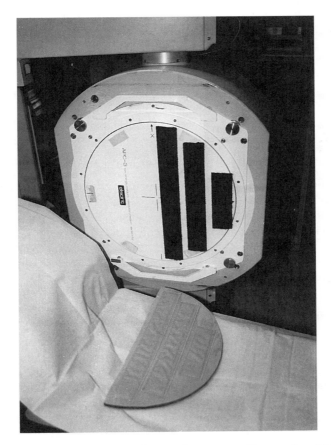

Figure 4-30. Lead shield with Velcro strips for attachment to collimator face. This shield is used to attenuate gallbladder and small bowel activity seen in ^{99m}Tc sestamibi studies.

2. After injection of the ^{99m}Tc sestamibi, the patient should be positioned supine on the imaging table. The patient's arms should be positioned above the head and strapped to the arm holder (see Fig. 4-26).

3. Cushions or a pillow should be placed under the patient's feet, as shown in Figure 4-27, to make the patient more comfortable and to reduce the likelihood of motion.

4. Rotate the gantry so that the detector is positioned anteriorly over the chest.

5. Move the table in or out of the gantry until the heart is positioned just above the lead shield, with most of the liver, small bowel, and gallbladder blocked from the field of view.

6. Adjust the table height and gantry radius of rotation to minimize patient-to-collimator separation over the range 45° right anterior oblique to 45° left posterior oblique, and rotate the gantry to the 45° right anterior oblique position.

7. The following are the recommended acquisition variables for the tomographic study with the use of a low-energy high-resolution collimator. If a low-energy all-purpose collimator is used, then the time per frame can be decreased by a factor of 2. The advantages of each collimator are low-energy high-resolution, higher resolution images and low-energy all-purpose, shorter acquisition time with decreased likelihood of patient motion.

   Single-head system: 180° circular orbit, 30–32 views at 40 seconds per view, approximately every 6° for step and shoot or continuous step and shoot rotations; 60–64 views at 20 seconds per view, approximately every 3° for continuous rotations; 64 × 64 word mode matrix.

   Dual-head system: 90° circular orbit per detector, 15–16 views per detector at 40–60 seconds per view, approximately every 6° for step and shoot or continuous step and shoot rotation; 30–32 views at 20–30 seconds per view, approximately every 3° for continuous rotations; 64 × 64 word mode matrix.

   Triple-head system: 120° circular orbit per detector, giving a total orbit of 360°; 20 views per detector at 30–40 seconds per view, approximately every 6° for step and shoot or continuous step and shoot rotations; 40 views per detector at 10–15 seconds per view, approximately every 3° for continuous rotations; 64 × 64 word mode matrix.

   Note: A circular orbit is preferred because a noncircular orbit may introduce artifacts.[11]

8. On completion of acquisition, replay the raw tomographic data and check image quality (inspect data for patient motion).

9. After completion of the study, instruct the patient when to return for the second study (depends on imaging protocol in use; see "Dose/Scan Interval").

10. For both the rest and stress studies, a first-pass left ventricular study may be performed while the patient is being injected with ^{99m}Tc sestamibi (see Procedure 4-10, "^{99m}Tc Sestamibi First-Pass Radionuclide Angiogram").

Computer Analysis

Perform uniformity and center-of-rotation corrections to the planar data. If possible, prefilter the planar data before back-projection. The optimal filter varies depending on how the filter algorithms have been implemented on the system. The most commonly used filters for ^{99m}Tc sestamibi studies are the Hann filter (sometimes called the Hanning filter) and the Butterworth filter. For a standard 40-cm field-of-view system with a pixel size of 6–7 mm/pixel for a 64 × 64 matrix, the Nyquist frequency is about 0.75 cycles/cm. For this type of system, the cutoff value for the Hann filter should be in the range of 0.4–0.6 cycles/cm (0.5–0.7 Nyquist or 0.25–0.35 cycles/pixel). For the Butterworth filter, the order should be in the range of 5 to 20, with cutoff values in the range of 0.2–0.4 cycles/cm.

The prefiltered data should then be reconstructed with a simple Ramp filter and a zoom of 2. One-pixel-thick transaxial slices should be generated and oblique reformatting performed to generate conventional long- and short-axis slices of the heart. Record the horizontal and vertical angular rotation of the heart used in generating the oblique slices, so that both stress and rest studies can be reconstructed in a similar manner.

Additional Analysis

In patients with myocardial infarction, the extent and severity of the infarct region can be determined with quantitative analysis of the short-axis slices. Briefly, this technique uses a fixed threshold value (60%) of counts in the short-axis circumferential profiles. From five representative slices (spanning the region from apex to base), the average radius of each slice is measured as well as the fraction of the counts in that slice that fall below the fixed threshold value. These 2 factors allow computation of the fraction of the myocardium that is underperfused. The ratio of minimum to maximum counts in the circumferential profile provides an index of the severity of the underperfused region.[4,12]

Additional Notes

1. Some patients may be unable to raise their arms above their head. If possible, ask them to raise only their left arm, with the right arm by their side. If this is not possible, acquire the SPECT study from 90° right lateral to 90° left lateral. The patient's arms should then be by the side and positioned posteriorly so that they are out of the field of view.
2. Artifacts produced by attenuation of photons by the breasts or the diaphragm may cause apparent perfusion defects. Suspected artifacts caused by the breast may be detected with a careful review of the anterior chest view and the rotating planar images.

Information on Film

Obtain hard copies of the stress and rest images displayed side by side. Images should be displayed using the orientation shown in Figure 4-28.[13]

Interpretation

Regions of decreased perfusion or absence of perfusion on a resting study usually represent acute or old myocardial infarction. Areas of decreased perfusion or absence of perfusion on the stress images, which are less severe on the rest images, may be due to transient ischemia. A constant deficit is usually due to myocardial infarction. The normal right ventricle is frequently visualized on the stress images. Visualization of the right ventricle on resting images is a sign of right ventricular hypertrophy. An increase in the size of the septum relative to the posterolateral wall is seen in asymmetric septal hypertrophy. Uniform widening of all the walls and increased tracer uptake are characteristic of concentric left ventricular hypertrophy. Although there is not the wealth of experience with ^{99m}Tc sestamibi as there is with ^{201}Tl, initial reviews have found little difference in the sensitivity and specificity of the two radiopharmaceuticals for the detection of coronary artery disease.[14]

Radiation Dosimetry

The estimated absorbed doses in organs and tissues of an average subject (70 kg) from an IV injection of 30 mCi (1,110 MBq) ^{99m}Tc sestamibi are shown in Table 4-14.[15]

Table 4-14. Absorbed Radiation Dose Estimates in a 70-kg Adult at Rest and During Stress After Intravenous Injection of 30 mCi (1,110 MBq) ^{99m}Tc Sestamibi[a]

Tissue	Absorbed Radiation Doses (Rest/Stress)	
	rad/30 mCi	mGy/1,110 MBq
Heart wall	0.5/0.5	5.1/5.1
Liver	0.6/0.4	5.8/4.2
Kidneys	2.0/1.7	20.0/16.7
Testes	0.3/0.3	3.4/3.1
Ovaries	1.5/1.2	15.5/12.2
Breasts	0.2/0.2	2.0/2.0
Thyroid	0.7/0.3	7.0/2.7
Stomach wall	0.6/0.5	6.1/5.3
Gallbladder wall	2.0/2.8	20.0/28.9
Small intestine	3.0/2.4	30.0/24.4
Upper large intestinal wall	5.6/4.5	55.5/44.4
Lower large intestinal wall	4.0/3.3	40.0/32.2
Urinary bladder wall	2.0/1.5	20.0/15.5
Total body	0.5/0.4	4.8/4.2

[a]Assumes a 2-hr voiding schedule.

References

1. Wackers FJ. The maze of myocardial perfusion imaging protocols in 1994. J Nucl Cardiol 1994; 1: 180–188.
2. Rocco TP, Dilsizian V, Strauss HW, Boucher CA. Technetium-99m isonitrile myocardial uptake at rest. II. Relation to clinical markers of potential viability. J Am Coll Cardiol 1989; 14: 1678–1684.
3. Cuocolo A, Pace L, Ricciardelli B, et al. Identification of viable myocardium in patients with chronic coronary artery disease: comparison of thallium-201 scintigraphy with reinjection and technetium-99m-methoxyisobutyl isonitrile. J Nucl Med 1992; 33: 505–511.
4. Gibbons RJ, Verani MS, Behrenbeck T, et al. Feasibility of tomographic ^{99m}Tc-hexakis-2-methoxy-2-methylpropyl-isonitrile imaging for the assessment of myocardial area at risk and the effect of treatment in acute myocardial infarction. Circulation 1989; 80: 1277–1286.
5. Christian TF, Schwartz RS, Gibbons RJ. Determinants of infarct size in reperfusion therapy for acute myocardial infarction. Circulation 1992; 86: 81–90.
6. Bilodeau L, Theroux P, Gregoire J, Gagnon D, Arsenault A. Technetium-99m sestamibi tomography in patients with spontaneous chest pain: correlations with clinical, electrocardiographic and angiographic findings. J Am Coll Cardiol 1991; 18: 1684–1691.
7. Marshall RC, Leidholdt EM Jr, Barnett CA. Single pass myocardial extraction and retention of a Tc-99m isonitrile vs. Tl-201 (abstract). Circulation 1987; 76 Suppl IV: IV-218.
8. Berman DS, Kiat H, Maddahi J. The new ^{99m}Tc myocardial perfusion imaging agents: ^{99m}Tc-sestamibi and ^{99m}Tc-teboroxime. Circulation 1991; 84 (Suppl. 3): 17–121.
9. Wackers FJ, Berman DS, Maddahi J, et al. Technetium-99m hexakis-2-methyoxyisobutyl isonitrile: human biodistribution, dosimetry, safety, and preliminary comparison to thallium-201 for myocardial perfusion imaging. J Nucl Med 1989; 30: 301–311.

10. Okada R, Glover D, Gaffney T, Williams S. Myocardial kinetics of technetium-99m-hexakis-2-methoxy-2-methylpropyl-isonitrile. Circulation 1988; 77: 491–498.

11. Maniawski PJ, Morgan HT, Wackers FT. Orbit-related variation in spatial resolution as a source of artifactual defects in thallium-201 SPECT. J Nucl Med 1991; 32: 871–875.

12. O'Connor MK, Hammel T, Gibbons RJ. In vitro validation of a simple tomographic technique for estimation of percentage myocardium at risk using methoxyisobutyl isonitrile technetium 99m (sestamibi). Eur J Nucl Med 1990; 17: 69–76.

13. ACC/AHA/SNM policy statement. Standardization of cardiac tomographic imaging. J Nucl Med 1992; 33: 1434–1435.

14. Sochor H. Technetium-99m sestamibi in chronic coronary disease: the European experience. Am J Cardiol 1990; 66: 91E–96E.

15. Package insert. Cardiolite. Kit for the preparation of technetium Tc-99m sestamibi. E.I. DuPont de Nemours Co., Sept. 1992.

99mTc Sestamibi First-Pass Radionuclide Angiogram

Summary Information

Radiopharmaceutical

    Adult dose: 30 mCi (1,110 MBq) ^{99m}Tc sestamibi.

    Pediatric dose: Minimal dose is 3 mCi (111 MBq), maximal dose is 20 mCi (740 MBq). Dose should be adjusted according to patient's weight (see Appendix A-3).

         Note: All injected doses should be in a volume of 0.2 ml or less.

Contraindications   A first-pass study is unlikely to be successful in a patient with tricuspid regurgitation or severe pulmonary hypertension.

Dose/Scan Interval   Computer acquisition should be started 1–2 seconds before the injection.

Views Obtained   Anterior view of the heart.

Indications

A first-pass flow study can be performed in conjunction with a rest or stress myocardial perfusion scan with ^{99m}Tc sestamibi. As with an equilibrium-gated RNA, it can be used for measurement of LVEF and to evaluate left ventricular regional wall motion. Its advantages over RNA include a short acquisition time and lower background activity. However, it has poorer resolution than RNA and is highly dependent on the delivery of a compact bolus to the left ventricle. Poor bolus injection or such clinical conditions as tricuspid regurgitation and severe pulmonary hypertension can invalidate the study.

Principle

A first-pass study evaluates the function of the heart during the short time (several seconds) that it takes the injected bolus to travel through the left ventricle. Because of the high activity and concentration of the injected bolus, extremely high count rates can be achieved (150–400 kcps). These count rates are required to provide statistically reliable data for calculation of LVEF. From data acquired over 4–7 cardiac cycles, an average LVEF is calculated by determining the minimal and maximal counts in the left ventricle during the passage of activity through the ventricle. Corrections are required for background activity and for abnormal beats. LVEFs calculated with this method have correlated well with those obtained with RNA[1] and contrast ventriculography.[2]

Patient Preparation

1. Draw 60 ml of saline into a 60-ml syringe, and attach it to a 40-inch extension set.
2. Place an 18-gauge IV catheter/needle set in an antecubital vein (preferably in the right arm), and attach the distal end of the extension set to the catheter. *Note:* Whenever possible, injections should be given via the right external jugular vein, because this technique produces a greater percentage of high-quality studies.[3]
3. Tape the catheter and the distal end of the extension set to the patient's arm. Check that all the connections are secure. See the arrangement shown in Figure 4-1.
4. Gently flush the extension set with 5–10 ml of saline to ensure good positioning of the catheter and flow through the injection site.
5. Acquisition on some gamma cameras requires an ECG trigger input. The ECG signal is recorded with the first-pass study as an aid in analysis of the cardiac cycles.

Before placement of the ECG electrodes, the skin should be prepared as follows:

1. Shave any superficial hair over the area of electrode placement.
2. With an alcohol-saturated gauze pad, clean the area to remove any oils.
3. Lightly abrade the skin with 200-grit emery paper.
4. Place three electrodes in the right and left midclavicular areas and below the heart, as shown in Figure 4-6.

Instrument Specifications

Multicrystal System

Gamma camera:	Scinticor SIM-400.
Collimator:	Medium-sensitivity collimator (18 mm).
Energy setting:	140 keV, 50% energy window.

Single-Crystal System

Gamma camera:	Large field-of-view system with high count rate capability (20% count loss greater than 150 kcps/maximal count rate greater than 400 kcps).
Collimator:	Low-energy high-sensitivity collimator (greater than 500 ct/min per μCi).
Energy setting:	140 keV, 20% energy window.
Additional items:	ECG gate may be required by some systems.
Computer system:	Acquisition requirements—dynamic acquisition with a 32 × 32 matrix and a frame rate of 30–40 frames per second (rest study) or 60–80 frames per second (stress study). Processing requirements—first-pass analysis software for left ventricle.

Imaging Procedure

Multicrystal System—Rest Study

1. The multicrystal system should be set to acquire 40 frames per second for 1,500 frames (37.5 seconds).

2. The patient should be standing upright with the chest against the collimator surface, as shown in Figure 4-31.
3. Inject a small 500 μCi (18.5 MBq) dose of ^{99m}Tc sestamibi into the side port of the extension set, and flush gently with 5–10 ml of saline. Check the position of the left ventricle on the persistence screen. Adjust the position of the patient and/or the detector so that the heart is located centrally in the field of view.
4. Before injection, ensure that the patient is comfortable and relaxed. Inject the ^{99m}Tc sestamibi into the side port closest to the catheter, as shown in Figure 4-1. (*Note:* Ensure that the needle of the injection syringe is positioned past the dead space at the top of the side port.) **Remove the empty syringe**.
5. Use the foot pedal to start acquisition on the computer. After 1–2 seconds, rapidly inject 60 ml of saline.
6. Ensure that the patient remains motionless until acquisition is complete and the system has performed dead-time correction.

Multicrystal System—Stress Study

1. The multicrystal system should be set to acquire 80 frames per second for 3,000 frames (37.5 seconds).
2. Position the patient upright with the chest against the collimator surface, as shown in Figure 4-32.
3. Inject a small 500 μCi (18.5 MBq) dose of ^{99m}Tc sestamibi into the side port of the extension set, and flush gently with 5–10 ml of saline. Check the position of the left ventricle on the persistence screen. Adjust the position of the patient and/or the detector so that the heart is located centrally in the field of view.

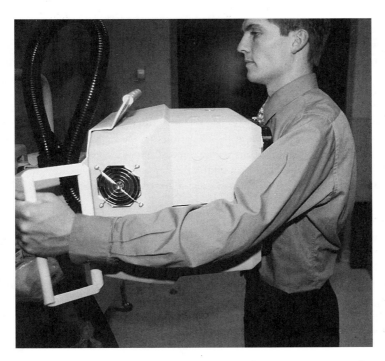

Figure 4-31. Patient in position for a resting first-pass study on a multicrystal system.

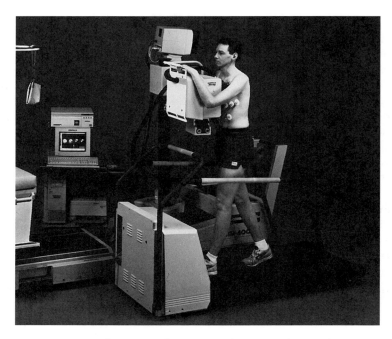

Figure 4-32. Patient in position for a stress first-pass study on a multicrystal system. (Courtesy of Scinticor, Inc.)

4. Place a small radioactive marker on the patient's chest medial to the right ventricle. The marker should be attached securely to the gantry with a wire or cable to ensure that marker is not left inadvertently on the patient when dismissed. Check that the marker is visible on the persistence screen, and note its approximate location on the screen. This is used to correct for patient motion during injection of the ^{99m}Tc sestamibi at peak exercise.

5. Before commencement of exercise, instruct the patient on the correct method to grip the detector head (see Fig. 4-32).

6. The patient should exercise as described in Procedure 4-7, "Stress Testing (Myocardial Perfusion Studies)." At peak exercise, inject the ^{99m}Tc sestamibi into the side port closest to the catheter, as shown in Figure 4-1. (*Note:* Ensure that the needle of the injection syringe is positioned past the dead space at the top of the side port.) **Remove the empty syringe**.

7. Check that the marker source is in the approximate location noted in step 4. Use the foot pedal to start acquisition on the computer. After 1–2 seconds, rapidly inject 60 ml of saline.

8. Ensure that the patient continues to exercise for another 90 seconds after injection.

Single-Crystal System—Rest Study

1. The acquisition should be set to acquire images in a 32 × 32 matrix at 30–40 frames per second for 30 seconds. If the system has a high count rate mode, ensure that this is turned on. Set zoom factor to 2.

2. Position the patient supine on the imaging table. The detector head should be positioned anteriorly over the heart, as shown in Figure 4-33.

3. If required, connect the ECG leads to the gating system and check the ECG signal to verify that the ECG trigger is being detected.

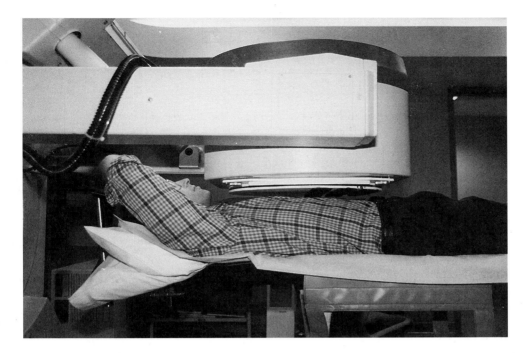

Figure 4-33. Patient in position for a resting first-pass study on a single-crystal system.

4. Inject a small, 500-µCi (18.5 MBq), dose of ^{99m}Tc sestamibi into the side port of the extension set, and flush gently with 5–10 ml of saline. Check the position of the left ventricle on the persistence screen. Adjust the position of the patient and/or the detector so that the heart is located centrally in the field of view.

5. Before the main injection, ensure that the patient is comfortable and relaxed. Inject the ^{99m}Tc sestamibi into the side port closest to the catheter. *Note:* Ensure that the needle of the injection syringe is positioned past the dead space at the top of the side port (Fig. 4-1). **Remove the empty syringe.**

6. Start acquisition on the computer. After 1–2 seconds, rapidly inject 60 ml of saline.

7. Ensure that the patient remains motionless until the acquisition is complete.

Note: Logistically, stress first-pass studies are not usually possible on single-crystal systems.

Computer Analysis

Most systems have semiautomated analysis programs for calculation of LVEF. The following general steps should be performed:

1. Using the raw data, draw a bolus ROI where activity is just starting to enter the right atrium from the superior vena cava, as shown in Figure 4-2.

2. Generate a time–activity curve from the bolus ROI. Obtain a hard copy of this display as verification of bolus quality. If possible, measure the full width at half maximum (FWHM) of the bolus peak. Bolus quality is defined as follows:

FWHM, sec	Quality
Less than 0.5	Excellent
0.5–1.0	Good
1.0–1.5	Adequate
Greater than 1.5	Delayed

3. The first-pass analysis software usually requests that the operator draw an approximate outline ROI around the left ventricle.
4. From this, the software generates a left ventricular time–activity curve and requests the user to select the lung phase of bolus transit and the left ventricular cycles to be analyzed (Fig. 4-34).
5. The user normally is requested to redraw the left ventricular ROI, based on the end-diastole and end-systole left ventricular images and on phase images of the left ventricle and outflow tract.
6. Based on this new ROI, the final report is generated, showing the average LVEF, cycles accepted and rejected, actual LVEF of individual cycles, and display of the final left ventricular ROI used.

Note: With stress first-pass studies, an additional step is required to correct for patient motion before analysis of the study. This should be performed by the system software, using the movement of the marker source as a reference point.

Note: Multicrystal gamma cameras usually achieve a maximal count rate greater than 300 kcps in a clinical study. Single crystal gamma cameras achieve approximately half this value. Note that maximal counts should be 150 kcps or higher for a good-quality study. Studies with maximal counts greater than 100 kcps, but less than 150 kcps, can be processed, but the count rate should be noted.

Information on Film

The following information should be recorded from the preceding analysis:

1. Maximal count rate achieved during acquisition
2. Bolus quality—display of the bolus and the ROI used to generate it

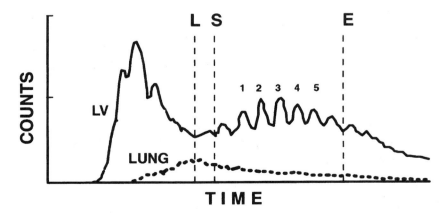

Figure 4-34. Time–activity curves from the left ventricle (LV) and the lungs. Markers L, S, and E are positioned at L, lung phase; S, start of LV phase; and E, end of LV phase. Cycles marked 1–5 have been selected for analysis.

3. Details of average and individual LVEF results for the selected cycles together with the cycle lengths of the displayed cycles and a display of the left ventricular ROI used.

Interpretation

In normal subjects, the LVEF should be approximately 60% (range 50–80%) at rest, increasing to 70% (range, 60–90%) with maximal exercise.[4] There should be no areas of abnormal wall motion (hypokinesis or dyskinesis). Abnormalities in cardiac function may be manifested as low-exercise LVEF and/or the presence of abnormalities in global and regional wall motion.

Radiation Dosimetry

The estimated absorbed doses in organs and tissues of an average subject (70 kg) from an IV injection of 30 mCi (1,110 MBq) ^{99m}Tc sestamibi are shown in Table 4-14.[5]

References

1. Wackers FJ, Berger HJ, Johnstone DE, et al. Multiple gated cardiac blood pool imaging for left ventricular ejection fraction: validation of the technique and assessment of variability. Am J Cardiol 1979; 43: 1159–1166.
2. Jengo JA, Mena I, Blaufuss A, Criley JM. Evaluation of left ventricular function (ejection fraction and segmental wall motion) by single pass radioisotope angiography. Circulation 1978; 57: 326–332.
3. Parker JA, Treves S. Radionuclide detection, localization and quantitation of intracardiac shunts and shunts between the great arteries. In: "Principles of Cardiovascular Nuclear Medicine," eds Holman BL, Sonnenblick EH, Lesch M. Grune & Stratton, New York, 1978, pp 189–218.
4. Upton MT, Rerych SK, Newman GE, Bounous EP Jr, Jones RH. The reproducibility of radionuclide angiographic measurements of left ventricular function in normal subjects at rest and during exercise. Circulation 1980; 62: 126–132.
5. Package insert. Cardiolite. Kit for the preparation of technetium Tc-99m sestamibi. E.I. DuPont de Nemours Co., Sept. 1992.

Myocardial Infarct Study

Summary Information

Radiopharmaceutical
  Adult dose: 20 mCi (740 MBq) ^{99m}Tc PYP administered intravenously.
  Pediatric dose: Adjusted according to patient's weight (see Appendix A-3).

Contraindications None.

Dose/Scan Interval Imaging should commence 3–4 hours after injection.

Views Obtained Anterior, left lateral, and 40°–50° LAO views should be obtained. SPECT images of the heart may be required.

Indications

Infarct imaging with ^{99m}Tc PYP is of limited value in the evaluation of patients with recent myocardial infarcts. In patients who present late (several days) after an infarct, ^{99m}Tc PYP imaging may be of some benefit in determining the size and location of the infarct, particularly if other clinical signs are inconclusive.[1] Occasionally, it may be of benefit in the evaluation of patients after cardiac operations when the diagnosis is complicated by the aftereffects of the operation.[2] A review of this technique by Parkey et al.[3] showed that ^{99m}Tc phosphate imaging is capable of detecting small transmural infarcts of 3 g or larger in mass.

Principle

In the mid-1970s, it was discovered that ^{99m}Tc PYP localized in areas of acute myocardial infarction.[4] The major mechanism of uptake is thought to be binding of the phosphate component of the radionuclide with calcium salt precipitates formed in the damaged cells. The most important determinants of ^{99m}Tc PYP uptake in the heart appear to be (1) the presence of necrotic tissue, (2) residual collateral blood flow to the necrotic tissue, and (3) time interval between occurrence of infarct and injection of ^{99m}Tc PYP.[3]

Patient Preparation

The patient should drink 2–3 glasses of water between the time of the injection and the scan.

Instrument Specifications

Gamma camera:	Any large field-of-view system can be used.
Collimator:	Low-energy high-resolution collimator.
Energy setting:	140 keV, 20% window.
Computer system:	Acquisition requirements—static acquisition (256 × 256 matrix), tomographic acquisition (64 × 64 matrix, 30–60 views).
	Processing requirements—no processing of planar views. Standard tomographic reconstruction software.

Imaging Procedure

1. Place the patient supine on the imaging table, with the detector positioned anteriorly and centered over the heart.
2. Acquire an anterior view of the heart for 1,000 kct on the computer (256 × 256 word mode matrix).
3. Repeat step 2, with the detector positioned in the left lateral and 40°–50° LAO positions.
4. After the LAO view, DO NOT move the detector until after the images have been checked by the nuclear medicine physician. In patients with an uptake pattern that is difficult to interpret, the physician may request either a tomographic acquisition or a "blood pool" image to aid in diagnosis (see "Additional Notes," following).

Computer Analysis

No analysis is required for the planar images.

Additional Notes

Tomographic Infarct Study

In some patients, the nuclear medicine physician may request that a tomographic study be performed to permit better differentiation of myocardial activity from surrounding activity in bone. In such cases, the study should be acquired and processed as for a ^{99m}Tc sestamibi scan.

Blood Pool Scan: Preparation and Imaging

In some patients, residual activity in the blood pool may hinder interpretation. In such cases, labeling of the blood pool and comparison of the blood pool image with the PYP image may assist in the differentiation of myocardial uptake from blood pool activity. For a blood pool scan, the adult dose is 10 mCi (370 MBq) of ^{99m}Tc-labeled RBCs. *Note:* Pyrophosphate from an infarct study will have coated RBCs; hence, it is not necessary to inject cold PYP for labeling purposes.

1. Place 10 mCi (370 MBq) of ^{99m}Tc pertechnetate in a volume of 1 ml into a 12-ml syringe.
2. Place 4 ml of heparinized saline in a 6-ml syringe.
3. Attach the 6- and 12-ml syringes to a 3-way stopcock.
4. Place a 21-gauge butterfly infusion set in an arm vein, and connect the syringes and stopcock to the infusion set, as shown in Figure 4-5.
5. Draw 6–10 ml of blood into the 12-ml syringe.
6. Draw 2 ml of heparinized saline through the stopcock into the 12-ml syringe. Push the rest of the heparinized saline through the butterfly infusion set.

7. Mix the blood, and let it stand for 10 minutes, then reinject it into the patient.
8. Acquire the LAO view for 1,500 kct on the computer (256 × 256 word mode matrix). This view should be acquired with the patient in the same position as for the LAO ^{99m}Tc PYP scan view.

Information on Film

On each computer film, check that the following information is recorded:

1. Patient name and clinic/hospital number.
2. Date, type of scan, and radiopharmaceutical used.
3. Time of each image after injection.

Interpretation

Any myocardial uptake of ^{99m}Tc PYP is considered abnormal. The following criteria are used to interpret the degree of uptake:

0 = No cardiac uptake.
1+ = Diffuse uptake—intensity is less than that of the ribs.
2+ = Focal or diffuse uptake—intensity equals that of the ribs.
3+ = Myocardial uptake—intensity is equal to that of the sternum.
4+ = Myocardial uptake—intensity is greater than that of the sternum.

Uptake at the 3+ level or higher is associated with an acute myocardial infarction. Focal or diffuse uptake at 2+ is associated with subendocardial damage, whereas diffuse uptake at this level may be due to chronic or unstable angina. Mild uptake (1+) may be seen in patients with cardiomyopathy, myocardial trauma, or skeletal muscle damage in the region of the heart. Possible causes of positive ^{99m}Tc PYP scans other than myocardial infarction are listed in Table 4-15.[1,5]

Radiation Dosimetry

The estimated absorbed doses in organs and tissues of an average subject (70 kg) from an IV injection of 20 mCi (740 MBq) ^{99m}Tc PYP are shown in Table 4-16.[6]

Table 4-15. Possible Causes of Positive ^{99m}Tc Pyrophosphate Scans Other Than Myocardial Infarction

Unstable angina
Left ventricular wall motion abnormalities
Left ventricular aneurysms
Cardiomyopathy
Rib fractures or skeletal muscle damage
Valvular calcification
Myocardial trauma
Persistent blood pool activity
Calcified costal cartilage
Skin lesions

Table 4-16. Absorbed Radiation Doses in a 70-kg Adult After Intravenous Administration of 20 mCi (740 MBq) ^{99m}Tc Pyrophosphate

Tissue	Absorbed Radiation Doses	
	rad/20 mCi	mGy/740 MBq
Heart wall		
Normal	0.15	1.5
Impaired	0.29	2.9
Kidneys	2.80	28.0
Skeleton	0.79	7.9
Bone marrow	0.56	5.6
Bladder		
2-hr void	1.95	19.5
4.8-hr void	4.60	46.0
Testes		
2-hr void	0.20	2.0
4.8-hr void	0.31	3.1
Ovaries		
2-hr void	0.19	1.9
4.8-hr void	0.31	3.1
Total body	0.17	1.7

References

1. Leppo J, Okada RD. Radionuclide imaging. In "Noninvasive Cardiac Imaging," eds Morganroth J, Paresi A, Pohost GM. Year Book Medical Publishers, Chicago, 1983, pp 179–199.
2. Righetti A, O'Rourke RA, Schelbert H, et al. Usefulness of preoperative and postoperative Tc-99m (SN)-pyrophosphate scans in patients with ischemic and valvular heart disease. Am J Cardiol 1977; 39: 43–49.
3. Parkey RW, Bonte FJ, Buja LM, Stokely EM, Willerson JT. Myocardial infarct imaging with technetium-99m phosphates. Semin Nucl Med 1977; 7: 15–28.
4. Bonte FJ, Parkey RW, Graham KD, Moore J, Stokely EM. A new method for radionuclide imaging of myocardial infarcts. Radiology 1974; 110: 473–474.
5. Wynne J, Holman BL, Lesch M. Myocardial scintigraphy by infarct-avid radiotracers. Prog Cardiovasc Dis 1978; 20: 243–266.
6. TechneScan PYP. Kit for the preparation of technetium Tc-99m pyrophosphate. Technical product data. Mallinckrodt Diagnostics, St. Louis. Revised Dec. 1980.

5

Endocrine System

Gregory A. Wiseman

Thyroid Scan
(^{99m}Tc Pertechnetate)

Summary Information

Radiopharmaceutical

Adult dose: 5 mCi (185 MBq) ^{99m}Tc pertechnetate administered intravenously.

Pediatric dose: Adjusted according to the patient's weight (see Appendix A-3).

Contraindications Uptake of ^{99m}Tc pertechnetate in the thyroid may be affected by thyroid medication and by foods or drugs containing iodine. Table 5-1 lists the medications that may affect the uptake of ^{99m}Tc pertechnetate. The most profound effects are from iodinated contrast materials. These may decrease uptake, from a few weeks (for excretory urography and cholecystography) to several months or even years (for bronchography and contrast myelography). The duration of the effect of many of these substances on thyroid uptake varies from patient to patient, and the limits given in Table 5-1 are only approximations.[1–4] In addition to the items in Table 5-1, previous nuclear medicine procedures using agents containing stannous ion may affect uptake for approximately 1 week.[5] If only qualitative images of the thyroid are important, then shorter time periods than those described in Table 5-1 may be sufficient to permit visualization of the gland.

Dose/Scan Interval Imaging should commence approximately 10-15 minutes after the injection.

Views Obtained Anterior, left anterior oblique, and right anterior oblique views of the thyroid gland are obtained as well as a 15-cm (the distance from the suprasternal notch to the aperture of the pinhole collimator) anterior view of the neck region.

Indications

Pertechnetate imaging of the thyroid gland is used to evaluate the size, shape, nodularity, and functional status of the thyroid gland. It is useful in assessing patients who have hyperthy-

Table 5-1. Substances and Drugs Known to Affect Thyroid Uptake

Substance	Name	Approximate Duration
Thyroid medications	Thyroxine	4–6 weeks
	Triiodothyronine	2 weeks
Antithyroid medications	Methimazole	4 weeks (primary effect lasts 2–3 days)
	Propylthiouracil	
	Mercazole (Europe)	
Iodine-containing products	Potassium iodide, povidone-iodine, Kelp, antitussives, iodine ointments (e.g., some sun tanning lotions), iodine tincture, iodoform	2–3 weeks
Radiographic contrast media	Intravenous water-soluble media	2–4 weeks
	Oral/fat-soluble media	2 months to 1 year

roidism, nodular goiter, solitary thyroid nodule and thyroiditis, and in screening of patients with suspected thyroid cancer (e.g., patients who received childhood irradiation to the face or neck area).

Principle

^{99m}Tc pertechnetate is trapped by the thyroid gland in a manner analogous to iodine. Hence, all conditions that influence or interfere with iodine uptake also affect uptake of pertechnetate by the thyroid. Unlike iodine, pertechnetate is not organified; thus, iodine and pertechnetate may give dissimilar results in certain conditions, notably chronic thyroiditis and occasionally with benign and malignant nodules.

Patient Preparation

Interview the patient with respect to the items listed in Table 5-1. If necessary, consult with a nuclear medicine physician before proceeding with the injection of ^{99m}Tc pertechnetate.

Instrument Specifications

Gamma camera:	Any large field-of-view system may be used.
Collimator:	Pinhole collimator with 5–6 mm aperture.
Energy setting:	140 keV, 15–20% window.
Analog formatter:	8 × 10 film, 105-mm (4-on-1) format.
Computer system:	Acquisition requirements—static (256 × 256 word mode matrix)
	Processing requirements—none.

Imaging Procedure

1. Imaging should commence 10–15 minutes after the injection.
2. Position the patient supine on the imaging table. Position the head in a head holder, as in Figure 5-1, with the neck extended.

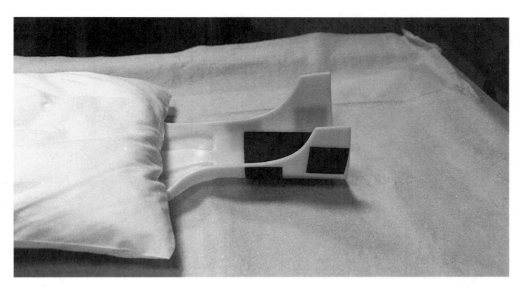

Figure 5-1. Head holder (adapted from a clip-on head restraint for SPECT imaging of the head).

3. The gamma camera and pinhole collimator should be positioned over the region of the neck, as in Figure 5-2. Move the detector away from the patient until the distance from the neck surface to the pinhole aperture is 15 cm.
4. Acquire an anterior view on the analog formatter and on computer (256 × 256 word mode matrix) for 250 kct. *Note:* The field of view should include the salivary glands, thyroid, and upper sternum.
5. Place ^{57}Co or ^{99m}Tc point source markers on the suprasternal notch, cricoid cartilage, and chin (Fig. 5-3) and acquire a 1-minute anterior image on the analog formatter and computer.
6. Remove the markers, and decrease the distance from the pinhole aperture to the patient's neck until the thyroid gland comfortably fills the field of view. Acquire an anterior view of the thyroid gland on the analog formatter and on computer (256 × 256 word mode matrix) for 250 kct.
7. Rotate the gantry ±30° to obtain the left and right anterior oblique views. These views should be acquired for the same time as the anterior view in step 6.
8. Check the images for activity along the midline between the two thyroid lobes. This activity may be due to activity in the esophagus. If present, have the patient drink a glass of water and repeat the anterior view.

Computer Analysis

None required.

Information on Film

Ensure that the following information is recorded on each film:

1. Patient name and clinic/hospital number
2. Date and time of ^{99m}Tc images after the injection
3. Type of scan and radiopharmaceutical
4. Orientation of each image and location of markers

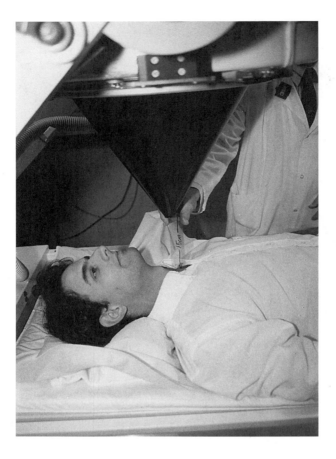

Figure 5-2. Pinhole collimator positioned 15 cm from the neck surface.

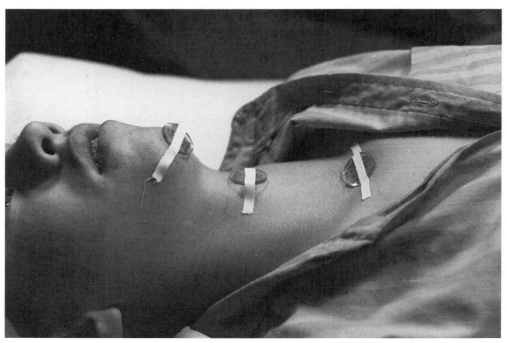

Figure 5-3. Placement of radioactive markers on the suprasternal notch, cricoid cartilage, and chin.

Interpretation

Normal

Normal scans show a butterfly-shaped area, with homogeneous uptake lying below and to either side of the cricoid cartilage.

Abnormal

An abnormal scan may show enlargement of the thyroid with areas of both increased and decreased nonhomogeneous uptake. Uptake may also be present sublingually along the thyroglossal duct and substernally.

Graves Disease

The scan shows diffuse enlargement of the gland with homogeneous uptake and an increased 24-hour ^{131}I uptake measurement.

Multinodular Goiter

The scan shows an enlarged thyroid with nonhomogeneous uptake.

Additional Notes

Palpation of the thyroid gland must be performed by the nuclear medicine physician for proper interpretation of the scan.

Radiation Dosimetry

The estimated absorbed doses in organs and tissues of an average subject (70 kg) from an IV injection of 5 mCi (185 MBq) ^{99m}Tc sodium pertechnetate are shown in Table 5-2.[6]

Table 5-2. Absorbed Radiation Dose Estimates in a 70-kg Adult After IV Administration of 5 mCi (185 MBq) ^{99m}Tc Pertechnetate

Tissue	Absorbed Radiation Dose	
	rad/5 mCi	mGy/185 MBq
Bladder wall	0.266	2.66
Stomach wall	1.25	12.5
Upper large intestinal wall	0.345	3.45
Lower large intestinal wall	0.305	3.05
Red marrow	0.095	0.95
Testes	0.045	0.45
Ovaries	0.11	1.10
Thyroid	0.65	6.50
Brain	0.07	0.70
Total body	0.06	0.60

References

1. Sarkar SD. In vivo thyroid studies. In "Diagnostic Nuclear Medicine," eds Gottschalk A, Hoffer PB, Potchen EJ. Williams & Wilkins, Baltimore, 1988, pp 756–768.
2. Schultz AL, Jacobson WE. The effect of propylthiouracil on the thyroid uptake of I^{131} and the plasma conversion ratio in hyperthyroidism. J Clin Endocrinol Metab 1952; 12: 1205–1214.
3. Greer MA. The effect on endogenous thyroid activity of feeding desiccated thyroid to normal human subjects. N Engl J Med 1951; 244: 385–390.
4. Pineda G, Clauria H, Rocha AFG, Harbert JC. The thyroid. In: "Textbook of Nuclear Medicine: Clinical Applications," eds Rocha AFG, Harbert JC. Lea & Febiger, Philadelphia, 1979, pp 1–50.
5. Montelibano EB, Ford DR Jr, Sayle BA. Altered ^{99m}Tc-pertechnetate distribution in a thyroid scan after ^{99m}Tc-Sn pyrophosphate administration. Clin Nucl Med 1979; 4: 277–282.
6. MIRD dose estimate report No. 8. Summary of current radiation dose estimates to normal humans from ^{99m}Tc as sodium pertechnetate. J Nucl Med 1976; 17: 74–77.

Ectopic Thyroid Scan (^{123}I/^{131}I)

Summary Information

Radiopharmaceutical

Adult dose: 400 µCi (14.8 MBq)^{123}I orally

or

100 µCi (3.7 MBq) ^{131}I orally.

Pediatric dose: Adjusted according to the patient's weight (see Appendix A-3).

Note: Obtain a written directive signed by the nuclear medicine physician before administering ^{131}I.

Contraindications   Pregnancy—a negative serum pregnancy test is required if the patient is a sexually active female less than 50 years of age and not using a reliable birth control method.

Uptake of ^{123}I and ^{131}I into normal and ectopic thyroid tissue is strongly affected by thyroid medication and by foods or drugs containing iodine. Table 5-1 lists the medications that may affect uptake of radioactive iodine. The most profound effects are from iodinated contrast materials. These may decrease uptake from a few weeks (for excretory urography and cholecystography) to several months or even years (for bronchography and contrast myelography).

The duration of the effect of many of these substances on thyroid uptake varies from patient to patient, and the limits given in Table 5-1 are only approximations.[1–4]

Dose/Scan Interval   Imaging should be performed approximately 6 and 24 hours after oral administration of ^{123}I and approximately 24 hours after oral administration of ^{131}I.

Views Obtained   Anterior neck, anterior, and/or posterior views of the chest are obtained for substernal thyroid; and anterior and/or posterior views of the pelvis, for struma ovarii. A whole-body scan may be requested by the nuclear medicine physician.

Indications

Ectopic thyroid tissue behaves in a manner similar to thyroid tissue with respect to its ability to trap and organify iodine. Hence, radioactive iodine can be used to assess the presence of ectopic functioning thyroid tissue such as lingual thyroid, substernal mass, and struma ovarii. Whenever possible, the use of ^{123}I is preferred to ^{131}I because of its lower radiation dose.

Note: The initial evaluation of a possible substernal or lingual thyroid should be performed using ^{99m}Tc pertechnetate (see Procedure 5-1, "Thyroid Scan [^{99m}Tc Pertechnetate]"), because this may provide the required information, avoiding the need to use ^{131}I.

Principle

Imaging of the thyroid gland is based on the fact that the production of thyroid hormones depends on the extraction of iodine from the blood and the organification and incorporation of the iodine into the thyroid hormones thyroxine and triiodothyronine. This is also true for functioning ectopic thyroid tissue.

Patient Preparation

Interview the patient with respect to the items listed in Table 5-1. If necessary, consult with a nuclear medicine physician before proceeding with administration of ^{123}I or ^{131}I.

Instrument Specifications

Gamma camera:	Any large field-of-view system may be used.
Collimator:	^{123}I—low-energy high-resolution collimator.
	^{131}I—high-energy collimator.
Energy setting:	^{123}I—159 keV, 15–20% window.
	^{131}I—364 keV, 15–20% window.
Analog formatter:	8 × 10 film, 70-mm (4-on-1 format).
Computer system:	Acquisition requirements—static (256 × 256 matrix).
	Processing requirements—none.

Imaging Procedure

1. Imaging should commence about 6 hours after administration of ^{123}I. If necessary, a repeat scan can be performed at 20–24 hours.
2. Imaging should commence 20–24 hours after administration of the ^{131}I.
3. The patient should be imaged supine on the imaging table, with the detector positioned anteriorly over the region of the neck (or pelvis, for struma ovarii). The region from the top of the head to the middle of the heart should be included in the field of view. Use a zoom of 1.5–2.0 to magnify this region to the full field of view of the gamma camera.
4. Acquire an image on the analog formatter and on computer (256 × 256 word mode matrix) for 10 minutes. Additional views (if required) should also be acquired for 10 minutes.
5. Place appropriate ^{57}Co or ^{99m}Tc point source markers on the patient (see "Additional Notes"). Adjust the energy window for the appropriate energy of the marker source, and acquire a 1-minute marker image on the analog formatter and computer (256 × 256 word mode matrix).

Additional Notes

1. The marker view should be obtained with the markers placed on the appropriate anatomic landmarks. For the neck region, mark the suprasternal notch, cricoid cartilage, chin, and any surgical scar (see Fig. 5-3). For the pelvis, mark the hips.

2. If required, a whole-body scan can be performed at 24 hours. Acquire anterior and posterior whole-body views at a scan speed of 10–15 cm/min on the analog formatter and on computer (1,024 × 256 matrix).

Computer Analysis

None required.

Information on Film

On each analog or computer film, ensure that the following information is recorded:

1. Patient name and clinic/hospital number
2. Date and time of images after administration of ^{123}I or [131]I
3. Type of scan and radiopharmaceutical
4. Orientation of each image, and location of the markers

Interpretation

Ectopic thyroid tissue is most commonly located sublingually or behind the sternum. Struma ovarii are located in the pelvic area.

Radiation Dosimetry

The estimated absorbed doses in organs and tissues of an average, 70-kg subject with a normal-functioning thyroid from oral doses of 400 μCi (14.8 MBq) [123]I and 100 μCi (3.7 MBq) [131]I sodium iodide are shown in Tables 5-3 and 5-4, respectively.[5]

Table 5-3. Absorbed Radiation Dose Estimates in a 70-kg Adult From Oral Administration of 400 μCi (14.8 MBq) [123]I Sodium Iodide

| | Absorbed Radiation Dose | | | | | |
| | rad/400 μCi Thyroid Uptake | | | mGy/14.8 MBq Thyroid Uptake | | |
Tissue	5%	15%	25%	5%	15%	25%
Thyroid	0.96	3.00	5.20	9.6	30.0	52.0
Stomach wall	0.10	0.09	0.08	1.0	0.92	0.84
Red marrow	0.012	0.012	0.012	0.12	0.12	0.12
Liver	0.012	0.011	0.011	0.12	0.11	0.11
Testes	0.005	0.005	0.005	0.05	0.05	0.05
Ovaries	0.014	0.014	0.014	0.14	0.14	0.14
Total body	0.010	0.011	0.012	0.10	0.11	0.12

Table 5-4. Absorbed Radiation Dose Estimates in a 70-kg Adult From Oral Administration of 100 μCi (3.7 MBq) ^{131}I Sodium Iodide

	Absorbed Radiation Dose						
	rad/100 μCi Thyroid Uptake				mGy/3.7 MBq Thyroid Uptake		
Tissue	5%	15%	25%		5%	15%	25%
Thyroid	26	80	130		260	800	1300
Stomach wall	0.17	0.16	0.14		1.7	1.6	1.4
Red marrow	0.014	0.020	0.026		0.14	0.20	0.26
Liver	0.020	0.035	0.048		0.20	0.35	0.48
Testes	0.008	0.009	0.009		0.08	0.09	0.09
Ovaries	0.014	0.014	0.014		0.14	0.14	0.14
Total body	0.024	0.047	0.071		0.24	0.47	0.71

References

1. Sarkar SD. In vivo thyroid studies. In "Diagnostic Nuclear Medicine," vol. 2, eds Gottschalk A, Hoffer PB, Potchen EJ. Williams & Wilkins, Baltimore, 1988, pp 756–768.
2. Schultz AL, Jacobson WE. The effect of propylthiouracil on the thyroid uptake of I^{131} and the plasma conversion ratio in hyperthyroidism. J Clin Endocrinol Metab 1952; 12: 1205–1214.
3. Greer MA. The effect on endogenous thyroid activity of feeding desiccated thyroid to normal human subjects. N Engl J Med 1951; 244: 385–390.
4. Pineda G, Clauria H, Rocha AFG, Harbert JC. The thyroid. In "Textbook of Nuclear Medicine: Clinical Applications," eds Rocha AFG, Harbert JC. Lea & Febiger, Philadelphia, 1979, pp 1–50.
5. Summary of current radiation dose estimates to humans from ^{123}I, ^{124}I, ^{125}I, ^{126}I, ^{130}I, ^{131}I, and ^{132}I as sodium iodide. J Nucl Med 1975; 16: 857–860.

^{131}I Thyroid Uptake Measurement

<hr>

Summary Information

Radiopharmaceutical

All doses of ^{131}I sodium iodide are administered orally. The exact activity administered depends on the type of uptake measurement and the presence of residual activity from previous ^{131}I uptake or scan procedures.

Standard uptake measurement:
Administered dose = 4-6 µCi (148–222 kBq) ^{131}I.

Residual thyroid remnant (post thyroidectomy):
Administered dose = 1 mCi (37 MBq) ^{131}I.

Total-body iodine scan (thyroid cancer):
Administered dose = 3 mCi (111 MBq) ^{131}I.

Pediatric dose:
Adjusted according to the patient's weight (see Appendix A-3).

If there is residual activity in the neck from previous ^{131}I scans or uptake studies, the doses for the standard uptake measurement may be increased using the regimen shown in Table 5-5. Residual neck activity is determined by a 1–3 minute uptake measurement over the neck before administration of the ^{131}I, as described in the section entitled "Procedure," following.

Note: A signed and dated written directive specifying the radioisotope and dose must be obtained from a nuclear medicine physician before doses greater than 30 µCi (1.11 MBq) ^{131}I can be administered.

Contraindications

Uptake of ^{131}I sodium iodide in the thyroid is strongly affected by thyroid medication and by foods or drugs containing iodine. Table 5-1 lists the medications that may affect uptake. The most profound effects are from iodinated contrast materials. These may decrease uptake from a few weeks (for excretory urography and cholecystography) to several months or even years (for bronchography and contrast myelography). The duration of the effect of many of these substances on thyroid uptake varies from patient to patient, and the limits given in Table 5-1 are only approximations.[1–5]

<hr>

Continues

Summary Information *(Continued)*

Dose/Scan Interval Uptake measurement can be performed at 4–6 hours and 20–24 hours for the standard uptake test. Uptake measurements for other indications (total-body iodine scan, residual or ectopic thyroid tissue, etc.) are generally performed at 24 or 48 hours after administration of the isotope.

Indications

^{131}I uptake measurements are of value in distinguishing between hyperthyroxinemia that is due to thyroiditis and Graves disease or toxic nodular goiter. It is also used in determining the appropriateness of a therapeutic dose of ^{131}I in patients with Graves disease, residual or recurrent thyroid carcinoma, or thyroid remnant after thyroidectomy.[6]

Table 5-5. Administered Dose as a Function of Residual Neck Activity Based on an Uptake Probe With a Sensitivity of 2,000 ct/min per μCi (54 ct/min per kBq) at 25 cm

Neck Activity ct/min	Suggested Dose	
	μCi	kBq
<250	4	148
250–525	4	148
525–825	6	222
825–1,100	8	296
1,100–1,375	10	370
1,375–2,050	16	592
2,050–2,750	20	740
2,750–3,400	26	962
3,400–4,100	30	1,110
4,100–4,800	36	1,332
4,800–5,500	42	1,554
5,500–6,500	50	1,850
6,500–7,900	60	2,220
7,900–9,600	75	2,775
9,600–14,000	100	3,700

Note: For doses greater than 30 μCi (1.11 MBq), the nuclear medicine physician will need to sign a written directive.

Principle

Iodine is an essential component in the production of the thyroid hormones triiodothyronine and thyroxine and is avidly extracted from the circulating blood. The degree to which the iodine is extracted from the blood and trapped in thyroid cells is a reflection of the functional status of the thyroid gland and amount of functioning thyroid tissue. Most papillary and follicular thyroid carcinomas concentrate radioiodine, and the ^{131}I tumor uptake measurement may be helpful in planning the ^{131}I therapy.

Patient Preparation

Interview the patient with respect to the items listed in Table 5-1. Patients receiving thyroid hormone replacement therapy should discontinue therapy several weeks before the study. In general, patients taking thyroxine (Synthroid) should be switched to triiodothyronine (Cytomel, 25 µg two or three times daily) 4 weeks before the study. The use of triiodothyronine should then be stopped 2 weeks before the study. If necessary, consult with a nuclear medicine physician before administering the [131]I.

Instrument Specifications

Uptake probe: 2 × 2-inch sodium iodide/photomultiplier tube assembly installed in a flat field lead collimator. The collimator should meet International Atomic Energy Agency (IAEA) specifications.[7] A measurement rod should be affixed to the side of the collimator to facilitate rapid and accurate determination of the neck-to-collimator distance.

Spectrometer/counter: Multichannel analyzer with scaler/rate meter.

Energy setting: 364 keV, 20–30% energy window, or integral counting with the lower discriminator set at 300 keV.

Additional items: Neck phantom—15 cm in diameter, 15 cm in height, with a hole for the standard. Distance from the edge of the phantom to the surface of the hole should be 0.5 cm.

Procedure

Dose Less Than 1 mCi: 37 MBq

1. Before administration of the ^{131}I dose, position the patient supine on the table to check for the presence of neck activity from previous studies.
2. The uptake probe should be positioned, as shown in Figure 5-4, with a probe-to-neck distance of about 25 cm. This distance should be set using the measurement rod attached to the side of the collimator and should be fixed for all uptake studies (both patient and standard). Count neck activity for 3 minutes, and record the total counts on the upper portion of the ^{131}I uptake worksheet (Fig. 5-5).
3. The administered dose of ^{131}I should be adjusted to account for neck activity using Table 5-5. Note that this table is based on an uptake probe with a sensitivity of 2,000 ct/min per µCi (54 ct/min per kBq) at 25 cm, as measured using a standard IAEA neck phantom

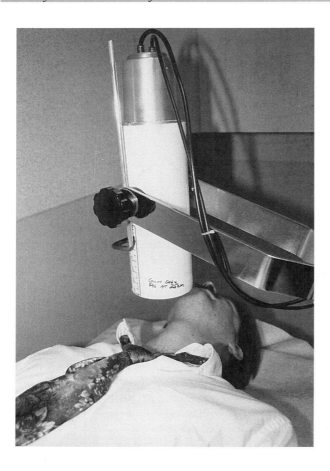

Figure 5-4. Uptake probe positioned over the region of the thryoid gland. *Note:* Neck extended and area free of clothing, jewelry, etc.

(Fig. 5-6). If the probe sensitivity differs, multiply the values for neck activity in Table 5-5 by the correction factor.

$$\text{Correction Factor} = \frac{\text{Measured Probe Sensitivity (ct/min/}\mu\text{Ci)}}{2,000}$$

4. Record the administered dose on the worksheet.
5. Place an identical dose of ^{131}I into a 5-ml vial for use as a standard.
6. Before measuring uptake in the patient, perform a 3-minute room background count and a 3-minute standard count.
7. To count the standard, place the vial containing the standard into a neck phantom and count for 3 minutes, as shown in Figure 5-6. The neck phantom should be as described under "Instrument Specifications" to conform to the standards proposed by the IAEA.[7]
8. At 6 and/or 24 hours after administration of the ^{131}I, position the patient for the uptake measurement as in steps 1 and 2. Acquire a 3-minute count over the neck.
9. Record the room background counts, patient counts, standard counts, and standard activity (microcuries or kilobecquerels) on the worksheet.
10. Perform correction for neck activity if it exceeds 250 ct/3 min. Otherwise, no background correction is required. *Note:* This value is based on an uptake probe with a sensitivity of 2,000 ct/min per μCi (54 ct/min per kBq) at 25 cm and may need to be adjusted for a given probe, as described in step 3.

I-131 UPTAKE : FOR STANDARD UPTAKE, ECTOPIC THYROID OR SUB-STERNAL MASS STUDY

Date and Time	TIME (hrs)	Decay Factor	Room Bkg. Cts	Neck Bkg. Counts	Patient Dose (uCi)	Standard (uCi)	Thyroid Counts	Thy-Bkg Counts	Thy-Bkg Cts / uCi	Standard Counts	Standard Cts / uCi	% Dose in Thyroid
	0	1.000										
	4	0.986										
	6	0.979										
	24	0.918										

Notes :
1. All counts (room bkd, neck bkg, thyroid and standard) should be for 3 minutes.
2. Perform background correction if the neck bkg. activity > 250 ct*(3 min). Otherwise no background correction is performed.
   *(Assumes that the uptake probe has a sensitivity of 2000 ct / min per uCi)
3. The % Dose in Thyroid is obtained from the equation : (Thy-Bkg cts/uCi) x 100 / (Standard cts/uCi).

I-131 UPTAKE : FOR TOTAL BODY IODINE SCAN OR RESIDUAL NECK SCAN STUDY

Date and Time	TIME (hrs)	Decay Factor	Thigh Bkg. Cts	Neck Bkg. Counts	Patient Dose (uCi)	Standard (uCi)	Thyroid Counts	Thy-Bkg Counts	Thy-Bkg Cts / uCi	Standard Counts	Standard Cts / uCi	% Dose in Thyroid
	0	1.000										

Notes :
1. All counts (neck bkg, thigh bkg, thyroid and standard) should be for 1 minute.
2. Background correction should always be performed : for neck bkg. > 100 ct*, multiply neck bkg. counts by the decay factor
   For neck bkg. < 100 cts : Thyroid-Bkg cts = Thyroid cts - Thigh cts
   For neck bkg. > 100 cts : Thyroid-Bkg cts = Thyroid cts - Thigh cts - Neck cts x Decay Factor
   *(Assumes that the uptake probe has a sensitivity of 2000 ct / min per uCi)
3. The % Dose in Thyroid is obtained from the equation : (Thy-Bkg cts/uCi) x 100 / (Standard cts/uCi).

Figure 5-5. Sodium iodide ^{131}I thyroid uptake worksheet.

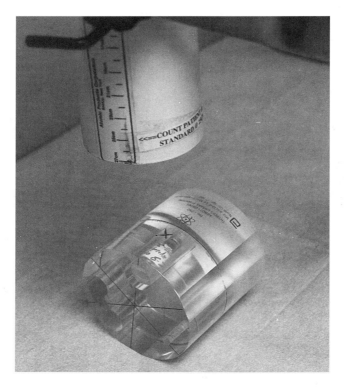

Figure 5-6. Probe positioned over neck phantom containing ^{131}I standard.

11. Calculate the decay-corrected activities of the patient and standard using the decay factors shown in column 2 of Figure 5-5 (e.g., corrected activity of the patient = administered activity × decay factor).
12. Divide the thyroid counts (background corrected) and standard counts by their respective activities to obtain counts per microcuries or counts per kilobecquerels.
13. Thyroid uptake is given by the following equation:

$$\% \text{ Dose in Thyroid} = \frac{\text{Thyroid ct per unit activity}}{\text{Standard ct per unit activity}} \times 100$$

Procedure

Dose Greater Than 1 mCi: 37 MBq

1. Before administration of the ^{131}I dose, position the patient supine on the table to check for the presence of neck activity from previous studies.
2. The uptake probe should be positioned, as shown in Figure 5-4, with a probe-to-neck distance of about 25 cm. This distance should be set using the measurement rod attached to the side of the collimator and should be fixed for all uptake measurements (both patient and standard). Count neck activity for 1 minute, and record the total counts on the lower portion of the ^{131}I uptake worksheet (see Fig. 5-5).
3. Administer the ^{131}I dose, and record the administered dose on the worksheet.
4. Place a known dose of ^{131}I in a 5-ml vial for use as a standard (measure and record standard activity using a dose calibrator).
5. Before measuring uptake in the patient, perform a 1-minute room background count and a 1-minute standard count.

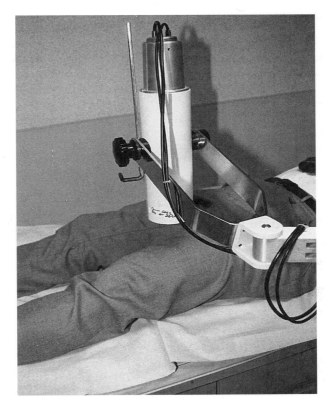

Figure 5-7. Thyroid uptake probe in position over the midsection of the thigh for measurement of background activity.

6. To count the standard, place the vial containing the standard in a neck phantom and count for 1 minute, as shown in Figure 5-6. The neck phantom should be as described under "Instrument Specifications" to conform to the standards proposed by the IAEA.[7]

7. At 24 hours after administration of the ^{131}I, position the patient for the uptake measurement as in steps 1 and 2. Acquire a 1-minute count over the neck.

8. Now, position the probe over the middle section of the thigh, as shown in Figure 5-7, and record the total counts for 1 minute.

9. Record the thyroid counts, thigh counts, standard counts, and standard activity (microcuries or kilobecquerels) on the worksheet (Fig. 5-5).

10. Background correction should always be performed as follows:
    a. If neck activity is greater than 100 ct/min before ^{131}I administration, multiply the neck counts by the appropriate decay factor shown in column 2 of Figure 5-5 and subtract from thyroid counts.
    b. Now, subtract thigh counts from thyroid counts to get the background correction thyroid counts.

11. Calculate the decay-corrected activities of the patient and standard using the decay factors shown in column 2 of Figure 5-5 (e.g., corrected activity of the patient = administered activity $\times$ decay factor).

12. Divide the background-corrected thyroid counts and standard counts by their respective activities to obtain counts per microcuries or counts per kilobecquerels.

13. Thyroid uptake is given by the following equation:

$$\% \text{ Dose in Thyroid} = \frac{\text{Thyroid ct per unit activity}}{\text{Standard ct per unit activity}} \times 100$$

Interpretation

Because of the wide variability in dietary iodine throughout the United States, no normal range can be applied, and each laboratory must establish a normal range for the population it serves. In our laboratory, the normal values are

24-hour ^{131}I: Uptake, normal range = 8–29%

6-hour ^{131}I: Uptake, normal range = 3–16%

Note: The 24-hour uptake can be predicted from the 6-hour uptake with the following equation:[6]

$$\% \text{ 24-Hour Uptake} = 73.2 \times \text{LOG}_{10} (\% \text{ 6-hour uptake}) - 55.7$$
$$(\text{e.g., } 17.5 = 73.2 \times \text{LOG}_{10} (10.00) - 55.7)$$

A chart for converting 6-hour uptake to 24-hour uptake is shown in Table 5-6.

Additional Notes

If an abnormally low uptake is recorded, question the patient again carefully about possible administration of medications or foods that affect thyroid uptake, checking back as far as 1 year.

Radiation Dosimetry

The estimated absorbed doses in organs and tissues of an average, 70-kg subject with a normal-functioning thyroid from an oral dose of 100 µCi (3.7 MBq) ^{131}I sodium iodide are shown in Table 5-4.[8]

Table 5-6. Conversion From 6-hour to 24-hour Uptake Values

6-hr Uptake %	24-hr Uptake %	6-hr Uptake %	24-hr Uptake %
10	17.50	52	69.91
12	23.30	54	71.11
14	28.20	56	72.27
16	32.44	58	73.38
18	36.19	60	74.46
20	39.54	62	75.50
22	42.57	64	76.51
24	45.33	66	77.49
26	47.88	68	78.44
28	50.23	70	79.36
30	52.43	72	80.26
32	54.48	74	81.13
34	56.40	76	81.98
36	58.22	78	82.80
38	59.94	80	83.61
40	61.57	82	84.39
42	63.12	84	85.16
44	64.60	86	85.91
46	66.01	88	86.64
48	67.37	90	87.35
50	68.66	92	88.05

References

1. Sarkar SD. In vivo thyroid studies. In "Diagnostic Nuclear Medicine," eds Gottschalk A, Hoffer PB, Potchen EJ. Williams & Wilkins, Baltimore, 1988, pp 756–768.

2. Schultz AL, Jacobson WE. The effect of propylthiouracil on the thyroid uptake of I^{131} and the plasma conversion ratio in hyperthyroidism. J Clin Endocrinol Metab 1952; 12: 1205–1214.

3. Greer MA. The effect on endogenous thyroid activity of feeding desiccated thyroid to normal human subjects. N Engl J Med 1951; 244: 385–390.

4. Pineda G, Clauria H, Rocha AFG, Harbert JC. The thyroid. In: "Textbook of Nuclear Medicine: Clinical Applications," eds Rocha AFG, Harbert JC. Lea & Febiger, Philadelphia, 1979, pp 1–50.

5. Thrall JH. Radiopharmaceuticals for endocrine imaging. In "Pharmaceuticals in Medical Imaging," eds Swanson DP, Chilton HM, Thrall JH. Macmillan, New York, 1990, pp 343–359.

6. Hayes AA, Akre CM, Gorman CA. Iodine-131 treatment of Graves' disease using modified early iodine-131 uptake measurements in therapy dose calculations. J Nucl Med 1990; 31: 519–522.

7. International Atomic Energy Agency: Consultants meeting on the calibration and standardization of thyroid radioiodine uptake measurements, November 28–30, 1960. Br J Radiol 1962; 35: 205–210.

8. Summary of current radiation dose estimates to humans from ^{123}I, ^{124}I, ^{125}I, ^{126}I, ^{130}I, ^{131}I, and ^{132}I as sodium iodide. J Nucl Med, 1975; 16: 857–860.

^{123}I Thyroid Scan and Uptake Measurement

Summary Information

Radiopharmaceutical

Adult dose: All doses of ^{123}I sodium iodide are administered orally. The standard uptake measurement requires an administered dose of 200 µCi (7.4 MBq) ^{123}I sodium iodide.

Pediatric dose: Adjusted according to the patient's weight (see Appendix A-3).

Contraindications   Uptake of ^{123}I sodium iodide in the thyroid is strongly affected by thyroid medication and by foods or drugs containing iodine. Table 5-1 lists the medications that may affect uptake. The most profound effects are from iodinated contrast materials. These may decrease uptake from a few weeks (for excretory urography and cholecystography) to several months or even years (for bronchography and contrast myelography). The duration of the effect of many of these substances on thyroid uptake varies from patient to patient, and the limits given in Table 5-1 are only approximations.[1–5]

Dose/Scan Interval   Uptake measurements can be performed at 4–6 hours and 20–24 hours after administration of ^{123}I. Note that with the short half-life of ^{123}I (13.2 hours), the 20–24 hour measurement may be inaccurate because of poor count statistics.

Views Obtained   Anterior view of the head, neck, sternum, and pinhole view of the thyroid.

Indications

^{123}I imaging of the thyroid gland is used to evaluate the size, shape, nodularity, and functional status of the thyroid gland. It is useful in assessing patients who have hyperthyroidism, nodular goiter, solitary thyroid nodule, and thyroiditis and in screening patients with suspected thyroid cancer (e.g., patients who received childhood irradiation to the face or neck area). ^{123}I sodium iodide uptake measurements are of value in distinguishing between hyperthyroxinemia due to thyroiditis from Graves disease or toxic nodular goiter, and they may also be of use in determining the appropriateness of a therapeutic dose of ^{131}I in patients with Graves disease, residual or recurrent thyroid carcinoma, or thyroid remnant after thyroidectomy.[6]

Principle

Iodine is an essential component in the production of the thyroid hormones thyroxine and triiodothyronine, and it is avidly extracted from the circulating blood. The degree to which the iodine is extracted from the blood and trapped in thyroid cells is a reflection of the functional status of the thyroid gland and amount of functioning thyroid tissue.

Patient Preparation

Interview the patient with respect to the items listed in Table 5-1. If necessary, consult with a nuclear medicine physician before proceeding with the administration of ^{123}I. Before administering the ^{123}I dose, check that the patient has not recently received ^{131}I for diagnostic or therapeutic purposes. If so, it may be necessary to obtain a background image of the neck region before the ^{123}I dose is administered. If ^{131}I background activity is present, the background image and all ^{123}I images should be acquired with a high-energy collimator.

Instrument Specifications

Gamma camera:	Any large field-of-view system can be used.
Collimator:	Low-energy all-purpose collimator and pinhole collimator (5–6 mm aperture). If residual ^{131}I activity is present, use only a high-energy collimator.
Energy setting:	159 keV, 20% window.
Analog formatter:	8 × 10 film, 9-on-1 format.
Computer system:	Acquisition requirements—static (256 × 256 matrix). Processing requirements—region of interest (ROI) analysis.

Imaging Procedure

1. If background activity is present in the patient from a previous administration of ^{131}I, acquire a 5-minute background image of the neck, as outlined in step 2, and eliminate acquisition of the pinhole image. Otherwise, proceed to step 3.
2. Ensure that the high-energy collimator is installed. A background image should be acquired with the patient supine on the imaging table, with the detector positioned over the region of the neck. The patient should be positioned with the head in a head holder, as shown in Figure 5-1, and with the neck extended. The region from the top of the head to the middle of the heart should be included in the field of view. Acquire a 5-minute image on the analog formatter and on the computer (256 × 256 matrix).
3. Imaging should commence 4–6 hours after administration of the ^{123}I.
4. A standard dose of ^{123}I (100 μCi [3.7 MBq]) should be placed in the neck phantom and positioned beside the patient's head, as shown in Figure 5-8.
5. Position the detector to include a region from the top of the head to the middle of the heart in the field of view. Acquire an image on the analog formatter and on the computer (256 × 256 word mode matrix) for 5 minutes.
6. Install the pinhole collimator, and set the distance from the pinhole aperture to the neck surface until the thyroid gland comfortably fills the field of view. Acquire a 10-minute anterior image on the analog formatter and on the computer (256 × 256 word mode matrix), as shown in Figure 5-2.
7. If required by the nuclear medicine physician, repeat steps 1–6 at 20–24 hours after administration of the ^{123}I.

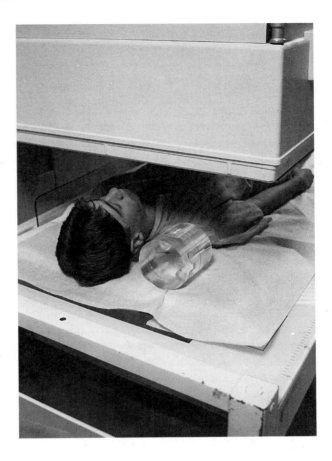

Figure 5-8. Patient and neck standard in position for scan and measurement of ^{123}I uptake.

Computer Analysis

1. Under ROI analysis, draw irregular ROIs over the thyroid, a background region immediately below the thyroid, and the standard. *Note:* If a background image was acquired, draw an irregular ROI over the thyroid on this image, and use this region for background correction.
2. Use the ^{123}I thyroid uptake worksheet (Fig. 5-9), and correct the thyroid counts for background activity. Calculate the percentage of uptake in the thyroid with the following equation:

$$\% \text{ Dose in Thyroid} = \frac{\text{Thyroid ct (background corrected)}}{\text{Standard ct} \times 2} \times 100$$

Note: The factor of 2 in the equation is the ratio of the patient dose to the standard dose. If the ratio is different, substitute the appropriate ratio in the equation.

Additional Notes

This procedure may be used in place of the standard ^{131}I uptake measurement with an uptake probe. Note that in some patients, insufficient activity may be present in the thyroid to give adequate image quality in the pinhole image.

If an abnormally low uptake is recorded, question the patient again carefully about possible administration of medications or foods that affect thyroid uptake, checking back as far as 1 year.

I-123 THYROID UPTAKE MEASUREMENT

Patient Name : _____

Clinic No. _____ Date : _____

Registration Desk : _____ Age : _____ Sex : ○ F ○ M

PATIENT CHECKLIST

CHECK IF PATIENT HAS RECEIVED ANY OF THE FOLLOWING SUBSTANCES, WITHIN THE INDICATED TIME PERIOD.

THYROID MEDICATION (e.g. SYNTHROID / CYTOMEL) - 4 to 6 weeks :	○ NO	○ YES
ANTI-THYROID MEDICATIONS (e.g. PROPYLTHIOURACIL) - 4 weeks :	○ NO	○ YES
X-RAY STUDY WITH WATER SOLUBLE CONTRAST MEDIA - 2 to 4 weeks :	○ NO	○ YES
X-RAY STUDY WITH ORAL / FAT SOLUBLE CONTRAST MEDIA - 2 to 12 months	○ NO	○ YES
LUGOL'S SOLUTION, BETADINE, KELP, IODIDES, TINCTURE of IODINE,		
ANTITUSSIVES, IODINE OINTMENTS (e.g. Coppertone), IODOFORM - 2 to 4 weeks :	○ NO	○ YES

IF THE ANSWER TO ANY OF THE ABOVE WAS "YES", PLEASE DESCRIBE BELOW THE SUBSTANCE, DATE AND TIME LAST TAKEN / ADMINISTERED, AND CONSULT WITH THE NUCLEAR MEDICINE PHYSICIAN BEFORE ADMINISTERING THE I-123 DOSE :

IS THE PATIENT BREASTFEEDING OR PREGNANT ? (ages 13-50) :   ○ NO   ○ YES --> check with Nuc. Med. physician before admin. of I-123 dose

---

I-123 PATIENT / STANDARD DOSE

I-123 DOSE (uCi) : _____ (nominal 200 uCi)   TIME ADMINISTERED : _____

I-123 STANDARD (uCi) : _____ (nominal 100 uCi)   TIME SCANNED : _____

I-123 UPTAKE CALCULATIONS

PATIENT :   Thyroid ROI = _____ cts (T)   Area (pixels) = _____ (TA)

Background ROI = _____ cts (B)   Area (pixels) = _____ (BA)

Thyroid - Background Counts = _____ cts (C) $\boxed{C = T - B \times (TA / BA)}$

STANDARD   Standard ROI = _____ cts (S)

% THYROID UPTAKE* = _____ % $\boxed{(C \times 50) / S}$

* Uptake calculation assumes that patient dose was TWICE standard dose !

Thyroid Uptake = _____ % @ _____ hours post administration

Figure 5-9. ^{123}I thyroid uptake worksheet.

Interpretation

Because of the wide variability in dietary iodine throughout the United States, no normal range can be applied, and each laboratory must establish a normal range for the population it serves. In our laboratory, the normal values are

Table 5-7. Absorbed Radiation Dose Estimates in a 70-kg Adult From Oral Administration of 200 μCi (7.4 MBq) of [123]I Sodium Iodide

	Absorbed Radiation Dose					
	mrad/200 μCi			mGy/7.4 MBq		
	Thyroid Uptake			Thyroid Uptake		
Tissue	5%	15%	25%	5%	15%	25%
Thyroid	480	1,500	2,600	4.8	15.0	26.0
Stomach wall	50	46	42	0.50	0.46	0.42
Red marrow	6	6	6	0.06	0.06	0.06
Liver	6	6	6	0.06	0.06	0.06
Testes	3	3	3	0.03	0.03	0.03
Ovaries	7	7	6	0.07	0.07	0.06
Total body	5	5	6	0.05	0.05	0.06

2-hour ^{123}I uptake, normal range = 8–29%
6-hour ^{123}I uptake, normal range = 3–16%

Note: The 24-hour uptake can be predicted from the 6-hour uptake with the following equation:[6]

% 24-hour uptake = 73.2 × LOG_{10} (% 6-hour uptake) − 55.7
(e.g., 68.66 = 73.2*LOG_{10} (50.0) − 55.7)

A chart for converting 6-hour uptake to 24-hour uptake is given in Table 5-6.

Radiation Dosimetry

The estimated absorbed doses in organs and tissues of an average, 70-kg subject with a normal-functioning thyroid from an oral dose of 200 μCi (7.4 MBq) [123]I sodium iodide are shown in Table 5-7.[7]

References

1. Sarkar SD. In vivo thyroid studies. In "Diagnostic Nuclear Medicine," vol. 2, eds Gottschalk A, Hoffer PB, Potchen EJ. Williams & Wilkins, Baltimore, 1988, pp 756–768.
2. Schultz AL, Jacobson WE. The effect of propylthiouracil on the thyroid uptake of I^{131} and the plasma conversion ratio in hyperthyroidism. J Clin Endocrinol Metab 1952; 12: 1205–1214.
3. Greer MA. The effect on endogenous thyroid activity of feeding desiccated thyroid to normal human subjects. N Engl J Med 1951; 244: 385–390.
4. Pineda G, Clauria H, Rocha AFG, Harbert JC. The thyroid. In: "Textbook of Nuclear Medicine: Clinical Applications," eds Rocha AFG, Harbert JC. Lea & Febiger, Philadelphia, 1979, pp 1–50.

5. Thrall JH. Radiopharmaceuticals for endocrine imaging. In: "Pharmaceuticals in Medical Imaging," eds Swanson DP, Chilton HM, Thrall JH. Macmillan, New York, 1990, pp 343–359.

6. Hayes AA, Akre CM, Gorman CA. Iodine-131 treatment of Graves' disease using modified early iodine-131 uptake measurements in therapy dose calculations. J Nucl Med 1990; 31: 519–522.

7. Summary of current radiation dose estimates to humans from ^{123}I, ^{124}I, ^{125}I, ^{126}I, ^{130}I, ^{131}I, and ^{132}I as sodium iodide. J Nucl Med 1975; 16: 857–860.

Neck/Total Body ^{131}I Scan

Summary Information

Radiopharmaceutical

Adult dose:
Total body iodine scan—3 mCi (111 MBq) ^{131}I sodium iodide administered orally.
Neck scan—1 mCi (37 MBq) ^{131}I sodium iodide administered orally.

Pediatric dose:
Adjusted according to the patient's weight (see Appendix A-3).

Note: A signed and dated written directive specifying the radioisotope and dose must be obtained from a nuclear medicine physician before the ^{131}I dose is administered.

Contraindications

Uptake of ^{131}I sodium iodide in normal and metastatic thyroid tissue is strongly affected by thyroid medication and by foods or drugs containing iodine. Table 5-1 lists medications that may affect neck and total body iodine scans. The most profound effects are from iodinated contrast materials. These may decrease uptake from a few weeks (for excretory urography and cholecystography) to several months or even years (for bronchography and contrast myelography). The duration of the effect of many of these substances on uptake in normal or metastatic thyroid tissue varies from patient to patient, and the limits given in Table 5-1 are only approximations.[1–5]

Dose/Scan Interval

For a neck scan, imaging begins 24 hours after administration of ^{131}I, and for a total-body iodine scan, 48 hours after administration.

Views Obtained

Neck scan:
Anterior planar image of the neck (including the face and upper chest).

Total-body iodine scan:
Anterior and posterior whole-body views. Also, anterior spot views of the anterior head, neck, and chest may be requested by the nuclear medicine physician.

Indications

Neck scans and total-body iodine scans are indicated in patients who have had a total or near-total thyroidectomy for thyroid carcinoma. Most thyroid cancers, with the exception of medullary carcinoma of the thyroid and anaplastic or poorly differentiated thyroid carcinoma, concentrate iodine. Hence, these scans can be used to determine the metastatic spread of the disease and/or the presence of any residual normal thyroid tissue. A neck scan is usually performed within 1–3 months after thyroidectomy to check for residual normal thyroid tissue and thyroid carcinoma in the neck. After this residual thyroid tissue has been ablated, a total-body iodine scan can be performed to check for metastatic disease.

Principle

The management of patients with thyroid carcinoma depends on the ability to detect any residual or recurrent tumor cells. Most papillary and follicular thyroid cancers are known to concentrate radioiodine, and in these cancers, the neck and total-body iodine scans can be used to reveal the extent of the metastatic spread of the cancer.

Patient Preparation

Interview the patient with respect to items listed in Table 5-1. A patient receiving thyroid hormone replacement therapy should discontinue the therapy several weeks before the study. In general, patients taking thyroxine (Synthroid) should be switched to triiodothyronine (Cytomel, 25 µg two or three times daily) 4 weeks before the study. The use of triiodothyronine should then be stopped 2 weeks before the study. Verify this with the patient. If necessary, consult with a nuclear medicine physician before proceeding with the administration of the ^{131}I.

Instrument Specifications

Whole-Body Images

Gamma camera:	Dual-head large field-of-view system.
Collimator:	High-energy collimator.
Energy setting:	364 keV, 15% window.

Spot images

Gamma camera:	Any large field-of-view system may be used.
Collimator:	High-energy collimator.
Energy setting:	364 keV, 15% window.
Analog formatter:	Whole-body views—8 × 10 or 11 × 14 film. Spot views—8 × 10 film, 105-mm (4-on-1) or 70-mm (9-on-1) format.
Computer system:	Acquisition requirements—whole-body (1,024 × 256 word mode matrix), static (256 × 256 word mode matrix). Processing requirements—ROI analysis of whole-body images.
Additional items:	Neck phantom—The phantom should conform to the IAEA standard for thyroid uptake measurements,[6] i.e., 15 cm in

diameter, 15 cm in height with a hole for the standard. The distance from the edge of the phantom to the surface of the hole should be 0.5 cm.

Imaging Procedure

Total-Body Iodine Scan

1. With the patient supine on the imaging table, acquire anterior and posterior whole-body images 48 hours after the administration of the ^{131}I. All images should be acquired on the analog formatter and also on the computer in a 1,024 × 256 word mode matrix. Acquisition time should be 20 minutes for a scan length of 200 cm (10 cm/min scan speed). A standard of 20–40 μCi (0.74–1.48 MBq) ^{131}I should be placed in the neck phantom and positioned in the field of view, ideally near the patient's feet, and imaged with the patient, as in Figure 5-10.
2. Record the administered dose of ^{131}I (decay-corrected to time of imaging) and ^{131}I activity in the standard.
3. Acquire a single anterior view of the neck and chest. The gamma camera should be centered on the thyroid bed, and the patient's neck should be extended. The image should be acquired for 15 minutes on the analog formatter and on the computer (256 × 256 word mode matrix).
4. Additional whole-body and spot views may be required at 72 hours after administration.

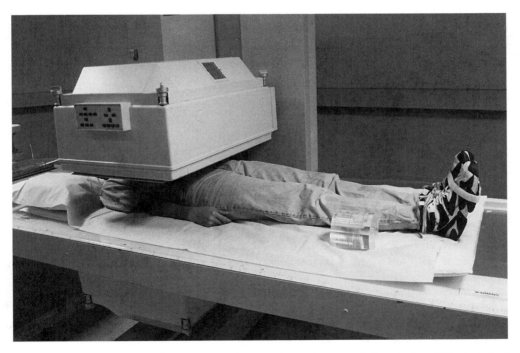

Figure 5-10. Neck phantom with standard positioned beside patient's feet during ^{131}I whole-body scan.

Neck Scan

1. With the patient supine on the imaging table, acquire a single anterior view of the neck and chest. The gamma camera should be centered on the thyroid bed, and the patient's neck should be extended to permit a close collimator-to-neck distance. The image should be acquired for 5 minutes on the analog formatter and on the computer (256 × 256 word mode matrix).
2. After the anterior spot view, acquire another 5-minute image with ^{131}I markers (1–2 μCi [37–74 kBq] per marker) placed on the cricoid cartilage, suprasternal notch, and chin (see Fig. 5-3).

Computer Analysis (Total-Body Iodine Only)

The whole-body images should be analyzed to determine the percentage of the whole-body dose and the percentage of the administered dose in any metastatic lesions present.

1. Under ROI analysis, draw ROIs around the entire anterior and posterior whole-body images and determine the total counts in the anterior (Ta) and posterior (Tp) images (Fig. 5-11).
2. Adjust image contrast so that the background counts are visible. Outline background ROIs (outside the body), as shown in Figure 5-11, and determine anterior (Ba) and posterior (Bp) background counts. These ROIs should be drawn at the level of the head or feet.
3. Determine the background-corrected anterior (Tca) whole-body counts with the following equation:

$$Tca = Ta - Ba \times \frac{\text{Whole-Body ROI (pixels)}}{\text{Background ROI (pixels)}}$$

   Repeat for the posterior (Tcp) whole-body counts.

4. Compute the whole-body geometric mean counts as

$$T = \sqrt{Tca \times Tcp}$$

5. For each lesion or organ, draw an ROI around the area of localized ^{131}I uptake on both anterior and posterior views. Draw a soft tissue background ROI using an area that has background activity similar to that of the lesion. Whenever possible, a contralateral or adjacent normal region should be selected for background, as in Figure 5-12.
6. Compute the geometric mean of the background-corrected anterior and posterior lesion counts, as in step 4.
7. Divide the result of step 6 by that of step 4 to determine the fraction of the whole-body activity present in the lesion.
8. Draw an ROI around the standard on both anterior and posterior views (see Fig. 5-12), and correct for background activity as in step 3.
9. Compute the geometric mean of the background-corrected anterior and posterior standard counts, as in step 4.
10. Apply decay correction to the standard and administered activities to give the true activities at the time of imaging. Multiply the results of step 9 by the ratio of administered-to-standard activities (decay-corrected).
11. Divide the result of step 6 by that of step 10 to determine the fraction of the administered dose in the lesion or organ.

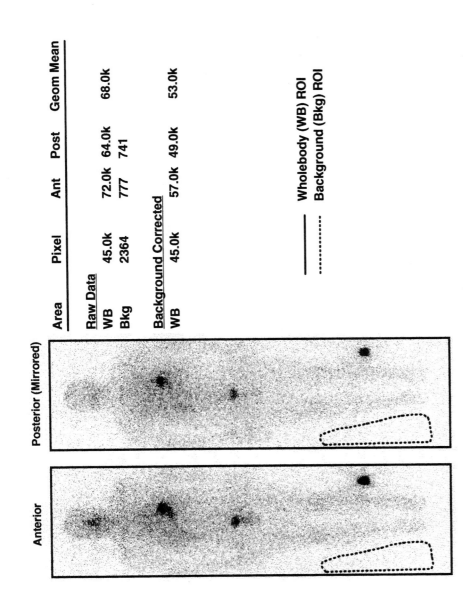

Area	Pixel	Ant	Post	Geom Mean
Raw Data				
WB	45.0k	72.0k	64.0k	68.0k
Bkg	2364	777	741	
Background Corrected				
WB	45.0k	57.0k	49.0k	53.0k

——————— Wholebody (WB) ROI

- - - - - - - Background (Bkg) ROI

Posterior (Mirrored)

Anterior

Figure 5-11. Anterior and posterior whole-body scans showing the placement of the whole-body ROIs and background ROIs. The posterior image has been mirrored to facilitate placement of the ROIs.

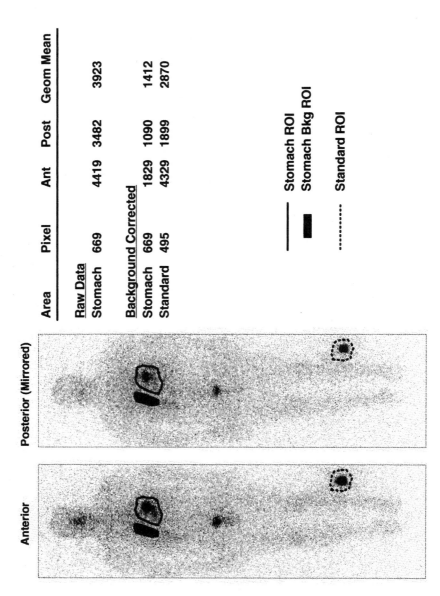

Area	Pixel	Ant	Post	Geom Mean
Raw Data				
Stomach	669	4419	3482	3923
Background Corrected				
Stomach	669	1829	1090	1412
Standard	495	4329	1899	2870

———— Stomach ROI

▬▬▬ Stomach Bkg ROI

--------- Standard ROI

Figure 5-12. Anterior and posterior whole-body scans showing ROIs over the stomach and appropriate background region, as well as ROIs over the standard. The posterior image has been mirrored to facilitate placement of the ROIs.

Information on Film

On each analog or computer film, ensure that the following information is recorded:

1. Patient name and clinic/hospital number
2. Date and time of each image after administration
3. Type of scan and radiopharmaceutical
4. Orientation of each image (e.g., anterior, posterior)
5. Results of analysis, showing all ROIs and computations

Interpretation

Normal

Neck scan:	There should be no significant accumulation of ^{131}I in the neck region, other than in the salivary glands and nasal sinuses. *Note:* Because of residual thyroid cells, there will be some ^{131}I localization in the region of the thyroid in all patients despite the surgical completeness of the thyroidectomy.
Total-body iodine scan:	^{131}I accumulation may be seen in the salivary glands, nasal sinuses, stomach, bowel, and bladder.

Abnormal

Neck scan:	Any focal areas of ^{131}I uptake, outside the thyroid remnant.
Total-body iodine scan:	Any areas of increased uptake other than normal areas. This uptake may be focal or it may be diffuse, particularly in the lungs.

Note: False-positive ^{131}I localization has occasionally been seen because of external contamination, esophageal activity, acute bronchitis, and diffuse bronchiectasis.[7]

Additional Notes

The nuclear medicine physician may request an ^{131}I uptake measurement in conjunction with the scan. Refer to Procedure 5-3.

Radiation Dosimetry

The estimated absorbed doses in organs and tissues of an average, 70-kg subject with a normal-functioning thyroid from an oral dose of 100 μCi (3.7 MBq) ^{131}I sodium iodine are shown in Table 5-4.[8]

References

1. Sarkar SD. In vivo thyroid studies. In: "Diagnostic Nuclear Medicine," eds Gottschalk A, Hoffer PB, Potchen EJ. Williams & Wilkins, Baltimore, 1988, pp 756–768.
2. Schultz AL, Jacobson WE. The effect of propylthiouracil on the thyroid uptake of I^{131} and the plasma conversion ratio in hyperthyroidism. J Clin Endocrinol Metab 1952; 12: 1205–1214.
3. Greer MA. The effect on endogenous thyroid activity of feeding desiccated thyroid to normal human subjects. N Engl J Med 1951; 244: 385–390.

4. Pineda G, Clauria H, Rocha AFG, Harbert JC. The thyroid. In: "Textbook of Nuclear Medicine: Clinical Applications," eds Rocha AFG, Harbert JC. Lea & Febiger, Philadelphia, 1979, pp 1–50.

5. Thrall JH. Radiopharmaceuticals for endocrine imaging. In "Pharmaceuticals in Medical Imaging," eds Swanson DP, Chilton HM, Thrall JH. Macmillan, New York, 1990, pp 343–359.

6. International Atomic Energy Agency: Consultants' meeting on the calibration and standardization of thyroid radioiodine uptake measurements, Vienna 1, Kaerntnerring, Austria, November 28–30, 1960. Br J Radiol 1962; 35: 205–210.

7. Bakheet S, Powe J, Hammami MM. The scope of false-positive pulmonary/mediastinal metastasis on radioiodine whole body imaging. Eur J Nucl Med 1994; 21 (Suppl.): S147.

8. Summary of current radiation dose estimates to humans from ^{123}I, ^{124}I, ^{125}I, ^{126}I, ^{130}I, ^{131}I, and ^{132}I as sodium iodide. J Nucl Med 1975; 16: 857–860.

Parathyroid Scintigraphy

Summary Information

Radiopharmaceutical

Adult doses: 1 mCi (37 MBq) of ^{99m}Tc sodium pertechnetate injected intravenously.
20 mCi (740 MBq) of ^{99m}Tc sestamibi injected intravenously.

Pediatric dose: Adjusted according to the patient's weight (see Appendix A-3).

Contraindications Any substance known to interfere with thyroid uptake of ^{99m}Tc pertechnetate can lead to difficulty in distinguishing between parathyroid lesions and normal surrounding tissue (see Table 5-1).

Particularly check whether the patient is taking thyroid medications or recently has had radiographic studies with iodinated contrast media. In such patients, check with the nuclear medicine physician to determine whether the ^{99m}Tc pertechnetate scan is to be performed.

Dose/Scan Interval

^{99m}Tc sodium pertechnetate: Imaging commences about 10 minutes after the injection.

^{99m}Tc sestamibi: Imaging commences immediately after the injection.

Views Obtained Obtain anterior views of the neck (thyroid region and sternum) with a pinhole collimator and anterior views of the chest and neck with a low-energy high-resolution collimator. Single photon emission computed tomography (SPECT) of the chest and neck is required in most patients, especially if no parathyroid tissue is seen in the neck, if suspicious uptake is seen in the chest, or for better localization of a parathyroid adenoma seen on the planar views.

Indications

Parathyroid scintigraphy is indicated for the localization of parathyroid adenomas in patients with hyperparathyroidism. Excessive secretion of parathyroid hormone is generally caused by a solitary adenoma.[1] Scintigraphy is used to localize accurately the parathyroid lesions and is most helpful in patients who have undergone previous neck operations.[2] Normal parathyroid glands usually are not visualized because of their small size.

Principle

Although ^{99m}Tc sestamibi was developed as a myocardial perfusion agent, it also localizes in various tumors. Several recent studies have shown its ability to localize in parathyroid adenomas.[3–5] After IV injection, ^{99m}Tc sestamibi appears to localize very rapidly (less than 5 minutes) in both parathyroid adenomas and thyroid tissue. Its washout from parathyroid adenomas appears to be slow, unlike from normal thyroid tissue, which is characterized by a relatively fast washout over 2–3 hours. For the initial images, ^{99m}Tc pertechnetate is required to permit subtraction of thyroid activity. Small adenomas or hyperplastic glands may not be visualized. The exact mechanism of ^{99m}Tc sestamibi localization in tumors is not known, but it may be related to intracellular mitochondrial accumulation.

Patient Preparation

None.

Instrument Specifications

Gamma camera:	Any large field-of-view system may be used.
Collimator:	Pinhole collimator with a 5–6 mm inset.
	Low-energy high-resolution collimator.
Energy setting:	140 keV, 15–20% window.
Analog formatter:	8 × 10 film, 70-mm (9-on-1) format.
Computer system:	Acquisition requirements—dynamic (128 × 128 word mode matrix), static (128 × 128 word mode matrix), SPECT (128 × 128 matrix).
	Processing requirements—image addition/subtraction, SPECT reconstruction.

Imaging Procedure

1. Check whether the patient is taking thyroid supplement or recently has had iodinated contrast medium. If so, confirm with the physician the need for the ^{99m}Tc pertechnetate scan. If it is not required, proceed with the ^{99m}Tc sestamibi injection.

2. Insert a 21-gauge butterfly infusion set into an antecubital vein. Inject 1 mCi (37 MBq) ^{99m}Tc pertechnetate and wait 10–15 minutes.

3. To reduce motion artifacts, place the patient on the imaging table with the head positioned in a head holder, such as in Figure 5-1. Position the gamma camera with the pinhole collimator at a distance of about 10 cm from the patient's neck surface, as in Figure 5-13, so that the thyroid and sternal region are in the field of view. Note that the thyroid should be positioned to fill the upper 1/3 to 1/2 of the field of view to permit visualization of the sternal region. If necessary, adjust the distance of the collimator from the patient to ensure that the appropriate part of the neck is visualized.

4. Acquire a 10-minute static acquisition on analog formatter. Acquire a dynamic study on computer (10 frames at 1 frame per minute, 128 × 128 matrix). Do not allow the patient to move.

5. Inject the ^{99m}Tc sestamibi and immediately acquire four 5-minute static acquisitions on an analog formatter. Acquire a dynamic study on computer (20 frames at 1 frame per minute, 128 × 128 matrix).

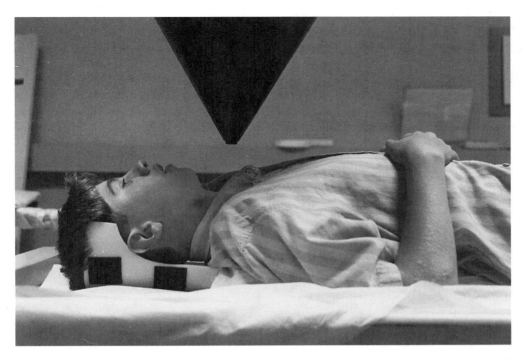

Figure 5-13. Gamma camera positioned over the neck to include thyroid and sternal region in the field of view. Note the use of the head holder to reduce motion artifacts.

6. Change to the low-energy high-resolution collimator, and position the gamma camera over the chest, with the thyroid in the upper part of the field of view. Using a magnification of 1.2–1.5, acquire a 10-minute static view of the chest from the bottom of the heart to the top of the salivary glands on an analog formatter (9-on-1, or 4-on-1 format) and on computer (128 × 128 matrix).

7. Increase the magnification to 2.0–2.5, and acquire a 10-minute static view of the neck and carotid arteries, with the neck extended as far back as possible to visualize the area behind the salivary glands.

8. In most patients, SPECT of the chest and neck region is required for localizing the parathyroid tissue. SPECT acquisition should commence immediately after completion of the planar images. *Note:* If SPECT imaging is not possible, oblique planar images should be acquired to better localize any uptake seen in the chest.

9. SPECT acquisition variables depend on the number of detector heads on the system.
   a. For a single-head system, acquire 60–64 views over 360° into a 128 × 128 word mode matrix at 30–40 seconds per view, using a high-resolution collimator and appropriate body contouring to minimize patient-to-collimator distance.
   b. For a dual-head or triple-head system, acquire views as in step 9a, with the time per frame reduced to 20 seconds per view. *Note:* The time per frame should be increased to 30–40 seconds for large patients (men greater than 100 kg, women greater than 80 kg) or if an ultrahigh-resolution collimator is used (collimator sensitivity less than 150 ct/min per μCi).

10. Delayed planar images should be acquired at 3–4 hours after injection (repeat steps 6 and 7).

Computer Analysis

On computer, first replay the sestamibi and pertechnetate pinhole studies and verify that no patient motion is present. If motion is present, either correct (by X/Y shift of the appropriate images) or eliminate these images from the analysis. Sum the sestamibi and pertechnetate images (Fig. 5-14A and B), and subtract a fraction of the summed pertechnetate image from the summed sestamibi image. The value of the fraction to subtract should be sufficient to eliminate the thyroid gland, thereby permitting better visualization of any parathyroid lesions (Fig. 5-14C). Check that there is no misalignment between the two summed images. If there is, realign the two images (by X/Y shift of one image). Figure 5-14 shows examples of undersubtraction, oversubtraction, correct subtraction, and misalignment between the sestamibi and pertechnetate studies. Display the pertechnetate, sestamibi, and subtraction images on the screen, and obtain a hard copy.

For SPECT studies, perform the following steps:

1. Apply uniformity and center-of-rotation correction to the data (on newer systems, this may be done automatically).
2. If possible, prefilter the planar data (a suggested filter is a Butterworth, order 10–12, cutoff at 0.4–0.5 Nyquist). Increase the cutoff frequency for dual- or triple-head systems.
3. Reconstruct 1-pixel-thick transaxial slices. The back-projection filter may be a Ramp or Ramp-Butterworth with a cut-off at 0.6–0.8 Nyquist.

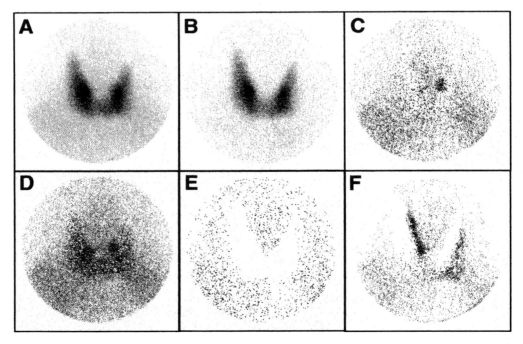

Figure 5-14. Parathyroid study. (**A**) ^{99m}Tc sestamibi image. (**B**) ^{99m}Tc pertechnetate image. (**C–F**) Subtraction images. (**C**) Correct subtraction. (**D**) Undersubtraction. (**E**) Oversubtraction. (**F**) Misalignment of the sestamibi and pertechnetate images.

Interpretation

Aberrant parathyroids can be located anywhere from the salivary glands to the top of the heart. A parathyroid adenoma will appear as a small focal area of increased uptake on the ^{99m}Tc sestamibi images. If the parathyroid is located outside of the thyroid area, it can be seen as an area of focal increased uptake without the use of computer subtraction. However, if the parathyroid is in the thyroid bed, it may be necessary to subtract the thyroid tissue to visualize it, or it may be visualized on the 3-hour image when thyroid activity has washed out. Interpretation may be more difficult in patients with multinodular goiters. In these patients, comparison with the pertechnetate scan and delayed images are particularly important for proper interpretation.

Radiation Dosimetry

The estimated absorbed doses in organs and tissues of an average subject (70 kg) from the administration of 20 mCi (740 MBq) of ^{99m}Tc sestamibi and 1 mCi (37 MBq) of ^{99m}Tc pertechnetate are given in Table 5-8.[6,7]

Table 5-8. Absorbed Radiation Dose Estimates in a 70-kg Adult at Rest After IV Injection of 20 mCi (740 MBq) of ^{99m}Tc Sestamibi and 1 mCi (37 MBq) of ^{99m}Tc Pertechnetate[a]

| | Absorbed Radiation Dose | | | |
| | ^{99m}Tc Sestamibi | | ^{99m}Tc Pertechnetate | |
Tissue	rad/20 mCi	mGy/740 MBq	rad/1 mCi	mGy/37 MBq
Thyroid	0.47	4.7	0.130	1.30
Liver	0.40	4.0	—	—
Gallbladder wall	1.33	13.3	—	—
Small bowel	2.00	20.0	—	—
Upper large intestine	3.60	36.0	0.068	0.68
Lower large intestine	2.80	28.0	0.061	0.61
Stomach wall	0.40	4.0	0.250	2.50
Heart wall	0.33	3.3	—	—
Kidneys	1.33	13.3	—	—
Bladder wall	1.33	13.3	0.053	0.53
Ovaries	1.00	10.0	0.022	0.22
Testes	0.27	2.7	0.009	0.09
Red marrow	0.33	3.3	0.019	0.19
Total body	0.33	3.3	0.014	0.14

[a]Assumes a 2-hr voiding schedule.

References

1. Heath H III, Hodgson SF, Kennedy MA. Primary hyperparathyroidism. Incidence, morbidity and potential economic impact in a community. N Engl J Med 1980; 302: 189–193.
2. Serpell JW, Campbell PR, Young AE. Preoperative localization of parathyroid tumours does not reduce operating time. Br J Surg 1991; 78: 589–590.
3. O'Doherty MJ, Kettle AG, Wells P, Collins RE, Coakley AJ. Parathyroid imaging with technetium-99m-sestamibi: preoperative localization and tissue uptake studies. J Nucl Med 1992; 33: 313–318.
4. Taillefer R, Boucher Y, Potvin C, Lambert R. Detection and localization of parathyroid adenomas in patients with hyperparathyroidism using a single radionuclide imaging procedure with technetium-99m-sestamibi (double-phase study). J Nucl Med 1992; 33: 1801–1807.
5. Palestro CJ, Tomas MB, Attie JN, et al. Parathyroid scintigraphy in primary hyperparathyroidism: thallium-201 and technetium-99m sestamibi (abstract). J Nucl Med 1994; 35: 15P.
6. MIRD/dose estimate report No. 8. Summary of current radiation dose estimates to normal humans from ^{99m}Tc as sodium pertechnetate. J Nucl Med 1976; 17: 74–77.
7. Package insert. Cardiolite. Kit for the preparation of technetium Tc99m sestamibi. E.I. duPont de Nemours Co., 1990.

Adrenal Medullary Scan (mIBG)

Summary Information

Radiopharmaceutical

Adult dose: 500–1,000 µCi (18.5–37 MBq) of [131]I mIBG injected intravenously

or

10 mCi (370 MBq) of [123]I mIBG injected intravenously.

Pediatric dose: Adjusted according to the patient's weight (see Appendix A-3).

Note: Metaiodobenzylguanidine (mIBG) is an analogue of norepinephrine, and theoretically a hypertensive crisis can be precipitated with rapid IV injection. Therefore, the IV injection of radiolabeled mIBG should be by slow infusion over a 20–30 second period.

Contraindications   Medications known or expected to interfere with the uptake of mIBG by the adrenal glands are listed in Table 5-10.

Dose/Scan Interval

[123]I mIBG: Imaging is performed 24 hours after the injection.

[131]I mIBG: Imaging is performed 24–72 hours after the injection.

Views Obtained   Anterior and posterior views of the chest and abdomen. Occasionally, views of the head and extremities are required. With [123]I mIBG, whole-body views should be obtained, and SPECT of the abdomen or other areas may be helpful.

Indications

Radioiodinated mIBG is a highly sensitive screening test for the localization of pheochromocytomas.[1,2] The technique is especially useful in patients in whom conventional anatomic imaging techniques may fail, such as extra-adrenal lesions and locally recurrent and metastatic tumors. In addition to being taken up by pheochromocytomas, radioiodinated mIBG may be used to image neuroblastomas, medullary thyroid carcinoma, paragangliomas, and carcinoid tumors (Table 5-9).[3–6] Lesions with high [131]I mIBG uptake may respond to treatment with large doses of this radiopharmaceutical.[7]

Principle

mIBG is synthesized from the guanidine portion of the antihypertensive drug guanethidine and the benzyl portion of the antiarrhythmic drug bretylium. This agent localizes in cate-

Table 5-9. ^{131}I-mIBG Tumor Imaging Results

Tumor	Tumors With ^{131}I-mIBG Uptake, %	Reference
Carcinoid	71 (67/94)	3
Pheochromocytoma	76 (16/21)	4
Paraganglioma	100 (3/3)	5
Medullary thyroid carcinoma	12 (2/17)	5
Small cell lung carcinoma	0 (0/4)	5

(Data from Khafagi et al.[9])

cholamine storage granules in adrenal medullary cells and adrenergic nerve endings. The mechanism of uptake appears to be primarily an active uptake-1 mechanism in the cell membrane. The mIBG is stored in granules from which it may be released and taken up again by the same mechanism.[8] Drugs that interfere with the study may do so by inhibiting the uptake-1 mechanism, depleting the storage granules, or inhibiting transport of the mIBG.

Patient Preparation

1. [131]I mIBG is an approved agent. However, [123]I mIBG is regulated as an investigational new drug (IND) by the Food and Drug Administration (FDA). Hence, for [123]I mIBG, the patient needs to sign a consent form before the study. The procedure should be fully explained to the patient.
2. Table 5-10 lists drugs known or expected to interfere with the uptake of radiolabeled mIBG.[9] The use of these drugs should be withdrawn for 2 weeks before the study, except for the antidepressants, whose use should be withdrawn 6 weeks before the study. *Note:* In patients with hypertension, blood pressure can be controlled with propranolol and phenoxybenzamine, if needed.
3. The thyroid gland should be adequately "blocked" before the administration of ^{123}I or [131]I mIBG. Patients should be given 10 drops of potassium iodide (Lugol solution) orally, 1–2 days before the injection of radiolabeled mIBG and for the duration of the scanning period.

Instrument Specifications

[131]I mIBG

Gamma camera:	Any large field-of-view system may be used.
Collimator:	High-energy collimator.
Energy setting:	364 keV, 15–20% window.
Analog formatter:	8 × 10 film, 70-mm (9-on-1) format.
Computer system:	Acquisition requirements—static (256 × 256 matrix). Processing requirements—none.

[123]I mIBG—Whole-Body/Planar Study

Gamma camera:	Whole-body views—dual-head large field-of-view system. Planar views—any large field-of-view system may be used.

Table 5-10. Drugs Known or Expected to Decrease mIBG Uptake

Drugs known to decrease mIBG uptake
    Antihypertensive/cardiovascular   Labetalol
                                              Reserpine
                                              Calcium channel blockers
    Antidepressants   Amitriptyline + derivatives
                                                Imipramine + derivatives
                                              Doxepin
                                            Amoxapine
                                              Loxapine
                                              Maprotiline
                                              Trazodone
    Sympathomimetics   Phenylephrine
                                              Phenylpropanolamine
                                              Pseudoephedrine, ephedrine
    Others   Cocaine

Drugs expected to affect mIBG uptake
    Adrenergic neurone blockers   Bethanidine, debrisoquine
                                              Bretylium
                                              Guanethidine
    Antipsychotics   Phenothiazines
                                              Thioxanthenes
                                              Butyrophenones
    Sympathomimetics   Amphetamine + related compounds
                                              Beta-sympathomimetics (systemic use)
                                              Dobutamine
                                              Dopamine
                                              Metaraminol

(Data from Khafagi et al.[9])

Collimator:	Low-energy high-resolution collimator.
Energy setting:	159 keV, 15–20% window.
Analog formatter:	Whole-body—8 × 10 or 10 × 14 film, 2-on-1 format.
	Planar views—8 × 10 film, 70-mm (9-on-1) format.
Computer system:	Acquisition requirements—static (256 × 256 matrix), whole-body (1,024 × 256 matrix).
	Processing requirements—none.

^{123}I mIBG—SPECT Study

Gamma camera:	SPECT—single-, dual-, or triple-head SPECT system with elliptical or body-contouring orbit.
Collimator:	Low-energy high-resolution or all-purpose collimator.
Energy setting:	159 keV, 15–20% window.
Computer system:	Acquisition requirements—SPECT (64 × 64 matrix).
	Processing requirements—SPECT reconstruction

Imaging Procedure

^{123}I mIBG

1. Acquire anterior and posterior whole-body images 24 hours after injection. Images should be acquired at a scan speed of 5 cm/min on the analog formatter and on the computer (1,024 × 256 word mode matrix).
2. Additional spot views of suspicious areas may be requested by the nuclear medicine physician. Spot views should be acquired for 1,000 kct or 20 minutes, whichever is shorter, on an analog formatter and on computer (256 × 256 word mode matrix).
3. If SPECT is required, the following acquisition variables should be used:

   Single-head system: Low-energy all-purpose collimator, 360° elliptical orbit, 64 × 64 word mode matrix. Acquire 60 views at 40 seconds per view with step-and-shoot mode or 120 views at 20 seconds per view with continuous mode. For a 40-cm field-of-view system, no zoom is required. For 50–60 cm field-of-view systems, zoom factor = 1.2.

   Dual- or triple-head system: Low-energy high-resolution collimators, 360° elliptical orbit, 64 × 64 word mode matrix. Acquire a total of 120 views at 15–20 seconds per view with either a step-and-shoot or continuous mode. For a 40-cm field-of-view system, no zoom is required. For 50–60 cm field-of-view systems, zoom factor = 1.2.

^{131}I mIBG

1. At 24 hours after injection, acquire anterior and posterior views of the abdomen and chest for 20 minutes per view.
2. As with ^{123}I mIBG, additional views of suspicious areas may be required. Most tumors are visible at 24 hours; however, a decrease in liver activity with time may allow better visualization of abdominal tumors at 48 or 72 hours.

Computer Analysis

None required for the planar or whole-body image data. SPECT data should be reconstructed as follows:

1. Apply uniformity and center-of-rotation correction to the data (on newer systems, this may be done automatically).
2. If possible, prefilter the planar data (possible filters are Butterworth, order 5–15, cutoff at 0.4–0.6 Nyquist, and Hann filter, cutoff at 0.7–0.9 Nyquist). Dual- and triple-head systems can use sharper filters (increase cutoff frequency).
3. Reconstruct 1-pixel-thick transaxial slices. The back-projection filter may be a Ramp or Ramp-Butterworth with a cutoff at 0.6–0.8 Nyquist.

Information on Film

On each analog and computer film, ensure that the following information is recorded:

1. Patient name and clinic/hospital number
2. Date, type of scan, and radiopharmaceutical
3. Time after injection
4. Orientation of each image (e.g., anterior, posterior)

Interpretation

The normal tracer distribution of radiolabeled mIBG includes faint uptake in the heart, liver, spleen, salivary glands, and occasionally, the colon. These regions of localization reflect the sympathetic innervation of the organs. Excretion of the tracer accounts for activity in the renal collecting system and urinary bladder. Normal adrenal glands are not usually identified with [131]I mIBG, but mild uptake can often be seen with the ^{123}I-labeled agent. Abnormal uptake in the adrenal gland generally is reflected by the asymmetry rather than by the amount of uptake. Suspected adrenal localization of tracer can be confirmed by injecting a small amount of ^{99m}Tc DTPA or ^{99m}Tc DMSA to show the kidneys. Abnormalities in other regions may be more difficult to characterize, and correlative scintigraphic or radiographic imaging is often necessary. Figure 5-15 shows the locations of pheochromocytomas found in a large surgical series[10] and indicates the need to scan the entire abdomen, chest, and neck.

[131]I mIBG imaging has an overall sensitivity of about 76% for the detection of pheochromocytomas.[4] This value increases to nearly 100% with [123]I mIBG, probably making it the most sensitive imaging procedure available for the detection of pheochromocytomas.[2] Table 5-9 summarizes the results obtained with ^{131}I-mIBG imaging in a variety of tumors.[3–5]

Radiation Dosimetry

Human dosimetry for mIBG labeled with both ^{123}I and ^{131}I has been assessed at the University of Michigan Medical Center (Table 5-11). These calculations were based on whole-body retention and tissue distribution data derived from rats. These data were then applied to the standard Medical Internal Radiation Dosimetry (MIRD) formulae. The assumption was made that thyroid uptake has not been blocked with potassium iodide.[11]

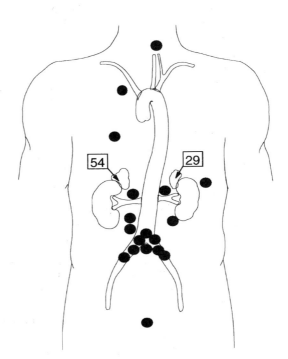

Figure 5-15. Distribution sites of pheochromocytomas seen in 100 patients; 17 patients had tumors in extraadrenal sites. (Adapted from Melicow,[10] with permission.)

Table 5-11. Absorbed Radiation Dose Estimates in a 70-kg Adult From IV Injection of 10 mCi (370 MBq) [123]I mIBG or 500 μCi (18.5 MBq) [131]I mIBG[a]

| | Absorbed Radiation Dose | | | |
| | [131]I mIBG | | [123]I mIBG | |
Tissue	rad/500 μCi	mGy/18.5 MBq	rad/10 mCi	mGy/370 MBq
Thyroid (unblocked)	17.5	175	22	220
Adrenal medulla	50.0	500	8.0	80
Heart wall	0.35	3.50	0.3	3.0
Liver	0.2	2.00	0.5	5.0
Spleen	0.8	8.00	1.4	14.0
Ovaries	0.5	5.00	0.6	6.0
Total body	0.05	0.50	0.2	2.0

[a]Estimated doses assume that thyroid uptake has not been blocked with potassium iodide.

References

1. Shapiro B, Copp JE, Sisson JC, et al. Iodine-131 metaiodobenzylguanidine for the locating of suspected pheochromocytoma: experience in 400 cases. J Nucl Med 1985; 26: 576–585.
2. Mozley PD, Kim CK, Mohsin J, et al. The efficacy of iodine-123-MIBG as a screening test for pheochromocytoma. J Nucl Med 1994; 35: 1138–1144.
3. Hoefnagel CA, Taal BG, Valdes Olmos RA. Role of [131I] metaiodobenzylguanidine therapy in carcinoids. J Nucl Biol Med 1991; 35: 346–348.
4. Swensen SJ, Brown ML, Sheps SG, et al. Use of ^{131}I-MIBG scintigraphy in the evaluation of suspected pheochromocytoma. Mayo Clin Proc 1985; 60: 299–304.
5. Von Moll L, McEwan AJ, Shapiro B, et al. Iodine-131 MIBG scintigraphy of neuroendocrine tumors other than pheochromocytoma and neuroblastoma. J Nucl Med 1987; 28: 979–988.
6. Shapiro B, Fig LM, Gross MD, Khafagi F. Radiochemical diagnosis of adrenal disease. Crit Rev Clin Lab Sci 1989; 27: 265–298.
7. McEwan AJ, Shapiro B, Sisson JC, Beierwaltes WH, Ackery DM. Radio-iodobenzylguanidine for the scintigraphic location and therapy of adrenergic tumors. Semin Nucl Med 1985; 15: 132–153.
8. Smets LA, Loesberg C, Janssen M, Metwally EA, Huiskamp R. Active uptake and extravesicular storage of m-iodobenzylguanidine in human neuroblastoma SK-N-SH cells. Cancer Res 1989; 49: 2941–2944.
9. Khafagi FA, Shapiro B, Fig LM, Mallette S, Sisson JC. Labetalol reduces iodine-131 MIBG uptake by pheochromocytoma and normal tissues. J Nucl Med 1989; 30: 481–489.
10. Melicow MM. One hundred cases of pheochromocytoma (107 tumors) at the Columbia-Presbyterian Medical Center, 1926–1976: a clinicopathological analysis. Cancer 1977; 40: 1987–2004.
11. Swanson DP, Carey JE, Brown LE, et al. Human absorbed dose calculations for iodine 131 and 123 labeled mIBG: A potential myocardial and adrenal medulla imaging agent. In: "Proceedings of the Third International Radiopharmaceutical Dosimetry Symposium." FDA 81-8166, Rockville, MD, 1981, pp 213–224.

Adrenal Cortical Scan (NP-59)

Summary Information

Radiopharmaceutical

Adult dose: 1 mCi (37 MBq) of ^{131}I-6-β-iodomethylnorcholesterol (NP-59). The dose should be injected intravenously over a 2–5 minute period.

Pediatric dose: None has been established.

Notes: 1. NP-59 is an IND, and its use requires physician-sponsored IND approval from the FDA. NP-59 is available from the University of Michigan Medical Center, Division of Nuclear Medicine.

2. NP-59 contains a solubilizing agent, Tween-80, which is a fatty acid ester. Thus, it should be injected slowly over a 2–5 minute period to prevent the endogenous release of histamine.

Contraindications None.

Dose/Scan Interval In general, imaging should commence 3–5 days after the injection (positive findings have been obtained as early as 24 hours after injection).

Views Obtained A posterior view of the abdomen that includes both adrenal glands is obtained. Occasionally, lateral views of the abdomen can be obtained for depth information and to assist in evaluating asymmetric uptake between the left and right adrenal glands.

Indications

NP-59 has a high affinity for the adrenal cortex and has been used to localize and identify abnormal adrenal function in adrenocorticotrophic (ACTH)-independent Cushing syndrome.[1] It also has been used in the evaluation of primary aldosteronism and hyperandrogenism.[2] In addition, the widespread use of abdominal computed tomography (CT) and magnetic resonance imaging (MRI) studies has resulted in NP-59 imaging being used to determine the functional nature of adrenal lesions found incidentally with such studies.[3]

Principle

NP-59 is an iodinated cholesterol analogue that is taken up in the adrenal cortex and some ovarian tumors. The uptake is due to cholesterol being the principal precursor for steroid hormone production.[4] After injection, NP-59 is absorbed into low-density lipoproteins and is eventually extracted by the adrenal cortex. Thus, the uptake of NP-59 reflects the processes of adrenocortical cholesterol uptake and so is affected by any drug or medication that alters cholesterol uptake by the adrenal cortex.[4]

Patient Preparation

1. NP-59 is regulated as an IND by the FDA. An IND approval from the FDA and approval of the institutional review board are required for all studies. In addition, the patient needs to sign a consent form before the study. The procedure should be explained fully to the patient.
2. Several drugs and dietary factors may alter the uptake of NP-59 by the adrenal cortex, including oral contraceptives, excessive salt intake, adrenocorticoids, and dexamethasone.[4] Drugs known to alter NP-59 uptake in the adrenal cortex are listed in Table 5-12. A complete medication history is required of all patients.
3. The thyroid gland should be "blocked" adequately before the administration of NP-59. The patient should be given 10 drops of potassium iodide (Lugol solution) orally 1–2 days before the injection of NP-59 and for 7–10 days afterward.
4. To diminish interference from bowel activity, the patient should be given 10 mg bisacodyl (Dulcolax) nightly for 3 days before the imaging study. Bisacodyl acts only on the colon and does not disturb the enterohepatic circulation of NP-59.[5]
5. Studies for hyperaldosteronism and hyperandrogenism require suppression of adrenal cortical function. The patient should be given 5 mg dexamethasone daily for 7 days before injection of NP-59 and thereafter daily until the end of the scanning period.
6. The patient should fast overnight or at least avoid fatty foods for 8 hours before injection.

Table 5-12. Drugs Known to Affect Adrenal Uptake of NP-59

Drugs and factors that decrease uptake
    Glucocorticoids
    Dexamethasone
    Metabolic inhibitors (e.g., aminoglutethimide)
    Antihypertensive agents
    Antagonists (e.g., spironolactone)
    Excessive salt intake
    Hypercholesterolemia
Drugs and factors that increase uptake
    Metabolic inhibitors (e.g., metyrapone)
    Exogenous adrenocorticotropic hormone
    All diuretics
    All oral contraceptives
    Cholesterol-lowering agents

(Adapted from Gross et al.,[4] with permission.)

Instrument Specifications

Gamma camera:	Any large field-of-view system may be used.
Collimator:	High-energy collimator.
Energy setting:	364 keV, 15–20% window.
Analog formatter:	8 × 10 film, 70-mm (9-on-1) format.
Computer system:	Acquisition requirements—static (256 × 256 matrix).
	Processing requirements—region of interest analysis.

Imaging Procedure

1. At 3, 5, and 7 days after injection, acquire a 20-minute posterior view of the abdomen on analog formatter and on computer (256 × 256 matrix). Occasionally, interfering activity may be seen in the large bowel despite bowel preparation. In such cases, administer an enema and repeat the scan.
2. If quantitation of percent uptake is required, perform the following procedures:
   a. Record the administered dose and the time of injection on the NP-59 uptake worksheet (Fig. 5-16).
   b. Acquire right and left lateral views for 10 minutes per view on computer (256 × 256 matrix). Lateral views need be acquired only once.
   c. In addition, a small aliquot (50 μCi/1.85 MBq) of the injected dose should be retained as a standard. Dilute the standard in 2–3 ml water, and place it in a small flat plastic flask (e.g., a tissue culture flask). Place the flask on the collimator surface, as in Figure 5-17, and obtain a 5-minute static acquisition (256 × 256 matrix). Place a disposable sheet under the flask in case of leakage. *Note:* The standard should be scanned immediately after the patient study. If quantitation is required on several days, rescan the same standard each day.

Computer Analysis

No computer analysis is required for a routine scan. If percent uptake of NP-59 in the adrenal glands is required, process the posterior and lateral images as described next:

1. Analysis requires knowledge of the millimeter per pixel calibration factor for the computer system. If this is not known, acquire an image (256 × 256 matrix) of two ^{57}Co markers placed 10 cm apart along the x-axis or y-axis of the collimator. Measure the separation between the markers in pixels, and compute the millimeter per pixel calibration factor with the following equation:

$$mm/pixel\ calibration\ factor = 100/separation\ in\ pixels$$

This factor should be in the range of 1.5–1.7 mm per pixel for a standard 40-cm field-of-view system.

2. From the left lateral view, measure the distance in pixels from the skin surface to the midpoint of the left adrenal gland. Convert this distance to millimeters by multiplying by the millimeter per pixel calibration factor. Compute the attenuation correction with the following equation:

$$Left\ Adrenal\ Correction\ Factor = e^{(0.011\ \times\ left\ adrenal\ depth\ in\ mm)}$$

Repeat for the right adrenal gland, using the right lateral view.

NP-59 ADRENAL UPTAKE MEASUREMENT

Patient Name : _____

Clinic No. _____   Date : _____

Registration Desk : _____   Age : _____   Sex : o F o M

NP-59 PATIENT / STANDARD DOSE

Pre-injection activity : _____ uCi   Standard activity : _____ uCi (S)

Post-inj. syringe act. : _____ uCi   Time : _____

Net injected activity : _____ uCi (P)   **Ratio of Patient Dose**

Injection Time :   _____   **/ Standard Dose :_____ (R) $\boxed{R = (P/S)}$

ADRENAL GLANDS : DEPTH CORRECTION

System Calibration Factor : _____ mm / pixel (256 x 256 matrix)

RIGHT ADRENAL GLAND	LEFT ADRENAL GLAND
Measured Depth : _____ pixels	Measured Depth : _____ pixels
_____ mm (D_R)	_____ mm (D_L)
Atten. Corr. Factor : _____ (CF_R)	Atten. Corr. Factor : _____ (CF_L)
$\boxed{CF_R = e^{(0.011 \times D_R)}}$	$\boxed{CF_L = e^{(0.011 \times D_L)}}$

CALCULATION OF % UPTAKE

Posterior View Right Adrenal	Adrenal ROI = _____ cts (RC) Area (pixels) = _____ (RA) Background ROI = _____ cts (BR) Area (pixels) = _____ (BA) Adrenal - Bkd Counts = _____ cts (R_{corr}) $\boxed{R_{corr} = RC - BR \times (RA / BA)}$
Posterior View Left Adrenal	Adrenal ROI = _____ cts (LC) Area (pixels) = _____ (LA) Background ROI = _____ cts (BL) Area (pixels) = _____ (BA) Adrenal - Bkd Counts = _____ cts (L_{corr}) $\boxed{L_{corr} = LC - BL \times (LA / BA)}$
Image of Standard	Standard ROI = _____ cts (SC) Adjusted to inj. dose = _____ cts (ID) $\boxed{\text{ID} = SC \times R \times 4 \text{ where} \\ R = \text{ratio of P/S doses}}$
% Uptake	% Uptake Right Adrenal = _____ % $\boxed{100 \times (R_{corr} \times CF_R) / \text{ID}}$ % Uptake Left Adrenal = _____ % $\boxed{100 \times (L_{corr} \times CF_L) / \text{ID}}$

Figure 5-16. Worksheet for the calculation of NP-59 adrenal uptake.

Note: If the adrenal glands are not visualized on the lateral views, adrenal depth can be inferred from kidney depth. This can be measured by ultrasound or from a lateral scan after injection of 100 μCi of ^{99m}Tc DMSA.

3. From the posterior view, draw background and adrenal ROIs, as in Figure 5-18. Determine the left adrenal counts (A_L) and left background counts (B_L), and compute the background-corrected left adrenal counts (A_{CL}) with the following equation:

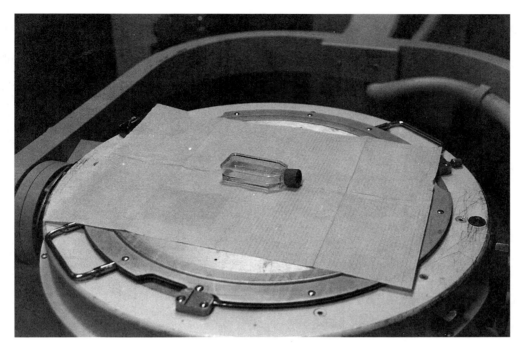

Figure 5-17. NP-59 standard in position on the collimator. A disposable sheet has been placed under the tissue culture flask in case of leakage.

$$A_{CL} = A_L - B_L \times \frac{\text{Left Adrenal ROI (pixels)}}{\text{Background ROI (pixels)}}$$

Repeat for the background-corrected right adrenal gland.

Figure 5-18. Regions of interest drawn over the left and right adrenal glands, with accompanying circumferential background ROIs.

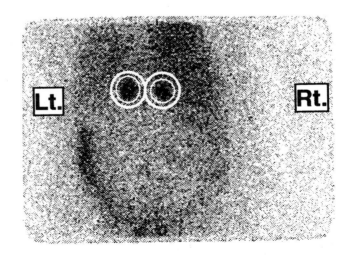

4. Multiply the background-corrected adrenal counts by their corresponding attenuation correction factors to obtain the attenuation-corrected counts.

5. From the image of the standard, draw an ROI around the flask and obtain total counts. Multiply by 4 to convert to total counts per 20 minutes, and then multiply by the ratio of patient-to-standard dose to obtain an estimate of total injected counts, as in the following equation:

$$\text{Total injected cts} = \text{Standard cts} \times 4 \times \frac{\text{Patient Dose (μCi)}}{\text{Standard Dose (μCi)}}$$

6. For the left adrenal gland, divide the results of step 4 by that of step 5 and multiply by 100 to obtain the percent uptake of NP-59, as shown in the following equation:

$$\%\text{Uptake (Left Adrenal)} = \frac{\text{Left adrenal cts (background and attenuation corrected)}}{\text{Total injected cts}} \times 100$$

7. Record the results on the worksheet (see Fig. 5-16). Repeat for the right adrenal gland.

Information on Film

On each analog and computer film, ensure that the following information is recorded:

1. Patient name and clinic/hospital number
2. Date, type of scan, and radiopharmaceutical
3. Time after injection
4. Orientation of each image (e.g., posterior, left lateral)

Interpretation

After intravenous injection of NP-59, significant activity is present in the liver and gallbladder and subsequently in the small bowel and large bowel. The uptake of NP-59 into normal adrenal glands is progressive over several days, with visualization optimum at 4–6 days after injection. The normal percent uptake of NP-59 is about 0.16% of the adminis-

Table 5-13. Absorbed Radiation Dose Estimates in a 70-kg Adult From IV Injection of 1 mCi (37 MBq) NP-59

Tissue	Absorbed Radiation Dose	
	rad/1 mCi	mGy/37 MBq
Adrenals	26.0	260
Liver	2.4	24
Ovaries	8.0	80
Testes	2.3	23
Total body	1.2	12

tered dose per adrenal gland (range, 0.073–0.26%).[6] Adrenal uptake of 0.3% or greater is abnormal. Asymmetry of 2:1 or greater is indicative of adenoma. NP-59 has a sensitivity of 81–100% in the identification of adrenal hyperplasia or adenomas in patients with Cushing's disease.[7]

Radiation Dosimetry

The estimated absorbed radiation doses in the organs and tissues of an average subject (70 kg) from IV injection of 1 mCi (37 MBq) NP-59 are shown in Table 5-13.[8]

References

1. Fig LM, Gross MD, Shapiro B, et al. Adrenal localization in the adrenocorticotrophic hormone-independent Cushing syndrome. Ann Intern Med 1988; 109: 547–553.
2. Miles JM, Wahner HW, Carpenter PC, Salassa RM, Northcutt RC. Adrenal scintiscanning with NP-59, a new radioiodinated cholesterol agent. Mayo Clin Proc 1979; 54: 321–327.
3. Kazerooni EA, Sisson JC, Shapiro B, et al. Diagnostic accuracy and pitfalls of [iodine-131] 6-beta-iodomethyl-19-norcholesterol (NP-59) imaging. J Nucl Med 1990; 31: 526–534.
4. Gross MD, Valk TW, Swanson DP, et al. The role of pharmacologic manipulation in adrenal cortical scintigraphy. Semin Nucl Med 1981; 11: 128–148.
5. Shapiro B, Nakajo M, Gross MD, et al. Value of bowel preparation in adrenocortical scintigraphy. J Nucl Med 1983; 24: 732–734.
6. Gross MD, Valk TW, Freitas JE, et al. The relationship of adrenal iodomethylnorcholesterol uptake to indices of adrenal cortical function in Cushing's syndrome. J Clin Endocrinol Metab 1981; 52: 1062–1066.
7. Goldsmith SJ. Endocrine system. In "Nuclear Medicine: Technology and Techniques," 3rd Edition, eds Bernier DR, Christian PE, Langan JK. Mosby-Year Book Inc., 1994, pp 222–251.
8. Gross MD, Shapiro B, Thrall JH, Freitas JE, Beierwaltes WH. The scintigraphic imaging of endocrine organs. Endocr Rev 1984; 5: 221–281.

111In Pentetreotide Scan

Summary Information

Radiopharmaceutical

Adult dose: 6 mCi (222 MBq) of ^{111}In pentetreotide injected intravenously.

Pediatric dose: Adjusted according to the patient's weight (see Appendix A-3).

Contraindications   Patients with moderate-to-severe renal failure will have a significantly slower clearance, and use of ^{111}In pentetreotide in these patients should be considered carefully.

Dose/Scan Interval   Imaging starts 4 hours after injection of the ^{111}In pentetreotide.

Views Obtained   At 4 hours, obtain anterior and posterior spot views of the area of interest, as requested by the nuclear medicine physician. Although the region to be imaged varies with the type of tumor, the following guidelines should be used for imaging the head and neck, thorax, and lower abdomen:

1. Head and neck views should include a single image of the left axilla, left cervical lymph node chain, and left lateral skull, and a corresponding image of the right axilla, lymph nodes, and skull.
2. Thoracic views should include anterior and posterior views, with a minimal amount of liver and spleen in the field of view.
3. Standard abdominal views should include the liver and spleen. Lower abdominal views should exclude the liver and spleen and include the inferior poles of the kidneys down to the proximal femur.
4. At 24 hours, repeat the spot views obtained at 4 hours, and also acquire anterior and posterior views of the thorax and upper and lower abdomen. SPECT imaging of the known or suspected region of the tumor will generally be requested by the nuclear medicine physician. Additional spot views may be required at 48 hours.

Indications

[111]In pentetreotide is a radiolabeled analog of the neuroendocrine peptide somatostatin. It localizes in tumors expressing somatostatin receptors, including—but not limited to—neuroendocrine tumors. It is used for the scintigraphic localization of the following tumors: carcinoid, islet cell carcinoma, gastrinoma, pheochromocytoma, small cell lung carcinoma, medullary thyroid carcinoma, neuroblastoma, paraganglioma, glucagonoma, pituitary adenoma, meningioma, VIPoma, and insulinoma.[1] Table 5-14 indicates the relative proportion of each type of tumor that has demonstrated uptake of ^{111}In pentetreotide.

Principle

Somatostatin is a neuroregulatory peptide that localizes primarily on tumor cells of neuroendocrine origin. Cell membrane receptors with a high affinity for somatostatin are present in the majority of neuroendocrine tumors, including carcinoids, islet cell carcinomas, and growth hormone producing pituitary adenomas.[2,3] A large number of binding sites have also been reported in other tumors such as meningiomas, breast carcinomas, astrocytomas, and small cell carcinomas of the lung.[4] [111]In DTPA-d-Phe-octreotide (pentetreotide) is a radiolabeled analog of somatostatin that retains many of the features of somatostatin, including its ability to bind to somatostatin receptor sites.[1]

Patient Preparation

The patient should be well hydrated before the ^{111}In pentetreotide is injected. Patients should drink two 8-oz glasses of water before injection and should be instructed to drink frequently for 24 hours after the injection (eight 8-oz glasses of water over 24 hours). The patient should be given one bottle of magnesium citrate laxative to take on the evening before the 24-hour and optional 48-hour imaging studies. If the patient is taking somatostatin therapeutically, it should be discontinued 48 hours or more before the scan. The patient should not take somatostatin until the study is completed or at least until after the imaging dose has been injected.

If the patient is being evaluated for an insulinoma tumor, place an IV catheter/needle set before injecting ^{111}In pentetreotide. A physician should be present, and a syringe containing an IV solution of 50% dextrose should be at the bedside in case of acute hypoglycemia after the injection of ^{111}In pentetreotide. Acute hypoglycemia is possible theoretically because pentetreotide may decrease glucagon levels to the degree that insulin from the tumor could significantly decrease blood levels of glucose.

Instrument Specifications

Gamma camera:	Planar views—any large field-of-view system may be used. Whole-body view—dual-head large field-of-view system.
SPECT:	Single-, dual-, or triple-head system with an elliptical or body contour orbit.
Collimator:	Medium-energy collimator.
Energy setting:	170 keV and 240 keV, 20% energy windows.
Analog formatter:	8 × 10 film, 105-mm (4-on-1) format—spot views.

Table 5-14. [111]In Pentetreotide Tumor Imaging Results

Tumor	Tumors With Uptake of [111]In Pentetreotide, %	Reference
Carcinoid	96 (69/72)	1
Pheochromocytoma	86 (12/14)	1
Medullary thyroid carcinoma	71 (20/28)	1
Paraganglioma	94 (50/53)	5
Small cell lung carcinoma	100 (34/34)	1
Insulinoma	61 (14/23)	1
Glucagonoma	100 (3/3)	1
Gastrinoma	100 (12/12)	1

Computer system: Acquisition requirements—static (256 × 256 matrix), SPECT (64 × 64 matrix).

Processing requirements—SPECT reconstruction.

Imaging Procedure

Planar Imaging

At 4 hours after injection, acquire anterior and posterior spot views of the suspected tumor region for 15 minutes per view on an analog formatter and on computer (256 × 256 word mode matrix). These views should be repeated at 24 hours after injection, and if requested by the nuclear medicine physician, at 48 hours.

SPECT Imaging

SPECT imaging is most helpful in the localization of intra-abdominal tumors. When requested, SPECT studies should be acquired using the following acquisition variables:

Single-head system: 360° elliptical orbit, 64 × 64 word mode matrix, 60–64 views at 30–40 seconds per view. No zoom for 40-cm field-of-view system. Zoom of 1.2 for 50–60 cm field-of-view systems.

Dual- or triple-head system: 360° elliptical orbit, 64 × 64 word mode matrix, with a total of 120 views at 15 seconds per view. No zoom for 40-cm field-of-view system. Zoom of 1.2 for 50–60 cm field-of-view systems.

Computer Analysis

No analysis required for planar/whole-body images. For SPECT studies, perform the following steps:

1. Apply uniformity and center-of-rotation correction to the data (on newer systems, this may be done automatically).
2. If possible, prefilter the planar data (possible filters are Butterworth, order 10, cutoff at 0.4–0.5 Nyquist, and Hann filter with cutoff at 0.8–0.9 Nyquist).
3. Reconstruct 1-pixel-thick transaxial slices. The back-projection filter may be a Ramp or Ramp-Butterworth with a cutoff at 0.6–0.8 Nyquist.

Information on Film

On each analog and computer film, ensure that the following information is recorded:

1. Patient name and clinic/hospital number
2. Type of scan and radiopharmaceutical
3. Date and time of each image after injection
4. Orientation of each image (e.g., anterior, posterior)

Interpretation

In normal subjects, ^{111}In pentetreotide accumulates in the pituitary gland, spleen, liver (especially in patients with low renal clearance), kidneys and urinary bladder, and minimally in the normal thyroid gland. At 24 hours, activity is seen in the gallbladder and in the small bowel. The colon may also be seen depending on the effectiveness of the laxative. Focal areas of increased uptake outside these regions may indicate the presence of tumor. *Note:* Bleomycin or external radiation of the lung may cause local pulmonary accumulation of ^{111}In pentetreotide, particularly along the pleura. Activity may also accumulate at sites of a recent operation. Transient accumulation has been noted in the nasal region and the lung hili in patients with viral infections of the upper respiratory tract.[1]

Table 5-15. Absorbed Radiation Dose Estimates in a 70-kg Adult After IV Injection of 6 mCi (222 MBq) of [111]In Pentetreotide

Tissue	Absorbed Radiation Dose	
	rad/6 mCi	mGy/222 MBq
Kidneys	10.83	108.3
Liver	2.43	24.3
Spleen	14.77	147.7
Uterus	1.27	12.7
Ovaries	0.98	9.8
Testes	0.58	5.8
Red marrow	0.69	6.9
Urinary bladder wall	6.05	60.5
Stomach	1.13	11.3
Small intestine	0.96	9.6
Upper large intestinal wall	1.16	11.6
Lower large intestinal wall	1.55	15.5
Adrenals	1.51	15.1
Thyroid	1.49	14.9

Radiation Dosimetry

The estimated absorbed doses in organs and tissues of an average subject (70 kg) from IV injection of 6 mCi (222 MBq) of ^{111}In pentetreotide are shown in Table 5-15.[6]

References

1. Krenning EP, Kwekkeboom DJ, Bakker WH, et al. Somatostatin receptor scintigraphy with [^{111}In-DTPA-D-Phen1]- and [123I-Tyr 3]-octreotide: the Rotterdam experience with more than 1000 patients. Eur J Nucl Med 1993;20:716–731.
2. Reubi JC, Kvols L, Krenning E, Lamberts SW. Distribution of somatostatin receptors in normal and tmor tissue.
3. Reubi JC, Hacki WH, Lamberts SW. Hormone-producing gastrointestinal tumors contain a high density of somatostatin receptors. J Clin Endocrinol Metab 1987; 65: 1127–1134.
4. Reubi JC, Kvols LK, Waser B, et al. Detection of somatostatin receptors in surgical and percutaneous needle biopsy samples of carcinoids and islet cell carcinomas. Cancer Res 1990; 50: 5969–5977.
5. Kwekkeboom DJ, van Urk H, Pauw BK, et al. Octreotide scintigraphy for the detection of paragangliomas. J Nucl Med 1993; 34: 873–878.
6. Package insert. OctreoScan. Kit for the preparation of Indium In-111 pentetreotide. Mallinckrodt Medical, Inc., St. Louis.

Gastrointestinal System

Brian P. Mullan

Salivary Gland Study

Indications

Salivary gland imaging (nuclear sialography) is indicated in the detection and evaluation of lesions involving the parotid, submandibular, and sublingual glands and in the evaluation of xerostomia (dryness of the mouth). The technique can be used to show alterations in secretory function and may be helpful in establishing the diagnosis of Warthin's tumor and in the evaluation of patients after radiotherapy to the head and neck.[1]

Principle

Several different ions, including the iodides and the pertechnetate ion, are actively trapped and secreted by the epithelial cells of the intralobular ducts, which are distributed uniformly throughout the three pairs of salivary glands. Gustatory stimulation, usually by means of citric acid, can be used to evaluate pertechnetate washout from the salivary glands.

Patient Preparation

The patient should fast for 2 hours before the study.

Instrument Specifications

Gamma camera: Any large field-of-view system can be used.

Collimator: Low-energy, high-resolution collimator.

Zoom factor:	Use a zoom of approximately 2.0–2.5 depending on the gamma camera field of view.
Energy setting:	140 keV, 20% energy window.
Analog formatter:	8 × 10 film, 70-mm (9-on-1) format.
Computer system:	Acquisition requirements—static (256 × 256 matrix), dynamic (64 × 64 matrix). Processing requirements—region of interest (ROI) analysis, curve generation.

Imaging Procedure

1. Before commencing the study, prepare a citric acid solution by mixing a 1:1 solution of lemon juice and water.[2] Draw 3 ml of the solution into a 3-ml syringe. Cut off the needle of a butterfly infusion set, and attach the tubing to the syringe, as shown in Figure 6-1.
2. With the detector facing horizontally, have the patient sit upright with the neck extended in front of the gamma camera.
3. Set the zoom factor on the gamma camera to include the head and neck in the field of view.
4. Inject 10 mCi (370 MBq) of ^{99m}Tc sodium pertechnetate intravenously.
5. Immediately after administration, obtain an anterior blood pool image of the head and neck for 500 kct on analog formatter and on computer (256 × 256 matrix).
6. At 10 minutes after the injection, obtain a 500-kct anterior view, and note the imaging time. Acquire left lateral and right lateral views of the head and neck for the same time.
7. To determine the washout of pertechnetate from the salivary glands, orient the patient to acquire an anterior view of the head and neck, as in step 2.
8. Set up and start the acquisition of a 20-minute dynamic study (64 × 64 word mode matrix, 40 frames at 30 seconds per frame) on a computer.
9. After 10 minutes, insert tubing into the patient's mouth and administer the citric acid solution. Have the patient hold the solution in the mouth for 30 seconds and then swallow. Ask the patient not to move the head during this process, because movement will affect ROI analysis of the dynamic study.
10. After completion of the dynamic study, repeat step 6, using the same time per frame as used for the 10-minute 500 kct anterior view. Label the views as "after citric acid."

Information on Film

On each analog and computer film, ensure that the following information is recorded:

1. Patient name and clinic/hospital number
2. Type of scan and radiopharmaceutical
3. Date and time of each image after injection and after citric acid
4. Orientation of each image (e.g., anterior, posterior, etc.)

Computer Analysis

With ROI analysis, select the dynamic study and draw irregular ROIs over each parotid and submandibular gland. The sublingual glands generally are too small for accurate analysis. Generate time–activity curves of the uptake and washout of pertechnetate from each gland. Mark on the curves the time of citric acid administration.

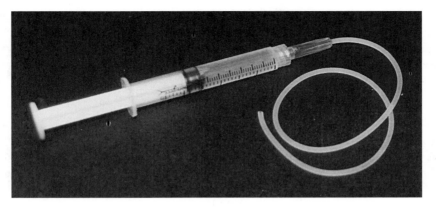

Figure 6-1. A 3-ml syringe and butterfly tubing containing a 1:1 solution of lemon juice and water.

Interpretation

In normal subjects, the uptake of the pertechnetate ion in all three sets of glands is rapid. The uptake should be uniform and symmetric. After administration of citric acid, a significant discharge of activity should occur, as shown in Figure 6-2.

Bilaterally decreased uptake and a blunted response to citric acid stimulation are often seen in certain types of vascular and connective tissue diseases (e.g., Sjögren's syndrome), in acute parotitis, and in some elderly persons. Unilaterally decreased uptake or absence of uptake may be seen in congenital aplasia or obstructive sialolithiasis and after surgical removal of a gland or radiotherapy to the head and neck.[3]

In general, this procedure is not capable of identifying salivary gland lesions. However, some tumors, such as Warthin's tumor, actively concentrate pertechnetate and appear as focal areas of increased uptake. Most metastatic lesions appear as cold areas, whereas benign lesions may show normal or decreased uptake.

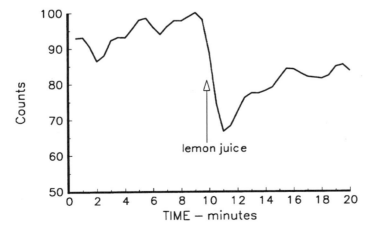

Figure 6-2. Uptake and washout of ^{99m}Tc pertechnetate from a normal parotid gland following citric acid stimulation.

Table 6-1. Absorbed Radiation Dose Estimates in a 70-kg Adult After Intravenous Administration of 10 mCi (370 MBq) ^{99m}Tc Sodium Pertechnetate

Tissue	Absorbed Radiation Dose	
	rad/10 mCi	mGy/370 MBq
Bladder wall	0.53	5.3
Stomach wall	2.50	25.0
Upper large intestinal wall	0.69	6.9
Lower large intestinal wall	0.61	6.1
Red marrow	0.19	1.9
Testes	0.09	0.9
Ovaries	0.22	2.2
Thyroid	1.30	13.0
Brain	0.14	1.4
Total body	0.14	1.4

Additional Note

If the initial views show considerable radioactivity in the mouth, ask the patient to drink a glass of water and then continue study.

Radiation Dosimetry

The estimated absorbed doses in organs and tissues of an average subject (70 kg) from the IV injection of 10 mCi (370 MBq) of ^{99m}Tc sodium pertechnetate are shown in Table 6-1.[4]

References

1. Klein RC. Salivary gland imaging. In "Manual of Nuclear Medicine Procedures," 4th Edition, eds Carey JC, Klein RC, Keyes JW. CRC Press, Baton Rouge, LA, 1983, pp 102–103.
2. Blue PW, Jackson JH. Stimulated salivary gland clearance of technetium-99m pertechnetate. J Nucl Med 1985; 26: 308–311.
3. Parret J, Peyrin JO. Radioisotope investigations in salivary pathology. Clin Nucl Med 1979; 4: 250–261.
4. MIRD Dose Estimate Report No. 8. Summary of current radiation dose estimates to normal humans from ^{99m}Tc as sodium pertechnetate. J Nucl Med 1976; 17: 74–77.

Esophageal Scintigraphy

Summary Information

Radiopharmaceutical

Adult dose: Each bolus contains 200 μCi (7.4 MBq) of ^{99m}Tc sulfur colloid added to
1. 10 ml of water (water bolus)
2. 0.7 g of gelatin and 2 ml of water (bolus 1)
3. 2 g of gelatin and 2 ml of water (bolus 2)

Pediatric dose: Adjusted according to patient's weight (see Appendix A-3).

Contraindications This study requires the cooperation of the patient and should not be performed in patients who are comatose or uncooperative.

Dose/Scan Intervals Imaging begins immediately after the radiolabeled bolus is placed in the patient's mouth.

Views Obtained Obtain a posterior view of the head, neck, and chest.

Indications

Esophageal scintigraphy is used in the evaluation of various esophageal disorders such as achalasia, scleroderma, diffuse esophageal spasm, nonspecific motor disorders, and Nutcracker's esophagus.[1–4] Esophageal scintigraphy can also be used to assess oropharyngeal function, particularly in stroke patients.

Principle

The complete esophageal scintigraphy study requires that the patient swallow three different boluses.[5] Bolus 1 is water, and boluses 2 and 3 are semisolid boluses of different viscosity (Fig. 6-3). Dynamic scintigraphy permits visualization of the transit of the bolus from the oral cavity through the esophagus to the stomach. It also permits measurement of transit time. Patients with the conditions listed under "Indications" may have delayed, fragmented, or absent esophageal transit of the boluses. Also, some patients exhibit reflux from the stomach into the esophagus (gastroesophageal reflux), and some stroke patients may aspirate activity into the lungs.

Patient Preparation

The patient should drink a glass of water immediately before the study to lubricate the mouth and to prepare for the study.

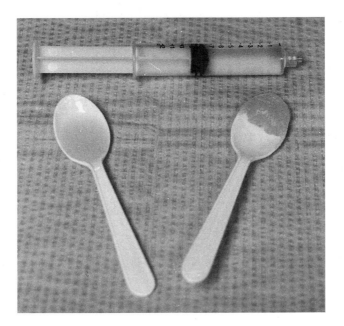

Figure 6-3. A 10-ml water bolus and semisolid boluses 1 and 2.

Bolus Preparation

Semisolid Boluses (Boluses 1 and 2)

1. For the two semisolid boluses, 0.7 g and 2.0 g of powdered gelatin (Jell-O Instant Pudding; General Foods Corp.), or an equivalent alternative, are required.
2. Weigh the required amount of gelatin powder, and transfer it to a 100-ml disposable plastic container.
3. Add 200 µCi (7.4 MBq) of ^{99m}Tc sulfur colloid in 0.1 ml to the gelatin powder, and place the plastic container in a suitable shielded area.
4. Add 2.0 ml of water to the container, and stir the contents with a spoon until the powder is completely dissolved.
5. Leave the gelatin to set for 5 minutes, after which it is ready to be used in the study.
6. After giving the dose to the patient, count the container and spoon and record the administered activity. Discard the spoon and plastic container in the radioisotope waste container.

Water Bolus

Draw 200 µCi (7.4 MBq) of ^{99m}Tc sulfur colloid in a volume of 0.5 ml or less into a 10-ml syringe. Next, draw enough water in the syringe to bring the total volume to 10 ml.

Instrument Specifications

Gamma camera:	Any large field-of-view system can be used.
Collimator:	Low-energy, all-purpose or low-energy, high-sensitivity collimator may be used.
Energy setting:	140 keV, 15–20% energy window.
Computer system:	Acquisition requirements—dynamic (64 × 64 matrix), static (256 × 256 matrix).

Processing requirements—ROI analysis, curve generation, image manipulation (condensed image generation).

Imaging Procedure

For each of the boluses, set up a two-phase dynamic acquisition. Phase 1 should acquire 128 frames at 0.25 seconds per frame. Phase 2 should acquire 96 frames at 1 second per frame. All data should be acquired in a 64 × 64 matrix (word or byte mode).

Note: A test run should be performed with 10 ml of nonradioactive water to lubricate the patient's mouth and to ensure that the patient understands the procedure.

1. ^{99m}Tc water bolus: The patient should be supine on the imaging table, with the camera positioned underneath the patient. This will eliminate the effect of gravity. The patient's mouth should be at the top of the field of view and the stomach at the bottom. Remove the needle and insert the tip of the syringe into the patient's mouth. Start the computer acquisition, and 1–2 seconds later, inject the 10 ml into the mouth, and ask the patient to swallow the entire bolus. The patient should be requested to perform dry swallows at 20, 40, 60, and 80 seconds. Record the times of the dry swallows on the worksheet (Fig. 6-4). Acquisition will take approximately 2 minutes. *Note:* Do not proceed with bolus 1 and 2 studies if more than 50% of the activity remains in the esophagus after the water bolus study. Ask the patient to drink a glass of water to clear the residual activity. If this fails, the study should be terminated.

2. Bolus 1 (0.7 g gelatin): The patient should be positioned upright with the back to the gamma camera, as shown in Figure 6-5. Again, the mouth should be at the top of the field of view and the stomach at the bottom. The patient should be instructed to turn the head to one side (this permits better visualization of the mouth and pharynx). Inform the patient that no mastication of the bolus is allowed. Give bolus 1 by spoon (Fig. 6-5), and have the patient swallow 1 second after computer acquisition begins. Dry swallows should be performed at 20, 40, 60, and 80 seconds. Give the patient a small cup of water (about 50 ml) to swallow at 100 seconds. This water bolus should be swallowed as quickly as possible and should not be sipped over a prolonged time. Record the times of the dry and water swallows on the worksheet (see Fig. 6-4).

3. Bolus 2 (2 g of gelatin): The procedure for bolus 2 is identical to that of bolus 1.

For stroke patients, anterior and posterior static images of the lungs should be acquired immediately after the bolus studies. Data should be acquired in a 256 × 256 word mode for 5 minutes. Additional static images should be acquired at 2 and 4 hours after the bolus studies.

Computer Analysis

Select the bolus study to be analyzed. If available, display the dynamic studies in a condensed image format.[6] This format condenses each 64 × 64 matrix image of the dynamic study by summing all rows so that a 64 × 64 matrix image is compressed into a 64 × 1 matrix. In this manner, x resolution is lost, but y resolution is retained, allowing 64 such compressed images to be stored in a 64 × 64 matrix (Fig. 6-6). Conventional analysis of the data requires placement of ROIs over the proximal, middle, and distal portions of the esophagus (Fig. 6-7) and generating time-activity curves. From either the curves or the condensed images, an estimate of bolus transit time can be obtained. For the static images of the lungs, adjust the contrast on the computer to permit better visualization of low levels of activity. Generate a hard copy of the lung images adjusted in this manner.

ESOPHAGEAL SCINTIGRAPHY

Patient Name : _____

Clinic No. _____   Date : _____

BOLUS TYPE	Time of dry swallows (secs)				50 ml water swallow
	20	40	60	80	100
Water Bolus					
Bolus 1					
Bolus 2					

Please record the actual times of the dry and wet swallows performed
by the patient for each bolus study

Notes : 1) Did the patient have difficulty initiating swallow of the bolus

      water bolus   o YES   o NO

      bolus 1   o YES   o NO

      bolus 2   o YES   o NO

  2) Please indicate if bolus could not be cleared from the esophagus

      water bolus   _____

      bolus 1   _____

      bolus 2   _____

  3) Please indicate any other problems encountered during the study

      _____

      _____

      _____

Technologist : _____

Figure 6-4. Esophageal scintigraphy worksheet.

Information on Film

On each computer film, ensure that the following information is recorded:

1. Patient name and clinic/hospital number
2. Date, type of scan, radiopharmaceutical, and bolus number (water, 1, or 2)
3. Time of dry swallows for the 3 boluses, and nonradioactive water swallow for boluses 1 and 2
4. Orientation of each image (e.g., posterior)

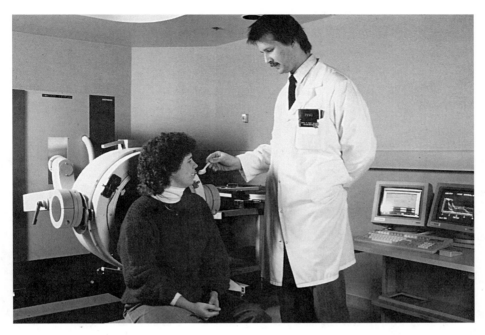

Figure 6-5. Position of patient for semisolid (bolus 1 and 2) studies.

Interpretation

In a normal subject, all three boluses should demonstrate smooth transit through the esophagus into the stomach in less than 10 seconds (see Fig. 6-6B). Occasionally, with the most viscous bolus (bolus 2), there may be some fragmentation or holdup, which should clear with repeated dry swallows. At the other extreme, in patients with achalasia, no progression of the bolus into the stomach may occur, despite repeated dry swallows and swallowing of additional glasses of water. In stroke patients, esophageal function may be normal, but oropharyngeal function may be abnormal. Delayed images in stroke patients can be helpful in determining aspiration of activity into the lungs.

Additional Notes

1. Many patients with esophageal disorders have difficulty in initiating swallowing and in swallowing at the prescribed times. Use the worksheet (see Fig. 6-4) to note any time that is different from the recommended times listed on the worksheet.
2. If the patient is nervous or worried, give additional glasses of water between esophageal studies to lubricate the mouth. Additional water may also be needed between studies if residual activity from the preceding study is seen.
3. Stroke patients require additional views at 5 minutes and at 2 and 4 hours after administration of the boluses.

Radiation Dosage

The estimated absorbed doses in organs and tissues of an average subject (70 kg) from the oral ingestion of 600 µCi (22.2 MBq) of ^{99m}Tc sulfur colloid are shown in Table 6-2.[7]

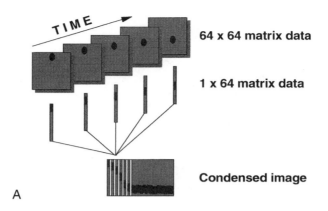

64 x 64 matrix data

1 x 64 matrix data

Condensed image

A

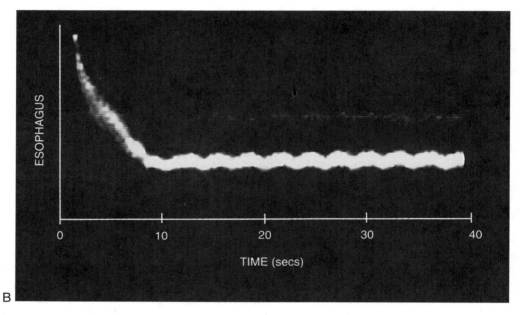

B

Figure 6-6. (A) Condensed image is created by compressing each 64 × 64 matrix image into a 1 × 64 matrix image and displaying the compressed images side-by side. (B) Condensed image showing regular progression of a water bolus through the esophagus of a normal patient.

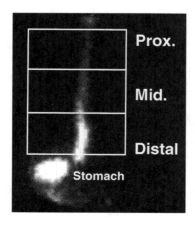

Figure 6-7. ROI analysis of esophageal transit, showing the placement of the proximal, mid, and distal ROIs on a posterior view of the esophagus and stomach.

Table 6-2. Absorbed Radiation Dose Estimates in a 70-kg Adult
From the Oral Administration of ^{99m}Tc Sulfur Colloid

Tissue	Absorbed Radiation Dose	
	rad/600 μCi	mGy/22.2 MBq
Stomach	0.084	0.84
Small intestine	0.156	1.56
Upper large intestine	0.288	2.88
Lower large intestine	0.198	1.98
Ovaries	0.058	0.58
Testes	0.003	0.03
Total body	0.011	0.11

References

1. Klein HA, Wald A. Esophageal transit scintigraphy. In "Nuclear Medicine Annual 1988," eds Freedman LM, Weissmann HS. Raven Press, New York, 1988, pp 79–124.
2. Datz FL. The role of radionuclide studies in esophageal disease. J Nucl Med 1984; 25: 1040–1045.
3. Taillefer R, Beauchamp G, Duranceau AC, Lafontaine E. Nuclear medicine and esophageal surgery. Clin Nucl Med 1986; 11: 445–460.
4. O'Connor MK, Byrne PJ, Keeling P, Hennessy TP. Esophageal scintigraphy: applications and limitations in the study of esophageal disorders. Eur J Nucl Med 1988; 14: 131–136.
5. Kim CH, Hsu JJ, O'Connor MK, et al. Effect of viscosity on oropharyngeal and esophageal emptying in man. Dig Dis Sci 1994; 39: 189–192.
6. Klein HA, Wald A. Computer analysis of radionuclide esophageal transit studies. J Nucl Med 1984; 25: 957–964.
7. Kit for the preparation of Technetium Tc 99m sulfur colloid. Technical product data. Amersham Healthcare, June 1993.

Gastroesophageal Reflux–Adults

Summary Information

Radiopharmaceutical

Administered dose: 300 μCi (11.1 MBq) of ^{99m}Tc sulfur colloid in a mixture of orange juice and dilute hydrochloric acid (total volume = 300 ml).

Contraindications   Recent gastrointestinal surgery, or conditons which prevent binder inflation.

Dose/Scan Interval   Imaging should be started within 10 minutes after ingestion of the ^{99m}Tc sulfur colloid.

Views Obtained   Obtain an anterior view of the stomach and esophagus.

Indications

The most accurate technique for the detection of gastroesophageal reflux is 24-hour pH monitoring. However, this test involves placement of an esophageal probe and is not practical or well tolerated in some patients. By comparison, radionuclide imaging is a simple noninvasive test that is well tolerated and has a sensitivity of 70–80% and a specificity of 93–100%.[1–3] It is indicated in patients with symptoms of gastroesophageal reflux, such as esophagitis, chest pain, and regurgitation.

Principle

To evaluate the integrity of the gastroesophageal sphincter, this test uses an acidified solution in conjunction with an abdominal binder to maximize the stress on the sphincter. This test permits quantitative evaluation of the degree of reflux into the esophagus by noting the activity in the esophagus relative to that in the stomach.

Patient Preparation

The patient should begin to fast at 8:00 PM the evening before the test. Explain the procedure fully to the patient. Question the patient about any recent abdominal operation that may cause discomfort with the abdominal binder.

Preparation of Radiolabeled Juice

Mix 300 μCi (11.1 MBq) of ^{99m}Tc sulfur colloid into a solution of 150 ml orange juice and 150 ml 0.1 N hydrochloric acid. Place the solution in a disposable cup. The entire volume should be administered to the patient.

Instrument Specifications

Gamma camera:	Any large field-of-view system can be used.
Collimator:	Low-energy, all-purpose collimator
Energy setting:	140 keV, 15–20% window for ^{99m}Tc.
Additional items:	Abdominal binder with sphygmomanometer (Model 14-390, W.M. Baum and Co., Copiague, NY).
Analog formatter:	Not required.
Computer system:	Acquisition requirements—static images (64 × 64 word mode matrix). Processing requirements—ROI analysis.

Imaging Procedure

1. Instruct the patient to drink the 300-ml solution containing the ^{99m}Tc sulfur colloid.
2. The patient should then be fitted with the abdominal binder, as shown in Figure 6-8. Ensure that the inflatable bladder is positioned over the stomach but below the costal margin.
3. Position the patient supine on the imaging table, with the gamma camera placed anteriorly. The gamma camera should be positioned so that the stomach is in the lower portion of the field of view.
4. Check the persistence image to ensure that no activity remains in the esophagus. If activity is present, give the patient 15 ml of water to clear the residual activity into the stomach.
5. Acquire a static view on the computer for 30 seconds (64 × 64 word mode matrix).
6. Inflate the abdominal binder to a pressure of 20 mm Hg, and repeat step 5.
7. Repeat step 5 at pressures of 40, 60, 80, and 100 mm Hg. Do not deflate the binder between the pressure levels.
8. After acquisition of the image at 100 mm Hg, deflate the binder and acquire a final postdeflation image.

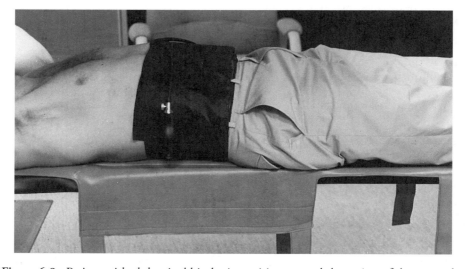

Figure 6-8. Patient with abdominal binder in position around the region of the stomach.

Additional Notes

1. As abdominal pressure increases, the stomach should appear to move up in the field of view. If the stomach moves down, the binder has been placed too high. In this case, deflate the binder, position it lower on the abdomen, and repeat steps 5–8.[4]
2. The images should be acquired as quickly as possible to minimize patient discomfort.
3. An increase in abdominal pressure of 20 mm Hg corresponds to an increase of about 5 mm Hg in pressure across the gastroesophageal sphincter.[4]

Computer Analysis

1. Review all the images. Adjust the contrast to set the maximum brightness to 5–10% of maximum, and check the images for activity in the esophagus.
2. On the first supine image (0 mm Hg), draw an ROI around the entire stomach and note stomach counts (S). Draw an ROI over the esophagus and a background ROI of equal size adjacent to it, as shown in Figure 6-9. Note the counts in the esophageal region (E) and background region (B), and record them on the worksheet (Fig. 6-10).
3. On subsequent images, draw the esophageal and background ROIs, and record the counts in these ROIs on the worksheet.
4. For each abdominal pressure, perform background correction and compute the gastro-esophageal reflux as shown in Figure 6-10.

Information on Film

On each computer film, ensure that the following information is recorded:

1. Patient name and clinic/hospital number
2. Date, type of scan, and radiopharmaceutical
3. Time/abdominal pressure of each image
4. Orientation of each image (e.g., anterior)

Interpretation

In normal subjects, the gastroesophageal reflux should be less than 5% at any pressure level. Reflux greater than 5% is considered abnormal and can usually be visualized on the static images.

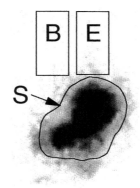

Figure 6-9. Image of the stomach and esophagus showing the placement of regions of interest around the stomach (S), esophagus (E), and background (B).

GASTROESOPHAGEAL REFLUX

Patient Name : _____

Clinic No. _____   Date : _____

Stomach Region of Interest (S)	Total Counts : _____ (S)

Abdominal Pressure	Esophageal Region		Background Region		Esoph - Bkg	GE Reflux
	Counts (EC)	Size (ES)	Counts (BC)	Size (BS)	Counts (EB)	(%)
0 mm Hg						
20 mm Hg						
40 mm Hg						
60 mm Hg						
80 mm Hg						
100 mm Hg						

Notes :

$$\text{Esoph - Bkg Counts (EB)} = EC - BC \times \frac{ES}{BS}$$

$$\% \text{ GE Reflux} = \frac{EB}{S} \times 100$$

Technologist : _____

Figure 6-10. Worksheet for recording gastric, esophageal, and background counts, and for calculation of gastroesophageal reflux.

Table 6-3. Absorbed Radiation Dose Estimates in a 70-kg Adult After Oral Administration of 300 μCi (11.1 MBq) of ^{99m}Tc Sulfur Colloid

Tissue	Absorbed Radiation Dose	
	rad/300 μCi	mGy/11.1 MBq
Stomach	0.04	0.42
Small intestine	0.08	0.78
Upper large intestine	0.14	1.44
Lower large intestine	0.10	0.99
Ovaries	0.03	0.29
Testes	0.00	0.03
Whole body	0.01	0.11

Radiation Dosimetry

The estimated absorbed doses in organs and tissues of an average subject (70 kg) from the oral ingestion of 300 μCi (11.1 MBq) of ^{99m}Tc sulfur colloid are given in Table 6-3.[5]

References

1. Seibert JJ, Byrne WJ, Euler AR, Latture T, Leach M, Campbell M. Gastroesophageal reflux—the acid test: scintigraphy or the pH probe? AJR 1983; 140: 1087–1090.
2. Le Luyer B, Texte D, Segond G, et al. Value of gastroesophageal scintigraphy for the detection of gastroesophageal reflux in infants. J Radiol 1983; 64: 693–697.
3. Blumhagen JD, Rudd TG, Christie DL. Gastroesophageal reflux in children: radionuclide gastroesophagography. AJR 1980; 135: 1001–1004.
4. Vitti RA, Malmud LS. Gastrointestinal system. In "Nuclear Medicine: Technology and Techniques" 3rd Edition, eds Bernier DR, Christian PE, Langan JK. Mosby Year Book, St. Louis, 1994, pp 302–334.
5. Kit for the preparation of Technetium Tc99m sulfur colloid. Technical product data. Amersham Healthcare, June 1993.

Gastroesophageal Reflux–Children

Summary Information

Radiopharmaceutical	Administered dose: 100–1,000 µCi (3.7–37 MBq) ^{99m}Tc sulfur colloid in milk or formula feed. The ^{99m}Tc sulfur colloid should be mixed to give a concentration of 5 µCi/ml (185 kBq/ml). The ingested volume of radiolabeled milk or formula will vary between 20 and 200 ml depending on the size of the child.
Contraindications	None.
Dose/Scan Interval	Imaging should commence during ingestion of the milk.
Views Obtained	Obtain a posterior view of the esophagus during ingestion of the milk/formula and an anterior or a posterior view of the stomach and esophagus after ingestion.

Indications

The most accurate technique for the detection of gastroesophageal reflux is 24-hour pH monitoring. However, this test involves placement of an esophageal probe and is not practical or well tolerated in some patients. By comparison, radionuclide imaging is a simple noninvasive test that is well tolerated and has a sensitivity of 70–80% and a specificity of 93–100%.[1–3] It is indicated in children with symptoms of gastroesophageal reflux, such as failure to thrive, gagging, and pneumonia that is due to aspiration.

Principle

Gastroesophageal reflux in children is a different entity from that seen in adults. Some reflux is common in many children, because of the different anatomic configuration of the gastroesophageal junction as compared with that of adults. Quantitation of the severity of reflux is based on both the severity and frequency of the reflux.[4] This procedure is more extensive than that used in adults, and in addition to the evaluation of gastroesophageal reflux, it provides some information on esophageal transit and gastric emptying.

Patient Preparation

The procedure should be performed at or close to the time that the child usually feeds. The child should not eat immediately before the study. Explain the procedure fully to the

291

parent or guardian. Request the parent or guardian to bring a change of clothing for the infant in case of vomiting or spillage of the radiolabeled milk.

Preparation of Radiolabeled Milk/Formula

Mix 1 mCi (37 MBq) of ^{99m}Tc sulfur colloid into 200 ml of milk or formula. Depending on the age of the child, place the radiolabeled milk in either a disposable bottle or cup. The child should consume a volume of milk consistent with the usual feeding habits.

Instrument Specifications

Gamma camera:	Any large field-of-view system can be used.
Collimator:	Low-energy, all-purpose or high-sensitivity collimator.
Energy setting:	140 keV, 15–20% window for ^{99m}Tc.
Additional items:	Lead sleeve to shield activity in the infant's bottle from the detector.
Analog formatter:	Not required.
Computer system:	Acquisition requirements—dynamic and static images (64 × 64 matrix) Processing requirements—ROI analysis, curve generation, and image summation.

Imaging Procedure

1. Place the patient in a sitting or semirecumbent position with the back to the gamma camera, as shown in Figure 6-11. The field of view should include the mouth, esophagus, and stomach.
2. Place the feeding bottle in the lead sleeve (to shield the detector), and allow the patient to begin feeding.
3. During the meal, acquire three dynamic acquisitions on computer to evaluate esophageal transit of the milk. Each study should be acquired for 100 seconds at 0.5 seconds per frame and stored in a 64 × 64 byte mode matrix. Acquisitions should be performed at the beginning, at the end, and half-way through the meal.
4. After completion of the meal, give the patient a small amount of unlabeled milk to clear the residual activity from the mouth and esophagus. Small infants should be burped. Note the volume of milk or formula consumed.
5. Now, reposition the patient supine on the imaging table, with the detector positioned either anteriorly or posteriorly over the stomach and esophagus.
6. Acquire a dynamic study on computer for 60 minutes at 3 seconds per frame into a 64 × 64 matrix.
7. At 1 hour, acquire anterior and posterior 5-minute static images of the lungs on computer (256 × 256 matrix) to check for aspiration.
8. Repeat step 7 at 2 hours and 24 hours (10-minute acquisition) to check for aspiration.

Additional Notes

1. If the infant was fed through a nasogastric tube, it is not necessary to acquire the early dynamic studies for evaluation of esophageal transit. The nasogastric tube should be removed before the 1-hour dynamic study, because activity in the tube may be mistaken for reflux.

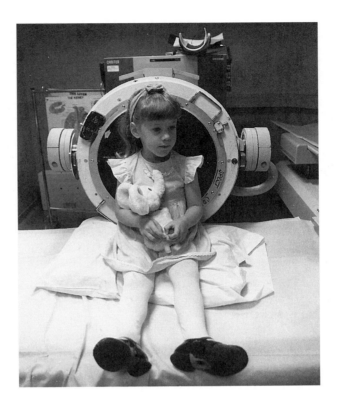

Figure 6-11. Patient in a sitting position with the detector positioned posteriorly over the esophagus.

2. Any abnormal foci of activity on the 1-, 2-, or 24-hour static images should be carefully evaluated to exclude contamination from vomit or regurgitation.

Computer Analysis

1. The three dynamic studies during feeding should be viewed in cine mode to evaluate esophageal transit.
2. On the 1-hour dynamic study, draw ROIs over the entire esophagus and over the upper half of the esophagus. Generate time-activity curves from these regions, and note the number of episodes of reflux. Obtain a hard copy of selected frames demonstrating reflux.
3. Reframe the 1-hour dynamic study by summing every 10 frames to condense the study from 1,200 to 120 frames. Draw an ROI around the stomach on the first image. Generate a time-activity curve of gastric activity over 1 hour.
4. Perform decay correction to the curve, and determine the fraction of activity remaining in the stomach at 1 hour. This is usually in the range of 50–70% of the initial value.[5]

Information on Film

On each computer film, ensure that the following information is recorded:

1. Patient name and clinic/hospital number
2. Date, type of scan, and radiopharmaceutical
3. Time and orientation of each image
4. A hard copy should be made of all ROIs and time–activity curves

Table 6-4. Absorbed Radiation Dose Estimates in a Pediatric Population After Oral Administration of 100 μCi (3.7 MBq) of ^{99m}Tc Sulfur Colloid

Tissue	Absorbed Radiation Dose, Rad per 100 μCi (mGy/ 3.7 MBq)				
	Newborn	1-Year-Old	5-Year-Old	10-Year-Old	15-Year-Old
Stomach	0.38 (3.83)	0.09 (0.93)	0.05 (0.51)	0.03 (0.31)	0.02 (0.22)
Small intestine	0.37 (3.72)	0.16 (1.64)	0.09 (0.90)	0.06 (0.58)	0.04 (0.36)
Upper large intestine	0.60 (5.96)	0.27 (2.67)	0.16 (1.64)	0.09 (0.90)	0.05 (0.54)
Lower large intestine	0.93 (9.27)	0.38 (3.80)	0.19 (1.94)	0.12 (1.20)	0.07 (0.72)
Ovaries	0.10 (0.99)	0.04 (0.42)	0.03 (0.33)	0.07 (0.72)	0.00 (0.01)
Testes	0.02 (0.18)	0.01 (0.07)	0.00 (0.03)	0.01 (0.11)	0.00 (0.01)
Thyroid	0.00 (0.02)	0.00 (0.01)	0.00 (0.00)	0.00 (0.00)	0.00 (0.00)
Total body	0.02 (0.20)	0.01 (0.11)	0.01 (0.06)	0.00 (0.04)	0.00 (0.02)

Interpretation

In normal infants, one or two episodes of reflux are not uncommon in the first 5 minutes.[3] Repeated episodes, particularly if the reflux extends into the upper esophagus, should be considered abnormal. The normal rate of gastric emptying varies with the volume of the meal and the position of the child. In preterm infants, infant formula empties with a half-life of about 50 minutes, whereas with older infants, it empties with a half-life of about 80 minutes.[6,7] Human milk empties more rapidly, with a half-life ranging from 25 minutes in preterm infants to 50 minutes in older infants.[6,7]

Radiation Dosimetry

The estimated absorbed doses in organs and tissues of children from newborn to 15 years old from the oral ingestion of 100 μCi (3.7 MBq) of ^{99m}Tc sulfur colloid are given in Table 6-4.[8]

References

1. Seibert JJ, Byrne WJ, Euler AR, et al. Gastroesophageal reflux—the acid test: scintigraphy or the pH probe? AJR 1983; 140: 1087–1090.
2. Le Luyer B, Texte D, Segond G, et al. Value of gastroesophageal scintigraphy for the detection of gastroesophageal reflux in infants. J Radiol 1983; 64: 693–697.
3. Blumhagen JD, Rudd TG, Christie DL. Gastroesophageal reflux in children: radionuclide gastroesophagography. AJR 1980; 135: 1001–1004.
4. Heyman S. Pediatric nuclear gastroenterology: evaluation of gastroesophageal reflux and gastrointestinal bleeding. In "Nuclear Medicine Annual 1985," eds Freeman LM, Weissmann HS. Raven Press, New York, 1985, pp 133–169.
5. Signer E. Gastric emptying in newborns and young infants: measurement of the rate of emptying using indium-113m-microcolloid. Acta Paediatr Scand 1975; 64: 525–530.
6. Cavell B. Gastric emptying in preterm infants. Acta Paediatr Scand 1979; 68: 725–730.
7. Cavell B. Reservoir and emptying function of the stomach of the premature infant. Acta Paediatr Scand (Suppl) 1982; 296: 60–61.
8. Castronovo FP Jr. Gastroesophageal scintiscanning in a pediatric population: dosimetry. J Nucl Med 1986; 27: 1212–1214.

Gastric Emptying (Solid/Liquid) Study

Summary Information

Radiopharmaceutical

Adult dose: Solid marker—1 mCi (37 MBq) of ^{99m}Tc sulfur colloid cooked in eggs.
Liquid marker—500 µCi (18.5 MBq) of ^{111}In DTPA mixed in milk.

Pediatric dose: Adjusted according to patient's weight (see Appendix A-3).

Contraindications   None.

Dose/Scan Interval   Imaging begins immediately after ingestion of the meal.

Views Obtained   The anterior view of the abdomen includes the stomach and small bowel. Dual-isotope acquisition is required for the ^{99m}Tc/^{111}In study.

Indications

The extended (up to) 4-hour gastric emptying procedure is designed for accurate assessment of solid and liquid emptying rates. It is particularly useful in patients who have undergone various surgical procedures for disease or abnormalities of the gastrointestinal system. The patient's symptoms may include nausea, vomiting, diarrhea, weight loss, and abdominal fullness and distention. *Note:* Although not as comprehensive an evaluation of gastric emptying, the combined gastric emptying/small bowel transit/colonic transit study (Procedure 6-6) provides a simpler, less expensive, and more useful assessment of overall gastrointestinal motility.

Principle

This test evaluates the stomach's rate of emptying by labeling the solid and liquid components of a meal with two different radiopharmaceuticals: ^{99m}Tc sulfur colloid bound to eggs and ^{111}In DTPA (diethylenetriamine pentaacetic acid) in milk.[1] Analysis of the activity remaining in the stomach over time permits estimation of the emptying half-time for both the solid and liquid phases.[2]

Patient Preparation

The use of all medications (with the exception of insulin and cardiac medications) should be discontinued for 48 hours before the study, unless indicated otherwise by the referring physician. The patient should fast beginning at 8:00 PM the evening before the study.

Meal Preparation

Meal Ingredients

1. 60 g egg substitute, uncooked (e.g., Eggbeaters)
2. 30 g chopped Canadian bacon (uncooked)
3. 20 g white bread
4. 60 ml lactose-free nutritionally complete formula (e.g., Sustacal)
5. 60 ml skim milk
6. 1 packet grape jelly
7. 1 pat (5–7 g) margarine

In addition, paper cups and plates, plastic utensils, and napkins are required.

Preparation: Mix 1 mCi (37 MBq) of ^{99m}Tc sulfur colloid with the raw egg substitute and Canadian bacon. Cook to a firm consistency in one half of the margarine. The remaining margarine and jelly should be spread on the bread. Mix the formula and skim milk, and add to 500 μCi (18.5 MBq) of ^{111}In DTPA. This meal has a caloric content of approximately 293 kcal. The meal composition is 25% protein, 57% carbohydrates, and 18% fat.

Note: In a patient who is allergic to eggs or milk, substitute mashed potatoes for the eggs and orange juice for the milk. These changes in the meal may alter the transit time.

Instrument Specifications

Gamma camera:	Any large field-of-view system can be used—if available, a dual-head system facilitates simultaneous anterior and posterior image acquisition.
Collimator:	Medium-energy collimator.
Energy setting:	140 keV, 15–20% window for ^{99m}Tc.
	247 keV, 15–20% window for ^{111}In.
Imaging table:	If available, a 45° inclined table provides a more physiologic arrangement for assessing gastric emptying.
	Computer system: Acquisition requirements—dual-isotope static (64 × 64 word mode matrix).
	Processing requirements—ROI analysis, time–activity curve generation.

Imaging Procedure

1. Explain the procedure fully to the patient.
2. Time zero is when the patient starts the meal. The liquid part of the meal should be taken at the end of the meal, if possible. The meal should be completed within 10 minutes.
3. After the patient has ingested the meal, position the patient supine on the inclined (45°) table, with the gamma camera positioned over the stomach and small bowel, as shown in Figure 6-12.
4. Acquire dual-isotope, static images (64 × 64 word mode, 2 minutes per image) immediately after positioning the patient and then at 5-minute intervals from time zero for the first hour. Thereafter, images should be acquired at 10-minute intervals for 4 hours.
5. The test is completed at 4 hours or when the stomach is empty. *Note:* Care should be taken to include the whole region of activity for the first two images and to center the stomach in the remaining images. The time required for the study is about 4.5 hours.
6. Note the times of the image acquisition on the gastric emptying worksheet (Fig. 6-13).

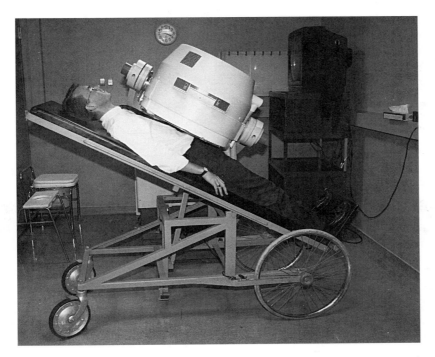

Figure 6-12. Gamma camera and patient position during gastric emptying study.

Note: If a dual-head system is available, acquire dual-head/dual-isotope images of the stomach. Anterior and posterior images permit calculation of the geometric mean of activity in the body and eliminate errors that are due to attenuation of activity as the meal moves from the fundus to the antrum.

Computer Analysis

1. Select the ^{111}In time zero static image. Under ROI analysis, outline all abdominal activity, even if it is outside the stomach. Record the ROI counts. Next, sequentially select all the ^{111}In images, outlining only activity in the stomach. For each image, record the ROI counts. Decay correction may be performed but is not essential for the ^{111}In data. Plot the counts versus time, and determine the half-time ($T_{\frac{1}{2}}$) from the emptying curve.

2. Select the ^{99m}Tc time zero static image, and repeat step 1. For each time point, multiply the ^{111}In counts by the crossover factor and subtract from the ^{99m}Tc counts (see "Additional Notes" for computation of the crossover factor). Apply decay correction to adjust all counts to their value at time zero. Plot the counts versus time, and determine the $T_{\frac{1}{2}}$ from the emptying curve.

3. For dual-head systems, process the posterior images as described in steps 1 and 2. For each time point, calculate the geometric mean of counts for ^{111}In and ^{99m}Tc as follows:

$$\text{Geometric Mean Counts} = (\text{Anterior Counts} \times \text{Posterior Counts})^{0.5}$$

4. Obtain a hard copy of the gastric emptying curves, the time zero images with their ROIs, and representative examples of ROIs and images over the scan duration.

GASTRIC EMPTYING - SOLID/LIQUID STUDY

Patient Name : _____ Sex : _____

Clinic No. _____ Date : _____

Gamma Camera : _____ Collimator : _____

In-111 to Tc-99m crossover factor : _____

TIME (min)	ACTUAL TIME hour/min	COMMENTS	TIME (min)	ACTUAL TIME hour/min	COMMENTS
0		start of meal	100		
5			110		
10			120		
15			130		
20			140		
25			150		
30			160		
35			170		
40			180		
45			190		
50			200		
55			210		
60			220		
70			230		
80			240		
90				end of study	

Comments : _____

_____

_____

Technologist : _____

Figure 6-13. Gastric emptying worksheet.

Information on Film

On each computer film, ensure that the following information is recorded:

1. Patient name and clinic/hospital number
2. Date, type of scan, radiopharmaceutical, and whether liquid or solid component of meal
3. Time of images after the meal
4. Orientation of each image (e.g., anterior)

Interpretation

Normal gastric emptying curves for solid and liquid phases are illustrated in Figure 6-14. Table 6-5 indicates the normal ranges in the nuclear medicine laboratory at the Mayo Clinic for the meal used. Values were determined in 20 normal volunteers (unpublished data).

Additional Notes

Note: Crossover of ^{111}In counts into the ^{99m}Tc energy window needs to be defined for each gamma camera-collimator combination. The crossover factor should be determined as follows:

1. Fill a plastic container with water to a depth of about 20 cm. The container should be 25–35 cm in width or diameter (e.g., plastic bucket). Inject approximately 100 µCi (3.7 MBq) ^{111}In into a 250-ml saline bag. Tape the saline bag to the side wall of the container. Position the container in front of the detector, as shown in Figure 6-15, oriented so that the saline bag is close to the collimator.
2. Acquire a dual-isotope study using settings identical to those used for the gastric emptying study. Images should be acquired in a 64 × 64 matrix for 5 minutes per image.
3. Rotate the container 180° so that the saline bag is now furthest away from the collimator face, and repeat step 2.

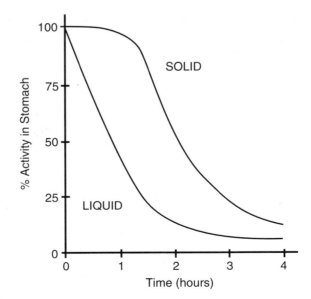

Figure 6-14. Normal gastric emptying curves for solid and liquid meals.

Table 6-5. Normal Ranges for Gastric Emptying Determined at the Mayo Clinic[a]

Meal	$t_{\frac{1}{4}}$[b]	$t_{\frac{1}{2}}$[b]	$t_{\frac{3}{4}}$[b]
Solid	99 (37–157)	129 (71–198)	164 (112–229)
Liquid	17 (10–30)	43 (33–75)	88 (72–137)

[a]$t_{\frac{1}{4}}$, $t_{\frac{1}{2}}$, and $t_{\frac{3}{4}}$ refer, respectively, to the times required for ¼, ½, ¾ of the radioactivity to leave the stomach.
[b]Median and 10–90% range in minutes.

4. Select the images acquired in step 2, and display the image acquired in the ^{111}In energy window. Using ROI analysis, outline the activity in the saline bag (the outline should not be too tight and should be drawn in a manner similar to that used for clinical gastric emptying studies) and determine the total ROI counts. Apply this ROI to the image acquired in the ^{99m}Tc energy window. Obtain the ratio of ^{99m}Tc/^{111}In counts.
5. Repeat step 4 for the second set of images, and obtain the average of the 2 ratios. This is the ^{111}In-to-^{99m}Tc crossover factor and should be in the range 0.75–1.25.

Radiation Dosimetry

The estimated absorbed doses in organs and tissues of an average subject (70 kg) from the oral ingestion of 1 mCi (37 MBq) of ^{99m}Tc sulfur colloid and 500 μCi (18.5 MBq) of ^{111}In DTPA are shown in Table 6-6.[3]

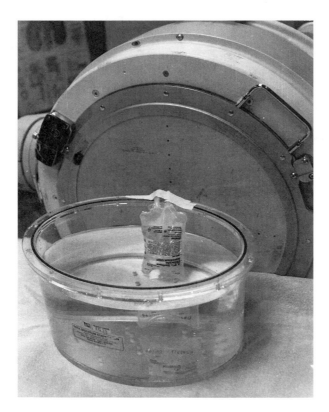

Figure 6-15. Setup for measurement of ^{111}In to ^{99m}Tc crossover factor.

Table 6-6. Absorbed Radiation Dose Estimates in a 70- kg Adult After Oral Administration of ^{99m}Tc Sulfur Colloid and ^{111}In DTPA

	Absorbed Radiation Doses			
	^{99m}Tc Sulfur Colloid		^{111}In DTPA	
Tissue	rad/1 mCi	mGy/37 MBq	rad/500 µCi	mGy/18.5 MBq
Stomach	0.14	1.40	0.09	0.90
Small bowel	0.25	2.50	0.49	4.90
Upper large intestine	0.40	4.00	1.30	13.0
Lower large intestine	0.33	3.30	1.30	13.0
Ovaries	0.09	0.90	0.26	2.60
Testes	0.01	0.05	0.019	0.19
Total body	0.02	0.20	0.04	0.40

References

1. Wright RA, Thompson D, Syed I. Simultaneous markers for fluid and solid gastric emptying: new variations on an old theme: concise communication. J Nucl Med 1981; 22: 772–776.
2. Malmud LS, Fisher RS. Scintigraphic evaluation of gastric emptying. In "Radionuclide Imaging of the G.I. Tract," ed Mettler F.A. Churchill Livingstone, New York, 1986, pp 35–52.
3. Harbert JC, Pollina R. Absorbed dose estimates from radionuclides. Clin Nucl Med 1984; 9: 210–221.

Gastric Emptying, Small Bowel Transit, and Colonic Transit Studies

---

Summary Information

Radiopharmaceutical

Adult dose: Solid marker—1 mCi (37 MBq) of ^{99m}Tc-labeled resin beads in egg.
Colonic marker—100 µCi (3.7 MBq) of ^{111}In-labeled resin beads in methacrylate-coated capsule.

Pediatric dose: No pediatric dose has been established.

Contraindications None.

Dose/Scan Interval

^{99m}Tc-labeled meal: Imaging begins immediately after ingestion of the meal.
^{111}In-labeled capsule: Imaging begins after the capsule clears the stomach.

Views Obtained Anterior and posterior views of the abdomen include the stomach and the small and large intestines. Dual-isotope acquisition is used for combined ^{99m}Tc and ^{111}In studies.

Indications

Symptoms such as nausea, vomiting, pain, and alterations in bowel movements that suggest an impairment of gastrointestinal motor function are relatively nonspecific; similar symptoms occur in functional gastrointestinal diseases as well as in organic motility disorders. Moreover, the severity of symptoms is subjective and often unrelated to the location of the abnormality within the gastrointestinal tract. Measurement of gastric emptying, small bowel transit, and colonic transit is helpful in the evaluation of such patients. These procedures help localize the region of the gastrointestinal tract that is abnormal and may assist the clinician in determining the most appropriate therapeutic approach.

Principle

^{99m}Tc-labeled resin beads in egg act as a solid residue. Their movement through the stomach and small bowel into the colon can be quantitated to give an index of gastric emptying

303

and small bowel transit time (SBTT).[1] For assessment of colonic transit, ^{111}In-labeled resin beads enclosed in a methacrylate-coated capsule are used. The methacrylate coating on the gelatin capsule is pH sensitive and dissolves on reaching the cecum. Assessment of its distribution in the colon at 4 and 24 hours gives an index of colonic transit time (CTT).[2,3]

Patient Preparation

1. In the United States, [99mTc]- and ^{111}In-labeled resin beads are not approved by the Food and Drug Administration (FDA). Hence, written informed consent must be obtained from all patients, because currently this study is performed on an investigational drug status.
2. The use of all medications (with the exception of insulin and cardiac medications) should be discontinued for 48 hours before the study, unless instructed otherwise by the referring physician. The patient should begin to fast at 8:00 PM the evening before the study.
3. Small plastic-coated [57]Co markers should be positioned on the inside of each iliac crest. Because reproducible positioning of these markers is critical, the patient's skin should be marked with indelible ink to facilitate repositioning of the markers each time the patient is imaged.
4. Remember to remove the [57]Co markers during the time intervals between image acquisitions, to prevent their loss.

Bead/Capsule Preparation

Preparation: Methacrylate Polymer

1. 125-ml wide-mouth storage flask with a ground-glass stopper
2. Magnetic stirrer and stirring bar
3. Acetone, 31 ml
4. Isopropyl alcohol, 46 ml
5. Dibutyl phthalate, 2 ml
6. Water, 1 ml
7. Methacrylate (Eudragit S100), 13 g

Prepare the solvent as a mixture of 4 parts acetone and 6 parts isopropyl alcohol. To the 77 ml of solvent in the wide-mouth flask, add 2 ml dibutyl phthalate and 1 ml water, mixing continually with the magnetic stirring bar. Very slowly add the methacrylate into the vortex of the stirring liquids (Fig. 6-16). It is essential to wet all the powder and to continue stirring until the powder has dissolved (about 30 minutes) and a clear, pale, straw-colored solution is formed. The methacrylate polymer is now ready for coating the capsule.

Preparation: Solid Marker ([99mTc]-Labeled Resin Beads in Egg)

1. 1 g resin beads (Amberlite IR-410, Sigma Chemical Co.)
2. 1 mCi (37 MBq) [99mTc] sodium pertechnetate in 0.1 ml saline

Wet about 1 g of the resin beads (Fig. 6-17) with saline. Add 0.1 ml saline solution containing 1 mCi (37 MBq) of [99mTc] sodium pertechnetate to the wetted beads (Fig. 6-18). The technetium ions bind to the beads, which are rinsed twice with normal

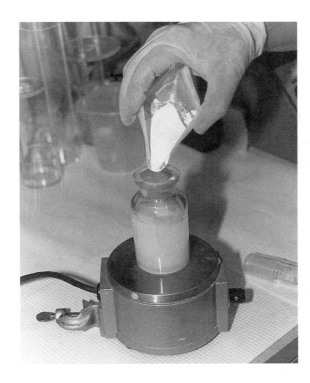

Figure 6-16. Preparation of the methacrylate solution.

saline and then with distilled water. Aspirate off the excess liquid, and mix the labeled beads with raw beaten eggs (2 eggs, remove 1 egg yolk).

Preparation: Colonic Marker (^{111}In-Labeled Methacrylate-Coated Capsule)

1. 750 mg resin beads (Amberlite IR-120, Sigma Chemical Co.)
2. 100 μCi (3.7 MBq) of ^{111}In indium chloride
3. Methacrylate polymer solution (Eudragit S-100)
4. 0–00 "medication" gelatin capsule
5. Fine thread or suture

Wet approximately 750 mg of the resin beads with a solution of 0.04 N HCl. Add ^{111}In indium chloride to the beads, and aspirate the excess solution. The indium cations bind to the beads, which should be rinsed twice with 0.04 N HCl and then with distilled water. Dry the beads in an oven for 10–15 minutes. Place a suture through one end of the capsule, and tie a small knot to ensure that the thread is secured inside the opened capsule. Place the dry beads in the gelatin capsule (Fig. 6-19). If the beads do not fill the capsule completely, add nonradioactive beads to fill the capsule. The beads must be dry so the gelatin capsule does not dissolve. After the beads are packed inside the capsule, close it with the capsule cap. Holding the string, dip the capsule completely into the flask containing methacrylate polymer, and make sure that the capsule is completely covered. Withdraw the capsule, and quickly dip it one more time to ensure a complete coating (Fig. 6-20). The polymer drop that hangs from the bottom of the capsule should be wiped off. Hang the capsule, and allow it to dry completely (about 1 hour) (Fig. 6-21). Clip off the suture close to the capsule. The capsule is ready for ingestion.

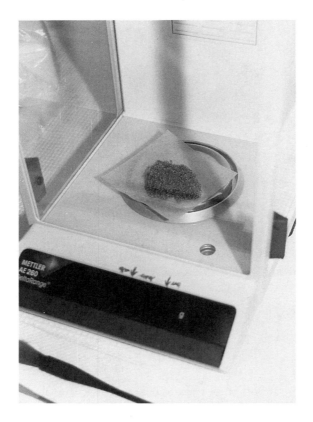

Figure 6-17. Amberlite IR-410 resin beads.

Meal Preparation

Gastric emptying and small bowel transit meal ingredients:

1. 2 eggs (without 1 of the egg yolks)
2. 1 slice of toast (brown bread)
3. 1 glass of skim milk (replace with 6 fl oz of water if patient refuses milk)

Estimated preparation time for the meal (including the preparation of ^{99m}Tc resin beads) is 27 minutes. The caloric content of meal is about 300 kcal.

Push Meal for Small Bowel and Colonic Transit Time Studies

This is an unlabeled meal designed to stimulate the gastroileal reflex and, thereby, to promote the propulsion of solid material from the ileum into the large intestine. The following are recommended push meals:

1. Hardee's	1 big roast beef sandwich
	1 regular order of french fries
	1 glass of water
2. Hardee's	1 chicken fillet sandwich
	½ order of french fries
	1 glass of water

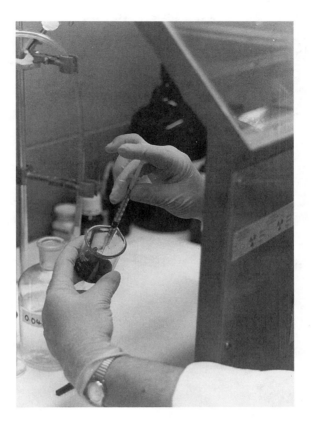

Figure 6-18. Addition of ^{99m}Tc pertechnetate to wetted beads.

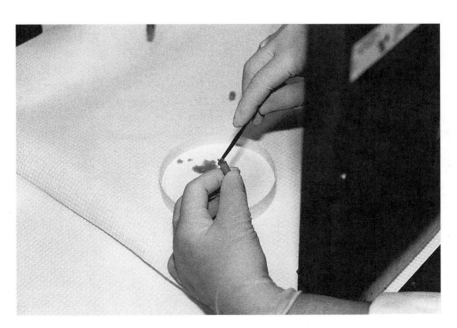

Figure 6-19. Pack the gelatin capsule with ^{111}In-labeled resin beads.

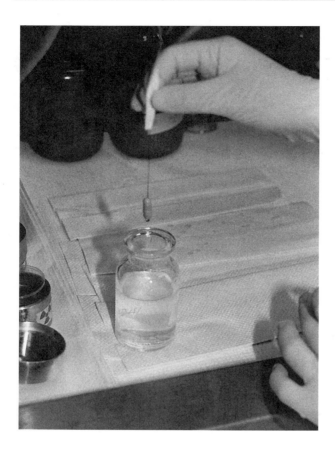

Figure 6-20. Gelatin capsule dipped in the methacrylate polymer solution.

3. McDonald's   1 hamburger
                 1 regular order of french fries
                 1 glass of water

One of these selections should be consumed between 3.5 and 4.0 hours after eating the radiolabeled egg meal. Each of these push meals has approximately 500 kcal. As an alternative, the patient should be asked to eat a "normal" dinner (approximately 500 kcal) consisting of both liquids and solids (e.g., turkey and mashed potatoes with milk or soda pop.)

Instrument Specifications

Gamma camera:	Any large field-of-view system can be used. Where available, a dual-head large field-of-view system should be used.
Collimator:	Low-energy, all-purpose collimator for gastric emptying and SBTT studies.
	Medium-energy collimator must be used for any study involving ^{111}In.
Energy setting:	140 keV, 15–20% energy window for ^{99m}Tc.
	247 keV, 15–20% energy window for ^{111}In during dual-isotope study

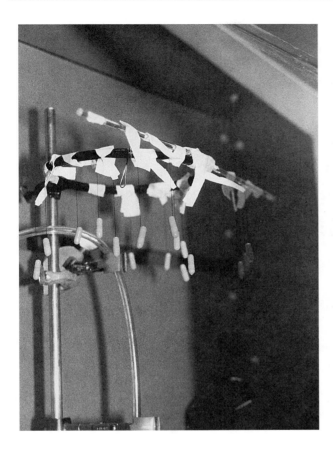

Figure 6-21. Polymer-coated capsules drying in air.

170 keV and 247 keV, 15–20% energy windows for study with only ^{111}In.

Computer system: Acquisition requirements—dual-isotope static (128 × 128 word mode matrix).

Processing requirements—ROI analysis, time–activity curve generation.

Imaging Procedure

Gastric Emptying

1. Install low-energy all-purpose collimator, and set energy window for 140 keV, with 15–20% energy window.
2. After the patient ingests the radiolabeled meal, position the patient upright in front of the gamma camera (Fig. 6-22). The field of view of the gamma camera should include the stomach and small bowel. Ensure that the ^{57}Co markers are in the field of view, because these aid in the interpretation of later images.
3. Acquire an anterior image on computer in a 128 × 128 word mode matrix for 2 minutes. Rotate the patient 180°, and acquire a posterior image for 2 minutes. On a dual-head system, simultaneously acquire the anterior and posterior images.

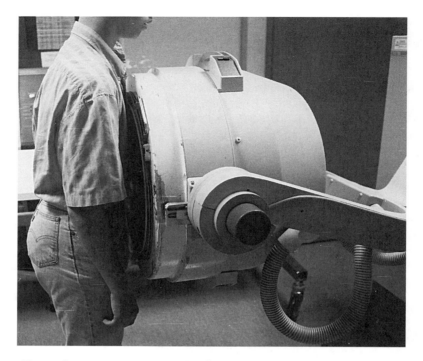

Figure 6-22. Patient positioned in front of the detector for anterior view.

4. Repeat steps 2 and 3 at 2 and 4 hours after ingestion of the radiolabeled meal.
5. Record whether the patient had any bowel movement or vomiting, and if so, at what time.

Gastric Emptying and Small Bowel Transit Time

1. All gamma camera variables/patient procedures are the same as for gastric emptying.
2. At 3.5–4.0 hours after ingestion of the radiolabeled meal, the patient should consume the push meal. Immediately after the push meal, the 4-hour images should be acquired, as for the 0- and 2-hour images.
3. An additional set of anterior and posterior images should be acquired at 6 hours after ingestion of the radiolabeled meal.
4. Record whether the patient had any bowel movement or vomiting, and if so, at what time.

Gastric Emptying Plus Small Bowel Transit Time
Plus Colonic Transit Time

1. Install a medium-energy collimator, and set the energy windows to acquire dual-isotope studies using the 140-keV peak for ^{99m}Tc and the 247-keV peak for ^{111}In.
2. The patient should swallow the methacrylate-coated capsule containing 100 μCi (3.7 MBq) ^{111}In resin beads. Water should be given before and with the capsule to aid in swallowing. Instruct the patient to continue fasting after ingesting the capsule. After the capsule has left the stomach (or 2 hours later, whichever comes first, as determined from a scout view), the patient should eat the radiolabeled meal.
3. As described, the small ^{57}Co markers should be taped to the iliac crests for the 2-, 4-, 6-, and 24-hour images. These markers are used to assist in distinguishing between the ascend-

ing colon and small bowel and between the descending colon and the rectosigmoid during ROI analysis of the images. *Note:* Ensure markers are retrieved after the study!

4. After ingesting the radiolabeled meal, the patient should be placed upright in front of the gamma camera and two dual-isotope images obtained (anterior, isotope A + isotope B; posterior, isotope A + isotope B). Acquisition time should be 2 minutes per image, and data should be stored in a 128×128 word mode matrix. The 2-hour images should be obtained as described.

5. At 3.5–4.0 hours after ingestion of the radiolabeled meal, the patient should consume the push meal. Immediately after the push meal, the 4-hour images should be acquired, as for the 0- and 2-hour images. The 6-hour images should be acquired as for the 4-hour images. Twenty-four-hour images should be acquired the next day. Patients can eat as they normally would between the 4- and 24-hour images.

6. It is important to ensure that all markers and all activity in the stomach, small bowel, and colon are included in the field of view of the gamma camera.

7. Record whether the patient had any bowel movement or vomiting, and if so, at what time.

Colonic Transit Time

1. Install a medium-energy collimator, and set the energy windows to acquire from the 170-keV and the 247-keV peak of ^{111}In.

2. The patient should swallow the methacrylate-coated capsule containing 100 µCi (3.7 MBq) of ^{111}In resin beads. Water should be given before and with the capsule to aid in swallowing. Instruct the patient to continue fasting after ingesting the capsule.

3. After the capsule has left the stomach (or 2 hours later, whichever comes first), the patient should eat a small breakfast. This breakfast should be identical to that used for gastric emptying studies, with the exception that no ^{99m}Tc-labeled resin beads are added to the eggs.

4. As described, the small ^{57}Co markers should be taped to the iliac crests for the 0-, 4- and 24-hour ^{111}In images. These markers are used to assist in correctly identifying the ascending colon, small bowel, descending colon, and rectosigmoid during ROI analysis of the images.

5. At 3.5–4.0 hours after ingestion of the breakfast meal, the patient should consume the push meal. Immediately after the push meal, the 4-hour images should be acquired with the patient upright in front of the gamma camera. Anterior and posterior images should be obtained for 2 minutes per image and stored in a 128×128 word mode matrix. Twenty-four-hour images should be acquired the next day. Acquisition variables should be the same as for the 4-hour images. Patients can eat as they normally would between the 4- and 24-hour images.

6. It is important to ensure that all markers and all activity in the stomach, small bowel, and colon are included in the field of view of the gamma camera.

Computer Analysis

On the computer, load into the display all the anterior images (both ^{99m}Tc and ^{111}In), and obtain a hard copy of this display. Repeat this process for the posterior images. This display is very useful in correctly determining the location of activity within the gastrointestinal tract. Process the anterior and posterior images as outlined later, using the worksheet shown in Figure 6-23.

Gastric Emptying

1. On the 0-hour images, ROIs should be drawn to include all activity in the field of view on both the anterior and posterior images. Record the ROI counts on the worksheet.

GASTRIC EMPTYING / SMALL BOWEL TRANSIT / COLONIC TRANSIT

Patient Name :   **Clinic No. :**   **Date :**

Technical Factors		Images Acquired	Time	Time Difference	Tc-99m Decay Corr. Factor	In-111 Decay Corr. Factor
System :		"0" hour		0.0	1.000	1.000
Collimator : O LEAP O MEGP		"2" hour				
In-111 to Tc-99m crossover factor :		"4" hour				
Administered meal/capsule	**Time**	"6" hour				
In-111 Capsule		"24" hour				
Tc-99m labelled meal						
Push meal						

ANALYSIS OF GASTRIC EMPTYING AND SMALL BOWEL TRANSIT TIME

Region of Interest	Image Number	Tc-99m Image Data			In-111 Image Data			Tc-99m crossover correct. geometric mean counts
		Ant cts	Post cts	G.M. cts	Ant cts	Post cts	G.M. cts	
STOMACH	"0" hour							
	"2" hour							
	"4" hour							
COLON	"6" hour							

To obtain the "Decay Corr G.M. cts", multiply the Tc-99m G.M. cts (GE/SBTT studies) by the Tc-99m decay corr. factor. For studies involving In-111, use the Tc-99m crossover corrected G.M. cts with the Tc-99m decay correction factor.

The 6 hour colon activity should be expressed as a percent of the total "0 hour" stomach activity.

Region of Interest	Image Number	Decay Corr G.M. cts	% Admin. Dose	% Act Emptied from Stomach
STOMACH	"0" hour		100	0
	"2" hour			
	"4" hour			
COLON	"6" hour			<- % Dose in Colon = SBTT

ANALYSIS OF COLONIC TRANSIT TIME

Colonic ROI's	4 hour colonic image cts			% Admin. Dose	24 hour colonic image counts				% Admin. Dose
	Ant cts	Post cts	G.M. cts		Ant cts.	Post cts	G.M. cts	DC/GM cts	
Ascending									
Transverse									
Descending									
Rectum/Sig.									
Total cts (include small bowel activity)				100	Total cts (include small bowel activity)				
GEOMETRIC CENTER (GC) = [As + 2 x Tr + 3 x Des + 4 x R/S] / 100 =					Stool Act. as % Admin Dose (4 hr - 24 hr) =				
					GC = [As + 2 x Tr + 3 x Des + 4 x R/S + 5 x Stool]/100 =				

Note : All calculations of the % Admin dose are done using the 4-hr total cts as the 100% value : this applies to counts from both the 4 and 24 hour images

FORM :GSBCT.FDB

Figure 6-23. Worksheet for calculation of gastric emptying (GE), SBTT, and CTT.

2. On the 2- and 4-hour images, outline only the stomach region, and enter the ROI counts on the worksheet. Enter the exact time interval between the 0-, 2-, and 4-hour images, and calculate the decay correction factor. Express counts in the 2- and 4-hour images as a percentage of the 0-hour counts.

Gastric Emptying and Small Bowel Transit Time

1. Analysis of the 0-, 2-, and 4-hour images should be performed as for the gastric emptying analysis described earlier.
2. In addition, on the 6-hour image, ROIs should be drawn around the colon (whatever segments are visible). In general, the colon is seen only on the 4- and 6-hour images. Enter the ROI counts in the worksheet, and apply decay correction. Express the decay-corrected colonic counts in the 6-hour image as a percentage of counts in the 0-hour image. This percentage is the SBTT index.

Gastric Emptying, Small Bowel Transit Time, and Colonic Transit Time

1. Analysis of the gastric emptying and SBTT is performed as described earlier with two exceptions: (1) If the ^{111}In capsule has clearly left the stomach, then include only the appropriate stomach and small bowel activity in the ROI. (2) Crossover correction must be applied to the ^{99m}Tc data if there is contamination from [111]In. The crossover correction factor varies depending on the width of the energy windows and on the gamma camera and collimator system used. See "Additional Notes" for computation of the crossover factor.
2. Analysis of CTT should be performed from the 4- and 24-hour ^{111}In images. All ^{111}In activity in the field of view must be included in the ROIs drawn on the 4-hour image, because this activity represents 100% of the administered dose.
3. ROIs should be drawn over the following five regions when activity is present in them: small bowel, ascending colon, transverse colon, descending colon, and rectum. These regions are created using the following criteria (Fig. 6-24):

Small bowel: Small bowel activity should be medial to the ascending colon. Normally, at 24 hours, little activity should be present in the small bowel; however, on occasion activity may be present in both the small bowel and stomach. All such activity should be included in the small bowel ROI.

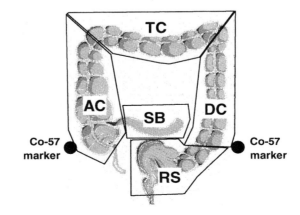

Figure 6-24. Placement of ROIs over the small bowel (SB), ascending colon (AC), transverse colon (TC), descending colon (DC), and rectosigmoid (RS).

Ascending colon: The ROI should be drawn to follow the medial border of the ascending colon to the transverse colon (i.e., the hepatic flexure is divided between the ascending colon ROI and the transverse colon ROI).

Descending colon: Draw as for the ascending colon, with the ROI dividing the splenic flexure.

Transverse colon: The segment between the ascending colon and the descending colon. Note that in some patients, the transverse colon may be U-shaped and descend into the pelvis.

Rectosigmoid: Generally, the rectosigmoid region is the segment of the left colon below the level of the [57]Co markers. Rectosigmoid activity appears more intense (hotter) on posterior than anterior images. This can help distinguish it from activity in the descending colon.

4. Express the anterior and posterior ROI counts as a percentage of the administered dose. The geometric center of the isotope distribution in the colon is calculated with the equation given in the worksheet (see Fig. 6-23). On the 24-hour images, all counts should be decay corrected. If the total colonic count at 24 hours is less than the total colonic counts at 4 hours, the difference is attributed to activity lost in the stool.

Colonic Transit Time

Analysis of a CTT study is identical to that described above for gastric emptying, small bowel transit, and colonic transit studies.

Caution: If the patient has vomiting or diarrhea (check the patient's medical chart), the activity lost needs to be accounted for in the calculations. To determine whether all activity is present, draw anterior and posterior ROIs over all ^{99m}Tc activity at time zero for gastric emptying and SBTT estimations and compute the geometric mean of the total counts. Likewise for CTT, draw anterior and posterior ROIs over all ^{111}In activity at 4 hours and compute the geometric mean of the counts. These are the 100% values. Now, draw ROIs over all activity visible at the times in question. Calculate total counts (with decay correction), and check that the values agree with the initial measurements (to within ±10%).

Obtain hard copies of the following:

1. Display of all anterior and posterior images, as described
2. ROIs used for calculations

Information on Film

On each computer film, ensure that the following information is recorded:

1. Patient name and clinic/hospital number
2. Date, type of scan, radiopharmaceutical(s)
3. Time of images after the meal
4. Orientation of each image (e.g., anterior)

Interpretation

Normal values for gastric emptying, SBTT, and CTT are as follows:[1–4]

Gastric emptying:	% Dose emptied from the stomach at 2 hours = 34% (range, 24–47%).
	% Dose emptied from the stomach at 4 hours = 98% (range, 56–100%).
Small bowel transit:	% Dose emptied from the small bowel at 6 hours = 41% (range, 11–70%).
Colonic transit:	Geometric mean of activity at 4 hours = 0.8–1.4.
	Geometric mean of activity at 24 hours = 1.7–4.0.

Additional Notes

Crossover of ^{111}In counts into the ^{99m}Tc energy window needs to be defined for each gamma camera-collimator combination. The crossover factor should be determined as follows:

1. Fill a plastic container with water to a depth of about 20 cm. The container should be 25–35 cm in width or diameter (e.g., a plastic bucket). Inject approximately 100 μCi (3.7 MBq) ^{111}In into a 250-ml saline bag. Tape the saline bag to the side wall of the container. Position the container in front of the detector, as shown in Figure 6-11, oriented so that the saline bag is close to the collimator.
2. Acquire a dual-isotope study using settings identical to those used for the gastric emptying, SBTT, and CTT studies. Images should be acquired in a 128 × 128 matrix for 5 minutes per image.
3. Rotate the container 180° so that the saline bag is now furthest away from the collimator face and repeat step 2.
4. Select the images acquired in step 2, and display the image acquired in the ^{111}In energy window. Using ROI analysis, outline the activity in the saline bag (the outline should not be too tight and should be drawn in a manner similar to that used for clinical gastric emptying studies) and determine the total ROI counts. Apply this ROI to the image acquired in the ^{99m}Tc energy window. Obtain the ratio of ^{99m}Tc/^{111}In counts.
5. Repeat step 4 for the second set of images, and obtain the average of the 2 ratios. This is the ^{111}In to ^{99m}Tc crossover factor and should be in the range of 0.75–1.25.

Radiation Dosimetry

The estimated absorbed doses in organs and tissues of an average subject (70 kg) from the oral administration of 1 mCi (37 MBq) ^{99m}Tc-labeled eggs and a 100 μCi (3.7 MBq) ^{111}In-labeled capsule are shown in Table 6-7.[3]

Table 6-7. Absorbed Radiation Dose Estimates in a 70-kg Adult From the Oral Administration of ^{99m}Tc and ^{111}In

| | Absorbed Radiation Dose | | | |
| | ^{99m}Tc-Labeled Amberlite | | ^{111}In-Labeled Amberlite | |
Tissue	rad/1 mCi	mGy/37 MBq	rad/100 μCi	mGy/3.7 MBq
Stomach	0.24	2.40	0.10	1.00
Small intestine	0.24	2.40	0.20	2.00
Upper large intestinal wall	0.40	4.00	0.45	4.50
Lower large intestinal wall	0.28	2.80	0.75	7.50
Ovaries	0.08	0.80	0.15	1.50
Testes	0.00	0.00	0.01	0.10
Red marrow	0.14	1.40	0.04	0.40
Total body	0.02	0.20	0.03	0.30

References

1. Camilleri M, Zinsmeister AR, Greydanus MP, et al. Towards a less costly but accurate test of gastric emptying and small bowel transit. Dig Dis Sci 1991; 36: 609–615.
2. Camilleri M, Colemont LJ, Phillips SF, et al. Human gastric emptying and colonic filling of solids characterized by a new method. Am J Physiol 1989; 257: G284–G290.
3. Von der Ohe MR, Camilleri M. Measurement of small bowel and colonic transit: indications and methods. Mayo Clin Proc 1992; 67: 1169–1179.
4. Camilleri M, Zinsmeister AR. Towards a relatively inexpensive, noninvasive, accurate test for colonic motility disorders. Gastroenterology 1992; 103: 36–42.

Colorectal/Neorectal Emptying Study

Summary Information

Radiopharmaceutical

Adult dose: 1 mCi (37 MBq) of ^{99m}Tc sulfur colloid in aluminum magnesium citrate (Veegum) gel.

Pediatric dose: None established.

Contraindications   None.

Dose/Scan Interval   Imaging begins immediately after placement of the gel.

Views Obtained   Obtain a right lateral view, with the patient sitting on a commode.

Indications

The purpose of this test is to evaluate colo/neorectal function and the emptying ability of the colo/neorectum in patients who have had a colectomy, mucosal rectectomy, or an ileal pouch-anal anastomosis. This procedure can also be used to evaluate colo/neorectal function and rectal emptying rates in patients without prior surgery.

Principle

Radioactive ^{99m}Tc sulfur colloid suspended in approximately 300 ml of aluminum magnesium silicate gel (Veegum) can be administered to the patient via a 16F transanal tube. From images taken before, during, and after evacuation of the artificial stool, it is possible to determine the emptying rate and relative percent emptying of the neorectal pouch.[1]

Patient Preparation

The patient needs to be limited to a liquid diet beginning at midnight before the day of the study. The patient also needs to change to a hospital gown before the study.

Veegum Preparation

In a 1,000-cc beaker, put 330 ml of water containing 1 mCi (37 MBq) of ^{99m}Tc sulfur colloid. The beaker should be heated to 37°C on a stirring platform with a magnetic stirring rod inside the beaker. Slowly add 25 g of aluminum magnesium silicate gel over a

20–25 minute period while constantly stirring to avoid lumping. This will give a 7.5% mixture of Veegum gel. The gel should be left to stir at 37°C for 15 minutes before it is used. Immediately before the procedure, draw the Veegum gel into 2 140-ml catheter syringes and attach a 16F transanal tube (Fig. 6-25).

Instrument Specifications

Gamma camera:	Any large field-of-view system can be used.
Collimator:	Low-energy, all-purpose collimator.
Energy setting:	140 keV, 15–20% energy window.
Computer system:	Acquisition requirements—dynamic (64 × 64 word mode matrix)
	Processing requirements—ROI analysis, curve generation.
Additional items:	Portable commode.

Imaging Procedure

1. The portable commode should be lined with a plastic bag to catch the gel when the patient evacuates it.
2. The nuclear medicine physician should fill the patient's lower bowel with the radioactive Veegum gel by inserting a 16F transanal tube to the level of the pouch and injecting the gel through the tube with the use of a 140-ml catheter syringe (injection time is approximately 15 minutes). If cramping should occur while filling, momentarily stop until the cramping subsides, then continue. The entire 300 ml should be injected, then the transanal tube should be removed. The patient will be asked to retain the gel until step 4.
3. Sit the patient on the commode in a right lateral position relative to the gamma camera (Fig. 6-26). Ensure that the patient is in a position comfortable for defecation. Acquire a preevacuation image on computer (3-minute static acquisition, 64 × 64 word mode matrix).

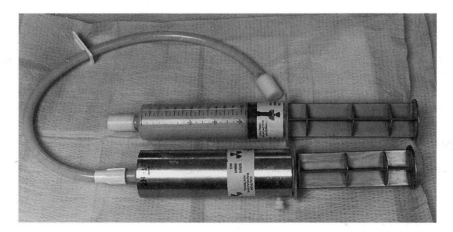

Figure 6-25. Veegum gel in 140-ml syringes. One syringe is enclosed in a lead sleeve with a 16F transanal tube attached.

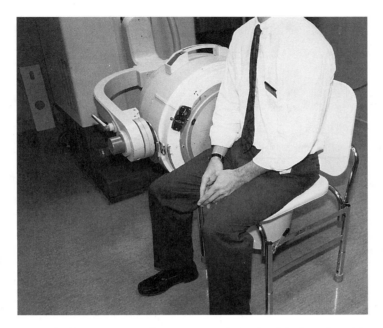

Figure 6-26. Patient seated on a commode in the right lateral position.

4. Set up a dynamic computer acquisition (64 × 64 word, 2 sec/frame, 120 frames). Start computer acquisition, and after about 10 seconds, ask the patient to empty the bowel.
5. After initial emptying, if the patient believes that he or she can empty more by leaning forward or any other way, have him or her do so. The patient should empty as much as possible before the final image. However, significant patient movement should be avoided, because this may move the rectal activity outside the ROI used in analysis.
6. Acquire a postevacuation image, as in step 3.

Computer Analysis

Select the dynamic study, and draw an ROI around the activity. Generate a time–activity curve showing the evacuation of the gel from the colo/neorectum. Obtain a hard copy of the time–activity curve and the ROI. Next, draw ROIs over the colo/neorectal pouch activity in the pre- and postevacuation images, and from the ratio of postevacuation-to-preevacuation ROI counts, compute the percent gel emptied.

Information on Film

On each computer film, ensure that the following information is recorded:

1. Patient name and clinic/hospital number
2. Date, type of scan, and radiopharmaceutical
3. Whether the image is pre- or postevacuation
4. Orientation of each image (e.g., right lateral)

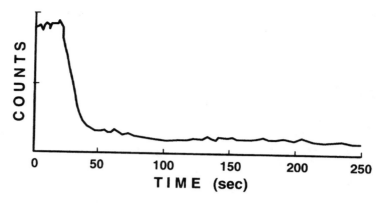

Figure 6-27. Normal anorectal emptying curve.

Interpretation

The normal range for normal subjects and ileal pouch patients is 48–72% (95% confidence interval).[1] If the pouch cannot contain the 300 ml of Veegum gel, a second region above the pouch may be visible. Quantitation of this area of small bowel can be compared with that of the pouch to get the relative amount of gel present above the pouch. Defecation should be completed in less than 90 seconds (median, 20 seconds) and should show an evacuation curve similar to that in Figure 6-27.

Radiation Dosimetry

The estimated absorbed doses in organs and tissues of an average subject (70 kg) from the rectal administration of 1 mCi (37 MBq) of ^{99m}Tc sulfur colloid are shown in Table 6-8.[1]

Table 6-8. Absorbed Radiation Doses in a 70-kg Adult From 1 mCi (37 MBq) ^{99m}Tc Veegum Gel

Tissue	Absorbed Radiation Dose			
	Minimum		Maximum	
	rad/1 mCi	mGy/37 MBq	rad/1 mCi	mGy/37 MBq
Rectal or neorectal	0.033	0.325	0.78	7.80
Ovaries	0.005	0.045	0.11	1.08
Small intestine	0.002	0.023	0.06	0.56
Bladder	0.002	0.017	0.04	0.41
Bone marrow	0.001	0.013	0.03	0.31
Testes	0.001	0.005	0.01	0.11
Total body	0.001	0.006	0.01	0.14

Doses are based on a 15-minute (minimum) and a 6-hour (maximum) residence time of the Veegum gel in the neorectum.

Reference

1. O'Connell PR, Kelly KA, Brown ML. Scintigraphic assessment of neorectal motor function. J Nucl Med 1986; 27: 460–464.

Anorectal Angle Study

Summary Information

Radiopharmaceuticals   No radiopharmaceutical is administered to the patient during this test. Instead, ^{99m}Tc pertechnetate is placed inside a balloon catheter to permit visualization of its position in the rectum. The following radioactive solutions are required:

1. 3-ml syringe containing 15 mCi (555 MBq) of ^{99m}Tc pertechnetate in 2 ml water
2. 50/60-ml syringe containing 5 mCi (185 MBq) of ^{99m}Tc pertechnetate in 40 ml water
3. (2 × 20 μCi (0.74 MBq) ^{99m}Tc markers, each attached to a strip of adhesive tape

Contraindications   None.

Dose/Scan Interval   Images may be taken immediately after the balloon is in place and filled.

Views Obtained   A right lateral view of the pelvis should be obtained. The patient should be lying in the left lateral decubitus position on the imaging table.

Indications

Anorectal continence is determined by several factors, including the anorectal angle, pressure level in the anal canal, rectal capacity, and the motility of the proximal colon and anal canal.[1] Of these, the anorectal angle is of central importance in maintaining anorectal continence.[2] Measurement of the anorectal angle is a useful indication of anorectal continence, particularly in patients who have undergone ileal pouch-anal anastomosis or other surgical procedures designed to maintain fecal continence.[3]

Principle

The anorectal angle is defined as the angle between the rectum and anal canal. It is formed by the anterior pull of the puborectalis muscle as it encircles the bowel at the anorectal junction (Fig. 6-28). Measurement of the anorectal angle is achieved by inserting a latex balloon formed around a semirigid catheter through the anal canal (details of the balloon are given in "Additional Notes"). The balloon-type apparatus is filled with water and ^{99m}Tc sodium pertechnetate. Images of the balloon filled with ^{99m}Tc sodium pertechnetate are

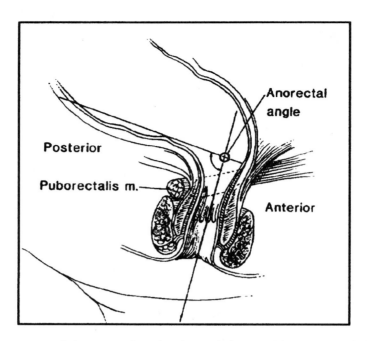

Figure 6-28. Diagram of the anorectal angle. The angle between the rectum and the anal canal is formed by the anteriorly directed pull of the puborectalis muscle. (From Barkel et al.,[4] with permission.)

taken under three conditions: at rest, while squeezing, and during attempted defecation. From analysis of these images, the angle of the anorectal junction can be obtained for each of these three conditions.[4]

Patient Preparation

The patient should change into a hospital gown before the test. The patient should lie on the imaging table in the left lateral decubitus position. The nuclear medicine physician inserts the balloon into the rectum. The position of the balloon in the rectum is shown in Figure 6-29.

Instrument Specifications

Gamma camera:	Any large field-of-view system may be used.
Collimator:	Low-energy, all-purpose collimator.
Energy setting:	140 keV, 15–20% energy window.
Computer system:	Acquisition requirements—static (64 × 64 word mode matrix). Processing requirements—software for measurement of distance and angle.
Additional items:	Balloon catheter (see "Additional Notes").

Imaging Procedure

1. Tape the two sealed ^{99m}Tc markers to the collimator face exactly 20 cm apart, and acquire a 15-second static image of the markers (64 × 64 word mode matrix).

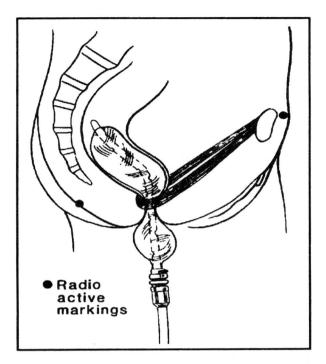

Figure 6-29. Diagram of the balloon device in place. Radioactive markers are taped to the skin over the pubis anteriorly and the coccyx tip posteriorly. (From Barkel et al.,[4] with permission.)

2. The two radioactive markers should then be taped to the skin over the pubis anteriorly and over the lip of the coccyx posteriorly (see Fig. 6-29).
3. After the balloon has been inserted into the rectum, 5 mCi (185 MBq) of ^{99m}Tc sodium pertechnetate in 40 ml of water should be injected into the catheter to fill the balloon (see Fig. 6-29). This permits good visualization of activity in the rectum and the region distal to the anal canal. The position of the balloon in the anal canal itself often is not well visualized because of the pressure of the anal canal. The 3-ml syringe containing 15 mCi (555 MBq) of ^{99m}Tc sodium pertechnetate should be injected into the catheter itself to permit visualization of the anal canal.
4. Three images should be acquired on computer (64 × 64 word mode matrix, 15 seconds per image) in the following order:
   a. Rest image—the patient is relaxed.
   b. Squeeze image—the patient contracts the sphincter muscles squeezing around the balloon.
   c. Defecation image—the patient strains to eject balloon (i.e., the Valsalva maneuver). The physician or nurse should hold the catheter to prevent actual expulsion.
5. After the three views are completed, withdraw the radioactive material into the 50/60-ml syringe and remove the catheter and balloon.
6. Dispose of the syringe in the radioactive waste bin. The catheter and balloon should be sterilized for future use.

Computer Analysis

Select the marker image and measure the distance (in pixels) between the two markers. Divide the distance by 20 to determine the pixels per centimeter calibration factor. On each of the three anorectal images, measure the angular flexion in the catheter (anorectal angle). Note the location of the flexion point (anorectal junction) and its displacement above or below an imaginary line joining the two skin markers. Convert this displacement to centimeters using the pixels per centimeter calibration factor.

Information on Film

On each computer film, ensure that the following information is recorded:

1. Patient name and clinic/hospital number
2. Date, type of scan, and radiopharmaceutical
3. Whether image is rest, squeeze, or defecation
4. Orientation of each image (e.g., right lateral)

Interpretation

In a normal patient in the decubitus position, the anorectal angle decreases from 105 ± 14° at rest to 88 ± 15° with squeezing, and 130 ± 11° with defecation. The anorectal junction should rise by approximately 1 cm with squeeze and should show little or no ascent with defecation.[4] The changes in the anorectal angle and junction between rest and squeeze images are shown in Figure 6-30.

Additional Notes

The balloon device is adapted from a design by Lahr et al.[5] It is constructed from a Penrose drain tube (16 cm long, 2.24-cm diameter latex sleeve) enclosing a 14F urinary catheter, a semirigid rubber catheter with an outside diameter of 5.33 mm (Fig. 6-31). The sleeve is tied off at either end with suture to form a balloon. A stopcock is attached to the end of

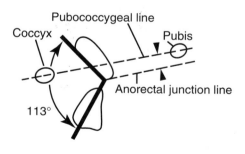

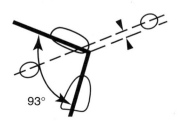

Figure 6-30. Diagrams of scintigraphic images: The resting anorectal angle is 113°, and the squeeze angle is 93° with ascended anorectal junction. (From Barkel et al.,[4] with permission.)

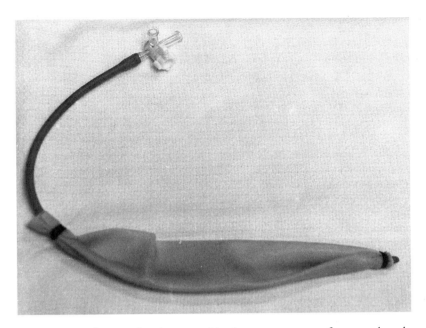

Figure 6-31. Balloon and catheter used in the measurement of anorectal angle.

the catheter. The balloon can be filled to a volume of 40 ml through the porthole in the catheter. The catheter itself can be filled to a volume of 2 ml.

Radiation Dosimetry

The estimated absorbed doses in organs and tissue of an average subject (70 kg) from the residence of 20 mCi (740 MBq) ^{99m}Tc sodium pertechnetate in the balloon for 15 minutes are shown in Table 6-9.[4]

Table 6-9. Absorbed Radiation Doses in a 70-kg Adult From the Residence of 20 mCi of ^{99m}Tc in the Anal Passage

Tissue	Absorbed Radiation Dose	
	rad/20 mCi	mGy/740 MBq
Rectum	0.784	7.84
Ovaries	0.066	0.66
Testes	0.006	0.06

References

1. Pemberton JH, Kelly KA. Achieving enteric continence: principles and applications. Mayo Clin Proc 1986; 61: 586–599.
2. Parks AG, Porter NH, Hardcastle J. The syndrome of the descending perineum. Proc R Soc Med 1966; 59: 477–482.
3. Cohen Z, McLeod RS, Stern H, et al. The pelvic pouch and ileoanal anastomosis procedure. Surgical technique and initial results. Am J Surg 1985; 150: 601–607.
4. Barkel DC, Pemberton JH, Pezim ME, et al. Scintigraphic assessment of the anorectal angle in health and after ileal pouch-anal anastomosis. Ann Surg 1988; 208: 42–49.
5. Lahr CJ, Rothenberger DA, Jensen LL, Goldberg SM. Balloon topography. A simple method of evaluating anal function. Dis Colon Rectum 1986; 29: 1–5.

Detection of Gastrointestinal Bleeding

Summary Information

Radiopharmaceutical

Adult dose:	20 mCi (740 MBq) of ^{99m}Tc-labeled red blood cells (in vitro labeling).
Pediatric dose:	Adjusted according to the patient's weight (see Appendix A-3).

Preparation of ^{99m}Tc-labeled red blood cells:

1. Withdraw 3 ml of blood from the patient, and label it with the UltraTag RBC kit or with an equivalent red blood cell labeling method.
2. The labeling procedure takes 20–30 minutes. Inject the red blood cells into the patient within 30 minutes after they have been labeled with ^{99m}Tc.

Contraindications   Barium contrast studies performed in the preceding 48 hours may cause attenuation of radioactivity from the gastrointestinal tract and obscure the site of bleeding. This procedure is best performed when the patient is actively bleeding.

Dose/Scan Interval   Imaging should be performed immediately after injection.

Views Obtained   An anterior view of the abdomen is the standard view for a gastrointestinal hemorrhage study. Upper and lower images of the abdomen may be required depending on the size of the patient and the size of the field of view of the gamma camera.

Indications

This procedure is indicated for patients in whom there is a question of active bleeding in the gastrointestinal tract.

Principle

The basic principle is to label the circulating blood so that extravasation at the bleeding site results in accumulation of radioactivity in the gastrointestinal tract.[1–3] The patient must be bleeding actively at the time of the study to localize the site of bleeding. Studies in dogs have indicated that the minimal detectable rate of bleeding is 0.1 ml/min.[4] It is likely that in clinical studies a bleeding rate 2 to 3 times this level would be required for the procedure to locate accurately the site of bleeding.[1]

Patient Preparation

None.

Instrument Specifications

Gamma camera:	Any large field-of-view system can be used.
Collimator:	Low-energy, all-purpose collimator.
Energy setting:	140 keV, 15–20% energy window.
Analog formatter:	8 × 10 film, 70-mm (9-on-1) format.
Computer system:	Acquisition requirements—dynamic (128 × 128 matrix).
	Processing requirements—none.

Imaging Procedure

1. Immediately after the injection, start a dynamic acquisition on computer (128 × 128 word mode matrix, 1 minute per frame, 60 frames). On an analog formatter, acquire a flow study for 9 frames at 2 seconds per frame.
2. After the flow study, set the analog formatter to acquire 1,000 kct images at 1 minute and 5 minutes after injection. Thereafter, acquire images every 5 minutes for 60 minutes, with the time per image set to that of the 5-minute image. After 1 hour, check with the nuclear medicine physician to see whether additional images should be acquired for 90 minutes.
3. If the early images are negative, then delayed images may be required by the nuclear medicine physician. For the delayed study, perform a dynamic acquisition on computer (128 × 128 word mode matrix, 1 minute per image, 20 images) and acquire a 1,000-kct static image on analog formatter (70-mm format).

Note: If a small field-of-view gamma camera is used, it may not be possible to include the entire abdomen in the field of view. In such cases, acquire the analog formatter flow study as described in step 1 and then set both the computer and analog formatter to acquire 2-minute static images, one of the upper abdomen and one of the lower abdomen, every 10 minutes for 60 minutes.

Computer Analysis

No computer analysis is required. However, the dynamic study should be played back as a movie to aid in determining the location of the site of bleeding.

Information on Film

On each analog and computer film, ensure that the following information is recorded:

1. Patient name and clinic/hospital number
2. Date and time after the injection

3. Type of scan and radiopharmaceutical
4. Orientation of each image (e.g., anterior)

Interpretation

In patients with a significant amount of active bleeding, visual inspection of the dynamic studies demonstrates increased accumulation of radiotracer in a distribution consistent with the large or small bowel. A review of the dynamic study in cine mode is useful in determining the location of the site of bleeding and in detecting small amounts of bleeding. With time and/or increased bleeding, the activity progresses along the lumen of the bowel (retrograde movement can occur).

Additional Notes

1. Poor labeling of the red blood cells may allow excretion of the pertechnetate through the stomach and kidneys, thus confounding interpretation.
2. If during the prescribed imaging time there is suggestion of a region of bleeding, the imaging sequence should be extended to look for further accumulation and movement of the tracer through the bowel. This dynamic imaging often aids in characterizing the exact location of the site of blood loss in the gastrointestinal tract.

Radiation Dosimetry

The estimated absorbed doses in organs and tissues of an average subject (70 kg) from an IV injection of 20 mCi of ^{99m}Tc-labeled red blood cells are shown in Table 6-10.[5]

Table 6-10. Absorbed Radiation Doses in a 70-kg Adult From ^{99m}Tc-Labeled Red Blood Cells

Tissue	Absorbed Radiation Doses	
	rad/20 mCi	mGy/740 MBq
Spleen	2.20	22.0
Bladder wall	0.48	4.8
Testes	0.22	2.2
Ovaries	0.32	3.2
Blood	0.80	8.0
Red marrow	0.30	3.0
Heart wall	2.00	20.0
Liver	0.58	5.8
Bone surfaces	0.48	4.8
Total body	0.30	3.0

References

1. Friedman HI, Hilts SV, Whitney PJ. Use of technetium-labeled autologous red blood cells in detection of gastrointestinal bleeding. Surg Gynecol Obstet 1983; 156: 449–452.
2. Gupta S, Luna E, Kingsley S, et al. Detection of gastrointestinal bleeding by radionuclide scintigraphy. Am J Gastroenterol 1984; 79: 26–31.
3. Robinson P. The role of nuclear medicine in acute gastrointestinal bleeding. Nucl Med Commun 1993; 14: 849–855.
4. Alavi A, Dann RW, Baum S, Biery DN. Scintigraphic detection of acute gastrointestinal bleeding. Radiology 1977; 124: 753–756.
5. UltraTag RBC Kit for the preparation of Technetium Tc [99m]-labeled red blood cells. Mallinckrodt Medical, St. Louis, MO. Revised January 1992.

99mTc Human Serum Albumin for Protein-Losing Gastroenteropathy

---

Summary Information

Radiopharmaceutical

Adult dose: 20 mCi (740 MBq) of 99mTc-labeled human serum albumin (HSA) injected intravenously

Pediatric dose: Adjusted according to the patient's weight (see Appendix A-3). *Note:* Because of the gastric accumulation of free pertechnetate, it is essential that less than 1% free pertechnetate be present in the 99mTc HSA preparation.

Contraindications 99mTc HSA is contraindicated in patients with known sensitivity to products containing HSA.

Dose/Scan Interval Imaging should commence within 1–2 minutes after the injection.

Views Obtained The liver and entire abdomen should be included in the field of view. Anterior views should be obtained.

Indications

Protein-losing enteropathy is a disorder involving the excessive loss of plasma protein in the gut. It can occur in such gastrointestinal diseases as Crohn's disease, ulcerative colitis, and ileocecal tuberculosis.[1] It has also been associated with more than 85 diseases, many unrelated to primary gastrointestinal disorders,[2] including lymphatic disorders, constrictive pericarditis,[3] congestive heart failure,[4] and nephrotic syndrome.[5] In an analogous manner to studies for the detection of gastrointestinal bleeding, 99mTc-labeled HSA can be used to qualitatively determine the location of protein loss in the gut. However, because of other confounding factors, the diagnosis of protein-losing enteropathy requires the quantitation of the degree of protein loss using procedures such as fecal alpha$_1$-antitrypsin measurement.[5]

Principle

The location and extent of protein loss anywhere in the gastrointestinal tract can be determined by imaging a radiolabeled plasma protein. 99mTc-labeled HSA is an ideal tracer for the detection of protein loss, because of its low false-positive index and short study time.[6]

333

Patient Preparation

Ask the patient to empty the bladder immediately before the scan.

Instrument Specifications

Gamma camera:	Any large field-of-view system can be used.
Collimator:	Low-energy all-purpose collimator
Energy setting:	140 keV, 15–20% energy window.
Analog formatter:	8 × 10 film, 70-mm (9-on-1) format.
Computer system:	Acquisition requirements—dynamic (128 × 128 matrix).
	Processing requirements—none.

Imaging Procedure

The patient should be positioned supine on the imaging table, with the gamma camera positioned anteriorly. Inject 20 mCi (740 MBq) of ^{99m}Tc HSA intravenously. Imaging should commence approximately 1 minute after the injection. Static images should be acquired at 1, 5, 10, 20, 30, and 60 minutes and at 2, 4, and 6 hours after injection, with 1,000 kct in the 1- and 5-minute images. All other images should be acquired for the same time as the 5-minute image. An additional image may be required at 24 hours after injection. If abnormal activity is seen in the gut, acquire a 5-minute static image over the thyroid to rule out the presence of free pertechnetate.

On computer, acquire a dynamic acquisition with the following variables: 128 × 128 matrix, 1 minute per view for 30 views. Additional static images (128 × 128 matrix, 750 kct per view) should be acquired at 1, 2, 4, and 6 hours after injection.

Computer Analysis

Play back the 30-minute dynamic acquisition as an aid in determining the origin of any abdominal activity seen on the analog images.

Information on Film

On each analog and computer film, ensure that the following information is recorded:

1. Patient name and clinic/hospital number
2. Date, type of scan, and radiopharmaceutical
3. Time of each image after injection
4. Orientation of each image (e.g., anterior)

Interpretation

Normal Scan

After the IV injection of ^{99m}Tc HSA, the blood pool should be visible immediately. This will become less evident with time because the ^{99m}Tc HSA does not remain in the intravascular space but diffuses into the extracellular compartments. In normal subjects, and in the absence of free pertechnetate, no activity should accumulate in the gut.[7]

Table 6-11. Absorbed Radiation Dose Estimates in a 70-kg Adult From 20 mCi (740 MBq) of ^{99m}Tc HSA

Tissue	Absorbed Radiation Dose	
	rad/20 mCi	mGy/740 MBq
Brain	0.19	1.9
Marrow	0.30	3.0
Kidneys	0.25	2.5
Bladder	0.66	6.6
Testes	0.32	3.2
Ovaries	0.33	3.3
Total body	0.29	2.9

Positive Scan

Abnormal activity may appear anywhere in the gut as early as 20 minutes after injection, although more typically it is 3–6 hours. The following issues should be considered in interpreting the scan:

1. The patient should not be actively bleeding (the patient should have a negative fecal blood loss test result), because the diagnosis of protein-losing enteropathy cannot be made in the presence of active bleeding.
2. If activity is seen in the stomach, it may be due to free pertechnetate. This can be confirmed by the presence of thyroid uptake in the neck scan and/or by the absence of alpha$_1$-antitrypsin in gastric juice (samples of gastric juice are obtained by nasogastric tube after an IV injection of alpha$_1$-antitrypsin).
3. If there is a known lesion in the gastrointestinal tract (from radiographic or other studies), this should be noted because it may aid in the interpretation of the image data.

Radiation Dosimetry

The estimated absorbed doses in organs and tissues of an average subject (70 kg) from an IV injection of 20 mCi (740 MBq) of ^{99m}Tc HSA are shown in Table 6-11.[8]

References

1. Greenberger NJ, Isselbacher KJ. Disorders of the alimentary tract. In "Harrison's Principles and Practice of Internal Medicine," eds Petersdorf RG, Adams RD, Braunwald E. McGraw-Hill, London, 1983, pp 1720–1738.
2. Waldmann TA. Protein-losing enteropathy and kinetic studies of plasma protein metabolism. Semin Nucl Med 1972; 2: 251–263.
3. Petersen VP, Hastrup J. Protein-losing enteropathy in constrictive pericarditis. Acta Med Scand 1963; 173: 401–410.

4. Davidson JD, Waldmann TA, Goodmann DS, Gordon RS Jr. Protein-losing gastroenteropathy in congestive heart failure. Lancet 1961; 1: 899–902.

5. Kluthe R, Liem HH, Nusslé D, Barandun S. Enteraler Plasmaeiweissverlust ("Proteindiarrhoe") beim nephrotischen Syndrom. Klin Wochenschr 1963; 41: 15–18.

6. Lan JA, Chervu LR, Marans Z, Collins JC. Protein-losing enteropathy detected by [99mTc]-labeled human serum albumin abdominal scintigraphy. J Pediatr Gastroenterol Nutr 1988; 7: 872–876.

7. Oommen R, Kurien G, Balakrishnan N, Narasimhan S. Tc-99m albumin scintigraphy in the localization of protein loss in the gut. Clin Nucl Med 1992; 17: 787–788.

8. Package insert. Technetium Tc 99m HSA Unit Dose. Medi-Physics, Paramus, NJ, Product number 4157, July 1987.

Detection of Meckel's Diverticulum

Summary Information

Radiopharmaceutical

    Adult dose: 5 mCi (185 MBq) of ^{99m}Tc sodium pertechnetate injected intravenously.

    Pediatric dose: Adjusted according to the patient's weight (see Appendix A-3).

Contraindications   None.

Dose/Scan Interval   Immediately after injection.

Views Obtained   The entire abdomen should be included in the field of view. Anterior and lateral views should be obtained.

Indications

A Meckel's scan may be indicated in patients with hematochezia (fresh blood in the stool), which can be caused by ectopic gastric mucosa in Meckel's diverticulum. The mucosa generally secretes hydrochloric acid, resulting in ulceration and bleeding in intestinal mucosa.[1]

Principle

The pertechnetate ion is actively trapped and secreted by gastric mucosa, primarily by the nonparietal cells in the stomach.[2] Meckel's diverticulum, which is a congenital outpouch in the distal ileum, may contain functioning gastric mucosa. Of the patients who present with symptoms, a high percentage (more than 50%) are found to have ectopic gastric mucosa.[1] Hence, it is possible to visualize and localize the aberrant mucosal tissue with a ^{99m}Tc sodium pertechnetate scan.[3]

Patient Preparation

The patient should fast for 3 hours before the study. If possible, the use of all drugs or procedures that may irritate the gastrointestinal tract should be stopped for 2–3 days before the study.[1] Potassium perchlorate should not be given, because it blocks uptake of the pertechnetate by the gastric mucosa. Ask the patient to empty the bladder immediately before the scan.

Instrument Specifications

Gamma camera:	Any large field-of-view system can be used.
Collimator:	Low-energy, all-purpose collimator.
Energy setting:	140 keV, 15–20% energy window.
Analog formatter:	8 × 10 film, 70-mm (9-on-1) format.
Computer system:	Acquisition requirements—dynamic (128 × 128 matrix).
	Processing requirements—none.

Imaging Procedure

1. Position the patient supine on the imaging table, with the gamma camera positioned anteriorly.
2. Inject 5 mCi (185 MBq) of ^{99m}Tc sodium pertechnetate intravenously.
3. When activity is visualized in the descending aorta, acquire a dynamic study on an analog formatter (9 frames at 5 seconds per frame).
4. Static images should then be acquired at 1, 5, 10, 15, 20, 25, and 30 minutes after injection, with 1,000 kct in the 1- and 5-minute images. All other images should be acquired for the same time as the 5-minute image.
5. On computer, acquire a dynamic acquisition with the following variables, 128 × 128 matrix, 1 minute per view for 30 views.
6. Additional lateral or oblique views may be required by the nuclear medicine physician.

Computer Analysis

Play back the 30-minute dynamic acquisition as an aid in determining the origin of any abdominal activity seen on the analog images.

Information on Film

On each analog and computer film, ensure that the following information is recorded:

1. Patient name and clinic/hospital number
2. Type of scan and radiopharmaceutical
3. Date and time of each image after injection
4. Orientation of each image (e.g., anterior)

Interpretation

Normal Scan

After the IV injection of ^{99m}Tc sodium pertechnetate, the blood pool is visible immediately, with gradual clearance of radioactivity from the blood and accumulation in the salivary glands, thyroid, and stomach. During the first 10 minutes, activity usually begins to appear in the stomach and increases in intensity, whereas the activity in the rest of the abdominal organs declines. As activity is secreted into the stomach lumen, it may travel down into the duodenum, followed by appearance in the jejunum and occasionally progressing as far as the ileum.

Table 6-12. Absorbed Radiation Dose Estimates in a 70-kg Adult From the Intravenous Administration of 5 mCi (185 MBq) of ^{99m}Tc Pertechnetate

Tissue	Absorbed Radiation Dose	
	rad/5 mCi	mGy/185 MBq
Bladder wall	0.265	2.65
Stomach wall	1.250	12.5
Upper large intestinal wall	0.340	3.40
Lower large intestinal wall	0.305	3.05
Red marrow	0.095	0.95
Testes	0.045	0.45
Ovaries	0.110	1.10
Thyroid	0.650	6.50
Brain	0.07	0.70
Total body	0.07	0.70

Positive Scan

A Meckel's diverticulum is typically seen as a small area of increased activity that appears simultaneously with the activity in the stomach, usually 10–20 minutes after injection. Activity in the diverticulum should persist throughout the study and parallel the pattern of uptake in the stomach. Meckel's diverticulum usually is located anteriorly in the right lower quadrant; and its apparent position may change as the patient is raised or turned or after voiding.

Additional Notes

In patients with a low acid output state (e.g., H2 receptor antagonists), visualization of the stomach and any ectopic mucosa may be poor. Pentagastrin may be used to stimulate gastric secretion, thereby increasing the uptake and secretion of ^{99m}Tc sodium pertechnetate from the gastric mucosa.[2] If used, pentagastrin should be injected subcutaneously (6 μg/kg body weight) immediately before injection of the pertechnetate.[4]

Radiation Dosimetry

The estimated absorbed doses in organs and tissues of an average subject (70 kg) from an IV injection of 5 mCi (185 MBq) ^{99m}Tc sodium pertechnetate are shown in Table 6-12.[5]

References

1. Sfakianakis GN, Conway JJ. Detection of ectopic gastric mucosa in Meckel's diverticulum and in other aberrations by scintigraphy: II. Indications and methods—a 10-year experience. J Nucl Med 1981; 22: 732–738.

2. O'Connor MK, O'Connell R, Keane FB, Byrne PJ, Hennessy TP. The relationship between technetium 99m pertechnetate gastric scanning and gastric contents. Br J Radiol 1983; 56: 817–822.

3. Sfakianakis GN, Conway JJ. Detection of ectopic gastric mucosa in Meckel's diverticulum and in other aberrations by scintigraphy: I. Pathophysiology and 10-year clinical experience. J Nucl Med 1981; 22: 647–654.

4. Treves S, Grand RJ, Eraklis AJ. Pentagastrin stimulation of technetium-99m uptake by ectopic gastric mucosa in a Meckel's diverticulum. Radiology 1978; 128: 711–712.

5. MIRD/Dose Estimate Report No. 8. Summary of current radiation dose estimates to normal humans from ^{99m}Tc as sodium pertechnetate. J Nucl Med 1976; 17: 74–77.

Liver/Spleen Scan

Summary Information

Radiopharmaceutical

Adult dose: 6 mCi (222 MBq) of ^{99m}Tc sulfur colloid or ^{99m}Tc albumin colloid injected intravenously.

Pediatric dose: Adjusted according to the patient's weight (see Appendix A-3).

Contraindications ^{99m}Tc albumin colloid is contraindicated in patients with known sensitivity to products containing HSA.

Does/Scan Interval Analog and digital images should be obtained 15–20 minutes after the injection.

Views Obtained

Planar liver scan: The following views should be obtained:
1. Anterior marker (lead strip marker)
2. Anterior
3. Posterior
4. Right anterior oblique
5. Right lateral
6. Left lateral

Planar spleen scan: Acquire views 1–6 and the following 3 additional views:
1. Right posterior oblique
2. Left anterior oblique
3. Left posterior oblique

Planar life-size liver scan: The following views should be obtained:
1. Anterior marker
2. Anterior
3. Posterior
4. Right lateral

Single photon emission computed tomography (SPECT) liver scan: Obtain tomographic images of the liver and spleen.

Indications

Various imaging techniques (ultrasonography, computed tomography [CT], magnetic resonance imaging) provide excellent anatomic information about the liver. Hence, liver/spleen scintigraphy is performed to assess the functional status of the liver, primarily in patients with cirrhosis, hepatitis, and metabolic disorders.[1] In patients with known lesions revealed by CT or ultrasonography (e.g., tumor, hematoma, cyst, abscess), liver/spleen scintigraphy may be used to assess further the nature of these lesions. Enlarged views of the liver (life-size liver scans) are useful in patients with known liver tumors who are receiving chemotherapy. The progress of treatment can be monitored by noting the change in tumor size on sequential scans. The images are acquired on film in a large format to facilitate simple measurement of lesion size from the film with a ruler.

Spleen imaging may be useful in the evaluation of infarcts or in the detection of residual splenic tissue after splenectomy.

Principle

After IV administration, ^{99m}Tc sulfur or albumin colloidal particles are cleared rapidly from the blood by the reticuloendothelial system, with a clearance half-life of 2–6 minutes, depending on particle size.[2] Uptake in the liver, spleen, and bone marrow is a function of blood flow and the functional capacity of the phagocytic cells. In normal subjects, 80–90% of the activity is in the liver, 5–10% is in the spleen, and the rest is in the bone marrow. After 15 minutes, only 5–10% of the injected activity remains in the blood. In patients with liver disease, disruption of normal hepatic blood flow may lead to nonuniform distribution of colloidal particles in the liver and/or increased uptake in the spleen and bone marrow.

Patient Preparation

No special preparation is required. However, if the patient is scheduled for other studies of the gastrointestinal tract, the liver/spleen imaging should be performed before barium or other contrast agents are administered, because they may cause photon-deficient artifacts in the images.

Instrument Specifications

Gamma camera:	Planar views—any large field-of-view system can be used. SPECT—single-, dual-, or triple-head system, preferably with elliptical/body contour orbit.
Collimator:	Low-energy, high-resolution collimator.
Energy:	140 keV, 15–20% energy window.
Analog formatter:	8 × 10 film, 70-mm format (9-on-1) for standard liver scans. 8 × 10 film, 1-on-1 format for life-size liver scans.
Computer system:	Acquisition requirements—static (256 × 256 matrix). Processing requirements—none for static views. SPECT reconstruction software.

Imaging Procedure

Planar Study—Standard Liver or Liver/Spleen Scan

1. The patient should be positioned supine on the imaging table. Position the gamma camera anteriorly, and acquire an image (1,000 kct per image) with standard-size reference markers. Figure 6-32 shows a lead strip (30 cm × 2 cm) positioned on the costal margin and a 10-cm lead circle marker taped to the camera head so that it is superimposed over

the image of the right lobe of the liver (*Note:* The marker disk should always be taped to the detector [rather than to the patient] to avoid parallax errors that are due to oblique orientation).

2. Acquire the anterior, posterior, right anterior oblique, and right lateral images (1,000 kct per image). Acquire the left lateral view for the same time as the right lateral view. For oblique views, the patient should be rotated 45°. For lateral views, the patient should be supine, with the detector facing horizontally.
3. For a spleen scan, acquire all images, as described in steps 1 and 2.
4. In addition, acquire left and right posterior oblique views and a left anterior oblique image (1,000 kct per image).
5. For computer acquisition, all images should be acquired in a 256 × 256 word mode matrix for 3 minutes per view.

Planar Study—Life-Size Liver Scan

1. Set an analog formatter for acquisition in a 1-on-1 format.
2. Acquire the anterior marker image, as in step 1. Label the marker image to indicate the 10-cm distance.
3. Acquire the anterior, posterior, and right lateral views (1,000 kct per view).

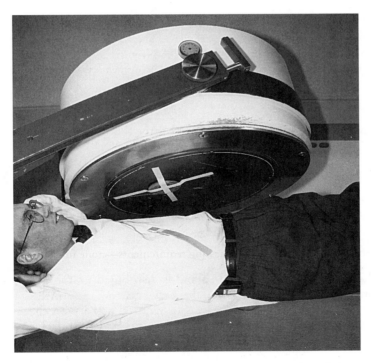

Figure 6-32. Lead strip marker in position over costal margin, and 10-cm lead disk attached to surface of collimator. The detector head has been moved away from the patient to better illustrate the position of the marker and disk.

SPECT Study

SPECT acquisition variables depend on the number of detector heads on the system.

1. For a single-head system, acquire 120–128 views over 360° into a 128 × 128 word mode matrix at 20 seconds per view, using a high-resolution collimator and, if available, appropriate body contouring to minimize the patient-to-collimator distance.
2. For a dual-head or triple-head system, acquire as in step 1, with the time per frame reduced to 15 seconds per view. Note: The time per frame should be increased to 20 seconds if an ultrahigh-resolution collimator is used (collimator sensitivity less than 150 ct/min per µCi).
3. Check that all loose clothing and straps are tucked away, because they may interfere with a body-contouring orbit.

Computer Analysis

SPECT Study

Perform the following steps:

1. Apply uniformity and center-of-rotation correction to the data (on newer systems, this may be done automatically).
2. If possible, prefilter the planar data (possible filters are Butterworth, order 10–12, cutoff at 0.4–0.6 Nyquist and Metz filter with a power of 3 and full width at half maximum [FWHM] of 6–10 mm).
3. Reconstruct 1-pixel-thick transaxial slices. The back-projection filter may be a Ramp or Ramp-Butterworth with a cutoff at 0.6–0.8 Nyquist.
4. Apply attenuation correction (Sorenson or Chang), with $\mu = 0.12$ cm^{-1}.

Information on Film

On each analog and computer film, ensure that the following information is recorded:

1. Patient name and clinic/hospital number
2. Date, type of scan, and radiopharmaceutical
3. Time of each image after injection
4. Orientation of each image (e.g., anterior, posterior)
5. Label marker image to show costal margin and 10-cm markers

Interpretation

In normal subjects, the radiolabeled colloid is distributed uniformly throughout the liver and spleen, with very faint uptake in the bone marrow. Any disease that disrupts liver blood flow or function may lead to areas of reduced activity on the liver scan. Tumors, cysts, and abscesses may be seen as single or multiple areas of decreased tracer uptake or absence of tracer uptake. Studies in patients with diffuse liver disease, such as cirrhosis and hepatitis, may show mild to severely irregular distribution with enlargement of the liver. In severe cases, the bone marrow is clearly visualized, and the tracer concentration in the spleen is greatly increased.

Table 6-13. Absorbed Dose Estimates in a 70-kg Adult From ^{99m}Tc Sulfur or Albumin Colloid

	Absorbed Radiation Dose	
Tissue	rad/6 mCi	mGy/222 MBq
Liver	2.04	20.4
Spleen	1.26	12.6
Bone marrow	0.17	1.65
Testes	0.01	0.08
Ovaries	0.03	0.34
Total body	0.11	1.13

Additional Notes

Attenuation artifacts may appear from female breast tissue overlaying the superior portion of the liver's right lobe. Breast shadow artifacts can be eliminated by taping the breast so that it is out of the way.

Radiation Dosimetry

The estimated absorbed doses in organs and tissues of an average subject (70 kg) from an IV injection of 6 mCi (222 MBq) of ^{99m}Tc sulfur colloid or ^{99m}Tc albumin colloid are shown in Table 6-13.[3,4]

References

1. Mettler FA. "Radionuclide Imaging of the GI Tract." Churchill Livingstone, New York, 1986, pp 83–182.
2. Datz FL. Gastrointestinal imaging. In "Clinical Practice of Nuclear Medicine," eds Taylor A Jr, Datz FL. Churchill Livingstone, New York, 1991, pp 317–360.
3. MIRD Dose Estimate Report No. 3. Summary of current radiation dose estimates to humans with various liver conditions from technetium 99m Tc-sulfur colloid. J Nucl Med 1975; 16: 108A–108B.
4. Package Insert. Microlite — kit for the preparation of Technetium Tc99m albumin colloid. Du Pont Merck Pharmaceutical Co, Billerica, MA, revised November 1991.

Liver Hemangioma Study

Summary Information

Radiopharmaceutical

Adult dose: 20 mCi (740 MBq) ^{99m}Tc-red blood cells (in vitro-labeled red blood cells).

Pediatric dose: Adjusted according to the patient's weight (see Appendix A-3).

Preparation of ^{99m}Tc-labeled red blood cells:

1. Withdraw 3 ml of blood from the patient, and label it with the UltraTag RBC kit or with an equivalent red blood cell-labeling method.
2. The labeling procedure takes 20–30 minutes. After preparation of the ^{99m}Tc red blood cells, reinject the radiolabeled cells within 30 minutes.

Contraindications None.

Dose/Scan Interval Imaging commences immediately after injection.

Views Obtained Obtain an anterior view of the liver and spleen and SPECT images of the liver and spleen.

Indications

Cavernous hemangiomas are the most common benign tumors of the liver. Generally, hemangiomas have a decreased blood flow but a large blood pool. Blood flow and blood pool studies of the liver using ^{99m}Tc-labeled red blood cells are reliable noninvasive techniques for the diagnosis of liver hemangiomas, with a specificity of nearly 100%[1,2] and a sensitivity that is highly dependent on lesion size.[3,4] Planar imaging is adequate for lesions of 3 cm or more. SPECT imaging is required for lesions less than 3 cm in diameter.[5,6]

Principle

Radiolabeled red blood cells circulating intravascularly can serve as a marker to identify hemangiomas. Hepatic hemangiomas are initially hypovascular, appearing as cold areas on the initial flow study. However, on delayed images taken at 20 minutes to 1 hour after injection, they are hypervascular and displayed as areas of increased activity within the liver. Planar imaging is adequate for large lesions; however, SPECT is required to visualize small lesions.

Patient Preparation

None.

Instrument Specifications

Gamma camera:	Planar views/flow study—any large field-of-view system may be used.
	SPECT—single-, dual-, or triple-head system, preferably with elliptical or body-contour orbit.
Collimator:	Planar flow study—low-energy, all-purpose collimator.
	Planar spot views/SPECT—low-energy, high-resolution collimator.
Energy setting:	140 keV, 15–20% energy window.
Analog formatter:	8 × 10 film, 70-mm (9-on-1) format.
Computer system:	Acquisition requirements—static (256 × 256 matrix), dynamic (64 × 64 matrix), SPECT (128 × 128 matrix). Processing requirements—none required for planar data. SPECT reconstruction software.

Imaging Procedure

Planar Study: Analog Formatter

Position the patient supine on the imaging table, with the gamma camera centered anteriorly over the liver. Start the analog formatter when activity is first visualized in the descending aorta. Record.

1. Flow study (5 seconds per image for 9 images).
2. Static images at 1, 5, 10, 15, 20, 25, and 30 minutes after injection with 1,000 kct per image for the initial 1- and 5-minute images. The time duration for the 5-minute image should then be used for subsequent images.
3. Delayed planar images may be required at 2–4 hours. Additional views (left anterior oblique or left lateral) may be required. The time per image should be as described in step 2.

Planar Study: Computer Acquisition

Start computer acquisition at the time of the injection. This is a 30-minute, 2-phase dynamic acquisition with the following variables:

1. Phase 1—60 frames at 1 second per frame, 64 × 64 word mode matrix
2. Phase 2—24 frames at 1 minute per frame, 64 × 64 word mode matrix

If delayed images are required, these should be acquired on computer in a 256 × 256 word mode matrix for 750–1,000 kct per image.

SPECT Study

SPECT of the liver should be performed after the 30-minute planar study is completed. The acquisition variables depend on the number of detector heads on the system.

1. For a single-head system, acquire 120–128 views over 360° into 128 × 128 word mode matrix at 20 seconds per view, using a high-resolution collimator and appropriate body contouring to minimize the patient-to-collimator distance.
2. For a dual-head or triple-head system, acquire views as in step 1, with the time per frame decreased to 12–15 seconds per view. Note: The time per frame should be increased to 20 seconds for big or obese patients (men more than 100 kg; women more than 80 kg) or if an ultrahigh-resolution collimator is used (collimator sensitivity less than 150 ct/min per μCi).
3. Check that all loose clothing and straps are tucked away, because they may interfere with a body-contouring orbit.

Computer Analysis

Planar Study

The dynamic acquisition should be replayed as an aid in determining the presence of any cold defects within the liver. The location of any suspected cold lesions on the initial flow study should be correlated with the later static views, on which these lesions should appear hot.

SPECT Study

Perform the following steps:

1. Apply uniformity and center-of-rotation correction to the data (on newer systems, this may be done automatically).
2. If possible, prefilter the planar data (possible filters are Butterworth, order 10–12, cutoff at 0.4–0.6 Nyquist and Metz filter with a power of 3 and FWHM of 6–10 mm).
3. Reconstruct 1-pixel-thick transaxial slices. Back-projection filter may be a Ramp or Ramp-Butterworth with a cutoff at 0.6–0.8 Nyquist.
4. Apply attenuation correction (Sorenson or Chang), with $\mu = 0.12$ cm^{-1}.

Information on Film

On each analog and computer film, ensure that the following information is recorded:

1. Patient name and clinic/hospital number
2. Date, type of scan, and radiopharmaceutical
3. Time of each image after injection
4. Orientation of each image (e.g., anterior)

Interpretation

Cavernous hemangiomas show a normal or decreased blood flow on the early flow study, and on the later images and on the SPECT images, they show a fill-in or hot spot pattern corresponding to increased blood pool activity (activity equal to the cardiac blood pool). The specificity of both planar and SPECT is close to 100%. Sensitivities of 93–100% have been reported for lesions more than 1.5 cm in diameter and 30–50% for smaller lesions.[5,6]

Radiation Dosimetry

The estimated absorbed doses in organs and tissues of an average subject (70 kg) from an IV injection of 20 mCi (740 MBq) ^{99m}Tc-labeled red blood cells are shown in Table 6-10.[7]

References

1. Brodsky RI, Friedman AC, Maurer AH, Radecki PD, Caroline DF. Hepatic cavernous hemangioma: diagnosis with 99mTc-labeled red cells and single-photon emission CT. AJR 1987; 148: 125–129.
2. Engel MA, Marks DS, Sandler MA, Shetty P. Differentiation of focal intrahepatic lesions with ^{99m}Tc-red blood cell imaging. Radiology 1983; 146: 777–782.
3. Kudo M, Ikekudo K, Yamamoto K, et al. Distinction between hemangioma of the liver and hepatocellular carcinoma: value of labeled RBC-SPECT scanning. AJR 1989; 152: 977–983.
4. Langsteger W, Lind P, Eber B, et al. Diagnosis of hepatic hemangioma with ^{99m}Tc-labeled red cells: single photon emission computed tomography (SPECT) versus planar imaging. Liver 1989; 9: 288–293.
5. Krause T, Hauenstein K, Studier-Fischer B, Schuemichen C, Moser E. Improved evaluation of technetium-^{99m}-red blood cell SPECT in hemangioma of the liver. J Nucl Med 1993; 34: 375–380.
6. Ziessman HA, Silverman PM, Patterson J, et al. Improved detection of small cavernous hemangiomas of the liver with high-resolution three-headed SPECT. J Nucl Med 1991; 32: 2086–2091.
7. UltraTag RBC—Kit for the preparation of technetium Tc 99m-labeled red blood cells, 068. Mallinckrodt, St. Louis. Revised January 1992.

Hepatic Artery Perfusion Study

Summary Information

Radiopharmaceutical
Adult dose: 5 mCi (185 MBq) of ^{99m}Tc macroaggregated albumin (MAA) injected through a hepatic artery catheter.
Pediatric dose: None established.

Contraindications None.

Dose/Scan Interval Immediately after injection.

Views Obtained Obtain an anterior view of the chest and abdomen, centered on the liver and spleen. Right lateral, left anterior oblique, and right anterior oblique views are also required.

Indications

^{99m}Tc MAA imaging can be used to assess the perfusion pattern from small-bore indwelling hepatic arterial catheters during chemotherapy and to ensure that catheter position is optimal.[1,2] The success of regional chemotherapy depends on precise delivery of the drug to the tumor-containing regions. This success may be compromised by several factors, including incorrect placement of the catheter, significant extrahepatic perfusion, and arteriovenous shunting, which reduces the exposure of the tumor to the drug and increases systemic toxicity. Significant changes in the degree of extrahepatic localization over time may also influence the chemotherapeutic regimen.

Principle

Successful regional hepatic arterial chemotherapy requires accurate placement of the catheter in the region containing the tumor. After injection through the catheter, macroaggregated particles of albumin, in the size range of 10–90 μm, are trapped in the first capillary bed encountered and, therefore, can be used as an indicator of the target region for the chemotherapeutic agent. Poor distribution of the ^{99m}Tc MAA in the target region (e.g. with lung uptake) may indicate impaired delivery of chemotherapeutic agents to that portion of the liver. If the catheter is positioned incorrectly, other extrahepatic uptake of the ^{99m}Tc MAA (e.g,. bowel activity) may be present.

Patient Preparation

The patient should have the chemotherapy catheter delivery system in position. A routine ^{99m}Tc sulfur colloid liver/spleen scan that was performed recently is often helpful for comparison. *Note:* A special needle may be required for puncture of the catheter infusion port.

Instrument Specifications

Gamma camera:	Any large field-of-view system can be used.
Collimator:	Low-energy, all-purpose collimator.
Energy setting:	140 keV, 15–20% energy window.
Analog formatter:	8 × 10 film, 70-mm (9-on-1) format.
Computer system:	Acquisition requirements—static (256 × 256 word mode matrix), dynamic (64 × 64 word mode matrix). Processing requirements—ROI analysis.

Imaging Procedure

1. Position the patient supine under the gamma camera, with the liver and spleen centered in the field of view.
2. With aseptic technique, administer 5 mCi (185 MBq) ^{99m}Tc MAA slowly. The total volume of ^{99m}Tc MAA should be 0.5–1.0 ml and should be injected over a 2-minute period through the hepatic catheter. Note: Assistance of the surgical or nursing staff should be sought to ensure correct injection of the ^{99m}Tc MAA.
3. After injection of the ^{99m}Tc MAA, the catheter should be flushed with normal or heparinized saline, as appropriate.
4. Immediately before injection, start the analog formatter (9 frames at 10 seconds per frame) and computer (64 × 64 word mode matrix, 30 frames at 3 seconds per frame).
5. After the injection, obtain the following views of the liver on analog formatter and on computer (256 × 256 word mode matrix) for 1,000 kct each:
   a. Anterior
   b. Left anterior oblique
   c. Right anterior oblique
   d. Right lateral

Reposition the detector over the lungs, and obtain anterior and posterior views for the same time as the anterior liver view in step 5a.

Computer Analysis

The dynamic flow study can be replayed as an aid in determining the route of ^{99m}Tc MAA into the liver and the origin of any extrahepatic activity. A simple index of extrahepatic shunting can be obtained from ROI analysis by obtaining the ratio of activity in the lungs to total activity in the abdomen and lungs.[3] This may be useful in tracking changes in the degree of shunting over time.

Information on Film

On each analog and computer film, ensure that the following information is recorded:

1. Patient name and clinic/hospital number
2. Type of scan and radiopharmaceutical
3. Date and time after injection
4. Orientation of each image (e.g., anterior, left anterior oblique)

Interpretation

The distribution of ^{99m}Tc MAA depends on the placement of the catheter, which may be selective. Hepatic regions not visualized on the ^{99m}Tc MAA scan represent areas not perfused by the catheter system. This can be intentional, depending on the selective nature of catheter placement. Radioactivity in the lungs indicates tumor arteriovenous shunting, which will reduce the exposure of the tumor to the drug and increase systemic exposure and toxicity. Other extrahepatic uptake (e.g., in the gut) may occur if the catheter is incorrectly positioned.

Additional Notes

^{99m}Tc MAA should be injected slowly over a 1–2 minute period. This is to simulate the flow rate during actual chemotherapy and to prevent streamlining of the flow, which potentially can alter the distribution of the radiotracer.

Radiation Dosimetry

No dosimetry is available for this procedure. A crude estimate of the dose to the liver can be obtained based on the doses that would be delivered from 5 mCi (185 MBq) ^{99m}Tc sulfur colloid and assuming that all the activity remains in the liver (see Table 6-13).

References

1. Kaplan WD, Ensminger WD, Come SE, et al. Radionuclide angiography to predict patient response to hepatic artery chemotherapy. Cancer Treat Rep 1980; 64: 1217–1222.
2. Bledin AG, Kantarjian HM, Kim EE, et al. 99mTc-labeled macroaggregated albumin in intrahepatic arterial chemotherapy. AJR 1982; 139: 711–715.
3. Ziessman HA, Thrall JH, Yang PJ, et al. Hepatic arterial perfusion scintigraphy with Tc-99m-MAA. Radiology 1984; 152: 167–172.

Hepatobiliary Scan

Summary Information

Radiopharmaceutical

Adult dose: 6 mCi (222 MBq) of ^{99m}Tc disofenin or ^{99m}Tc mebrofenin injected intravenously.

Pediatric dose: Adjust according to the patient's weight (see Appendix A-3).

Contraindications   None.

Dose/Scan Interval   Analog images should be obtained starting 1 minute after injection. Computer acquisition should be started at the time of injection.

Views Obtained   The anterior view of the abdomen includes the liver and small bowel. Oblique views (right anterior oblique, left anterior oblique, or right lateral) may be required in some patients.

Indications

Hepatobiliary scintigraphy with ^{99m}Tc iminodiacetic acid (IDA) compounds is useful in evaluating the patency of the common bile duct and the cystic duct. This test is very sensitive and specific for acute cholecystitis. Because IDA compounds are extracted by hepatocytes and excreted unconjugated into the bile, hepatocyte function and biliary drainage can be evaluated. This test may also be helpful in evaluating patients with jaundice or abdominal pain and after hepatic/biliary operations.[1–3] This is not a test for cholelithiasis (gallstones), because many patients with cholelithiasis have normal hepatobiliary function.

Principle

Biliary tract scintigraphy can be performed with either ^{99m}Tc disofenin or ^{99m}Tc mebrofenin. Both of these agents are iminodiacetic acid derivatives that are cleared rapidly from the blood by the hepatocytes and excreted in the bile in high concentrations. In normal fasting subjects, peak liver uptake occurs about 10 minutes after injection, with visualization of the hepatic duct and gallbladder after 20–40 minutes. In normal subjects, about 9% of the disofenin and 1% of the mebrofenin are excreted in the urine in the first 2 hours. Increased serum levels of bilirubin increase renal excretion and may lead to visualization of the kidneys in some patients.[4]

Patient Preparation

The patient should fast for a minimum of 4 hours before the study. A false-positive study (nonvisualization of the gallbladder) may result if the patient has eaten recently.

Note: If amino acids or lipid solutions are being given intravenously to a patient who has not eaten for 24 hours, sincalide (a synthetic analog of cholecystokinin) should be given, as described later.

Note: If tube feeding is used in the patient (Osmolite, Ensure, Vital, etc.), it should be discontinued 4 hours before the study. It is not necessary to give sincalide to these patients.

Note: If the patient has received morphine within 4 hours before the IDA study, inform the nuclear medicine physician, because morphine may result in delayed visualization of the bowel that is due to constriction of the sphincter of Oddi. The study will need to be interpreted with this in mind.

Note: If necessary, the effects of morphine may be reversed with the IV administration of 0.8 mg naloxone hydrochloride (naloxone is a competitive opiate antagonist).[5]

Note: With patients on long-term fasting, a sincalide infusion can be given before the IDA agent is injected. The sincalide infusion should be confirmed with the nuclear medicine physician before infusion. The sincalide causes gallbladder contraction, thereby decreasing cystic duct bile statis, and enhancing visualization of the gallbladder.

Cholecystokinin Infusion

To reconstitute sincalide (Kinevac, Squibb), add 5 ml of sterile water to the vial and shake it for 1 minute (see instructions on the package insert). This gives a concentration of 1 µg/ml. The administered dose is 0.02 µg/kg body weight, giving a dose of 1.4 µg for a 70-kg adult. Infuse the sincalide over a 2-minute period, approximately 30 minutes before injection of the IDA tracer.

Instrument Specifications

Gamma camera:	Any large field-of-view gamma camera system can be used.
Collimator:	Low-energy, all-purpose or high-resolution collimator.
Energy setting:	140 keV, 15–20% energy window.
Analog formatter:	8 × 10 film, 70-mm (9-on-1) format.
Computer system:	Acquisition requirements—dynamic (64 × 64 word mode matrix).
	Processing requirements—none.

Imaging Procedure

The patient should be positioned supine on the imaging table, with the gamma camera positioned anteriorly.

Analog Formatter

Images of the liver should be obtained at 1, 5, 10, 15, 20, 25, 30, 45, and 60 minutes after injection, with 1,000 kct in the 1- and 5-minute images. All other images should be acquired for the same time as the 5-minute image. In patients in whom the gallbladder is not visualized by 60 minutes, morphine may be administered or additional images may be necessary at 2 and 4 hours. If the small bowel or gallbladder is not visualized on these images, the nuclear medicine physician may request an additional image at 24 hours to assess common bile duct patency. At 24 hours, an additional anterior oblique or lateral view may be required to aid distinction between radioactivity in the gallbladder and bowel.

Computer Acquisition

Immediately after injection, computer acquisition should be performed using a 64×64 word mode matrix, with 30 seconds per frame for 120 frames. If the gallbladder is not visualized after 1 hour, morphine may be used to stimulate contraction of the sphincter of Oddi and promote filling of the gallbladder. When delayed imaging is required, the use of morphine should allow the study to be completed in 90 minutes rather than in 4 hours. After morphine administration, additional images should be acquired at 1, 5, 10, 15, 20, and 30 minutes after the injection of morphine. The nuclear medicine physician will determine when morphine is required. See "Additional Notes" for a complete procedural guide on the use of morphine.

Computer Analysis

The dynamic study should be replayed in cine mode as an aid in determining the exact location of activity, particularly in distinguishing between activity in the gallbladder and the common bile duct or cystic duct.

Information on Film

On each analog and computer film, ensure that the following information is recorded:

1. Patient name and clinic/hospital number
2. Date, type of scan, and radiopharmaceutical
3. Time of each image after injection and after administration of morphine (if administered)
4. Orientation of each image (e.g., anterior)

Interpretation

In normal subjects, the radiotracer is distributed homogeneously in the liver by 1–5 minutes after the injection, with the gallbladder, common bile duct, and intestinal tract being visualized by 1 hour. In females, the dome of the right lobe of the liver may be attenuated by the right breast. An abnormal pattern may show any of the following: focal hepatic defects seen during the parenchymal phase, persistent nonvisualization of the gallbladder up to 4 hours after the injection, reflux of tracer into the stomach, or pooling of tracer outside the biliary tract or intestinal tract.

Additional Notes

Use of Morphine During Hepatobiliary Imaging Studies

Morphine is a controlled substance, and written documentation is required for its use. Morphine is commonly supplied in a 10-ml vial, with a concentration of 1 mg/ml. The usual dosage of morphine sulfate when used for hepatobiliary imaging procedures is 0.04 mg/kg of body weight. This should be diluted in 10 ml of normal saline and administered intravenously over 3 minutes. The morphine injection is stored in glass ampules. Special filter needles (Monoject, 18-gauge × 1.5 inches) should be used when drawing the morphine solution into the syringe to minimize the chance for removing glass particles along with the solution. The IV injection of morphine in low doses is usually well tolerated and without complications, and it will not aggravate symptoms. Possible contraindications for use of this morphine-assisted technique are hyperamylasemia, a history of opiate addiction, or rarely, allergy to morphine. Also, it is contraindicated in patients in whom the physician does not want the clinical symptoms obscured by morphine.

After completion of the study, any unused portion of the morphine should be discarded in the sink, and the disposal should be witnessed by another healthcare worker (e.g., prescribing physician, nuclear medicine/pharmacy technologist, nurse). The technologist and the healthcare worker witnessing the disposal of the controlled substance should both sign their name on the morphine administration record. This record should also be signed by the nuclear medicine physician. One copy should be retained in nuclear medicine unit, and the second one should be sent to the dispensing pharmacy (procedures for dealing with morphine may vary depending on local regulations for controlled substances).

Radiation Dosimetry

The estimated absorbed doses in organs and tissues of an average subject (70 kg) from an IV injection of 6 mCi (222 MBq) of ^{99m}Tc disofenin or ^{99m}Tc mebrofenin are shown in Table 6-14.[6,7]

Table 6-14. Absorbed Radiation Doses in a 70-kg Adult From the Intravenous Injection of ^{99m}Tc Mebrofenin or ^{99m}Tc Disofenin

| | Absorbed Radiation Doses | | | |
| | rad/6 mCi | | mGy/222 MBq | |
Tissue	Mebrofenin	Disofenin	Mebrofenin	Disofenin
Liver	0.29	0.18	2.9	1.8
Gallbladder wall	0.83	0.84	8.3	8.4
Small intestine	1.79	1.08	17.9	10.8
Upper large intestinal wall	2.84	2.10	28.4	21.0
Lower large intestinal wall	2.18	1.50	21.8	15.0
Urinary bladder wall	0.17	0.53	1.7	5.3
Ovaries	0.61	0.45	6.1	4.5
Testes	0.03	0.04	0.30	0.40
Red marrow	0.20	0.09	2.00	0.90
Total body	0.12	0.09	1.2	0.9

References

1. Kim EE, Moon TY, Delpassand ES, Podoloff DA, Haynie TP. Nuclear hepatobiliary imaging. Radiol Clin North Am 1993; 31: 923–933.
2. Ziessman HA. Scintigraphy in the gastrointestinal tract. Curr Opin Radiol 1992; 4: 105–116.
3. Drane WE. Nuclear medicine techniques for the liver and biliary system. Update for the 1990s. Radiol Clin North Am 1991; 29: 1129–1150.
4. Stadalnik RC, Matolo NM, Jansholt AL, Vera DR. Clinical experience with ^{99m}Tc-disofenin as a cholescintigraphic agent. Radiology 1981; 140: 797–800.
5. Patch GG, Morton KA, Arias JM, Datz FL. Naloxone reverses pattern of obstruction of the distal common bile duct induced by analgesic narcotics in hepatobiliary imaging. J Nucl Med 1991; 32: 1270–1272.
6. Package insert. Choletec—kit for the preparation of technetium Tc ^{99m} mebrofenin. Squibb Diagnostics, New Brunswick, NJ, revised March 1987.
7. Package insert. Hepatolite—kit for the preparation of technetium Tc ^{99m} Disofenin. DuPont, Billerica, MA, January 1994.

Hepatobiliary Scan With Gallbladder Ejection Fraction

Summary Information

Radiopharmaceutical

Adult dose: 6 mCi (222 MBq) ^{99m}Tc disofenin or ^{99m}Tc mebrofenin injected intravenously.

Pediatric dose: Adjusted according to the patient's weight (see Appendix A-3).

Contraindications   Check that the patient does not have a known sensitivity to HSA.

Dose/Scan Interval   Analog and digital images should be acquired over the first 60 minutes, as for a conventional hepatobiliary scan. At 60–90 minutes after the injection, depending on the time of gallbladder filling, the infusion of sincalide should be started and the second series of analog and computer images should be acquired.

Views Obtained   The anterior view of the abdomen is optimized to visualize the gallbladder and liver.

Indications

In patients without gallstones, motility disorders of the gallbladder or of the cystic duct may be associated with recurrent chronic biliary pain. Gallbladder motility has previously been assessed by measuring the gallbladder response to cholecystokinin with cholecystography. However, this radiographic procedure provides only a qualitative index of gallbladder function. Hepatobiliary agents provide a noninvasive and quantitative method for assessing gallbladder and cystic duct contractility.

Principle

Hepatobiliary scintigraphy with the quantification of gallbladder ejection fraction can be performed with either ^{99m}Tc disofenin or ^{99m}Tc mebrofenin. Both of these agents are iminodiacetic acid derivatives that are cleared rapidly from the blood by the hepatocytes and excreted into the bile and gallbladder in high concentrations. After the gallbladder has filled with radioactivity, the rate of gallbladder emptying and the fraction of activity emptied in response to a known stimulus such as cholecystokinin can be used as a measure-

361

ment of contractility.[1,2] The administration of cholecystokinin should be performed as an infusion rather than as a slow bolus to mimic the physiologic response to food.[3]

Patient Preparation

The patient should fast for a minimum of 4 hours before the study. A false-positive study (nonvisualization of the gallbladder) may result if the patient has recently eaten.

Cholecystokinin Infusion

Withdraw 25 ml saline from a fresh 250-ml saline bag. Add 25 ml 5% w/v HSA USP solution (0.05 g/ml) to the saline bag to give a 0.5% w/v HSA solution. A synthetic analog of cholecystokinin called sincalide is used. To reconstitute the sincalide (Kinevac, Squibb) vial, add 5 ml of sterile water. This gives a concentration of 1 µg/ml. The administered dose is 0.02 µg/kg per hour. Draw the required dose of sincalide into a syringe, and inject it into the 250-ml 0.5% w/v HSA solution. Set the infusion pump to infuse the sincalide-HSA solution at a rate of 250 ml/hr.

Instrument Specifications

Gamma Camera:	Any large field-of-view system can be used.
Collimator:	Low-energy, all-purpose or low-energy, high-resolution collimator.
Energy setting:	140 keV, 15–20% energy window.
Analog formatter:	8 × 10 film, 70-mm (9-on-1) format.
Computer system:	Acquisition requirements—dynamic (64 × 64 word mode matrix).
	Processing requirements—ROI analysis, curve generation.

Imaging Procedure: Part I

The patient should be positioned supine on the imaging table.

Analog Formatter

Anterior images of the liver should be obtained at 1, 5, 10, 15, 20, 25, 30, 45, and 60 minutes after injection, with 1,000 kct in the 1- and 5-minute images. All other images should be acquired for the same time as the 5-minute image. In patients in whom the gallbladder is not visualized or adequately filled after 60 minutes, imaging may be continued for 90 minutes before sincalide infusion.

Computer Acquisition

Immediately after injection, computer acquisition should be performed using a 64 × 64 word mode matrix, with 30 seconds per frame for 120 frames.

Imaging Procedure: Part II

Approximately 60–90 minutes after injection of the IDA agent and/or when gallbladder uptake is significant with minimal liver activity, the sincalide infusion should be started.

Ensure that the gamma camera is positioned for optimal visualization of the gallbladder. The patient and camera position should remain unaltered for the remainder of the study.

Analog Formatter

A second series of images of the gallbladder/liver should be obtained with 1,000 kct per image for the first image. Images should then be acquired every 5 minutes for 70 minutes. All other images should be acquired for the same time as the first image.

Computer Acquisition

A second dynamic computer acquisition should be started, with 140 frames at 30 seconds per frame in a 64 × 64 word mode matrix.

Sincalide Infusion

Infusion of the sincalide-HSA solution should commence 5 minutes after the start of the second computer acquisition. Infusion should be continued for 45 minutes only.

Computer Analysis

1. Play back the 140 images from the second computer acquisition as a dynamic study, and check for patient motion. If no motion is present, proceed to step 2. If motion is present, apply motion correction to the data. The most appropriate motion correction algorithms for this type of study are those based on the diverging squares method.[4,5] Check the corrected data to ensure that motion has been reduced to an acceptable level.
2. Draw ROIs over the gallbladder and over an adjacent area of liver for background correction. The gallbladder ROI should include the entire gallbladder. The background ROI

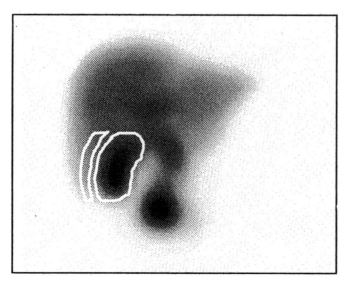

Figure 6-33. Anterior view of liver and gallbladder showing placement of ROIs over the gallbladder and background regions.

should be lateral to the gallbladder and over the liver, as shown in Figure 6-33. Neither ROI should include small bowel activity. From these ROIs, generate time–activity curves.

3. After adjustment for differences in the sizes of the ROIs, subtract the background curve from the gallbladder curve. Perform decay correction on the subtracted curve. Normalize the output curve so that the highest curve value is set to 100%.

4. The gallbladder ejection fraction can be read directly from the curve, or it can be obtained by viewing curve statistics and obtaining the minimal curve value. A typical gallbladder ejection fraction curve is shown in Figure 6-34. The gallbladder ejection fraction is calculated with the following equation:

$$\% \text{ Ejection Fraction} = \frac{\text{Initial Gallbladder ct} - \text{Final Gallbladder ct}}{\text{Initial Gallbladder ct}} \times 100$$

5. From the computer, obtain a hard copy of the gallbladder showing the placement of the ROIs, the raw gallbladder and background curves, and the final normalized gallbladder curve (with decay and background correction).

Information on Film

On each analog and computer film, ensure that the following information is recorded:
1. Patient name and clinic/hospital number
2. Date, type of scan, and radiopharmaceutical
3. Time of each image after injection and start and end of sincalide infusion
4. Orientation of each image (e.g., anterior)

Interpretation

Normal gallbladder ejection fraction is more than 40%.

Additional Notes

A bolus injection of sincolide may be given to the patient prior to the hepatobiliary study, if necessary (e.g., in cases of prolonged fasting.) This does not preclude the use of the sincolide-HSA infusion to measure gallbalder ejection fraction.

Radiation Dosimetry

The estimated absorbed doses in organs and tissues of an average subject (70 kg) from an IV injection of 6 mCi (222 MBq) of ^{99m}Tc disofenin or ^{99m}Tc mebrofenin are shown in Table 6-14.[6,7]

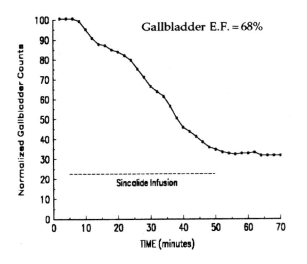

Figure 6-34. Example of normal gallbladder ejection fraction curve.

References

1. Yap L, Wycherley AG, Morphett AD, Toouli J. Acalculous biliary pain: cholecystectomy alleviates symptoms in patients with abnormal cholescintigraphy. Gastroenterology 1991; 101: 786–793.
2. Ziessman HA, Fahey FH, Hixson DJ. Calculation of a gallbladder ejection fraction: advantage of continuous sincalide infusion over the three-minute infusion method. J Nucl Med 1992; 33: 537–541.
3. Eisner RL, Noever T, Nowak D, et al. Use of cross-correlation function to detect patient motion during SPECT imaging. J Nucl Med 1987; 28: 97–101.
4. Cooper JA, Neumann PH, McCandless BK. Detection of patient motion during tomographic myocardial perfusion imaging. J Nucl Med 1993; 34: 1341–1348.
5. Sarva RP, Shreiner DP, Van Thiel D, Yingvorapant N. Gallbladder function: methods for measuring filling and emptying. J Nucl Med 1985; 26: 140–144.
6. Package insert. Choletec—kit for the preparation of technetium Tc [99m] mebrofenin. Squibb Diagnostics, New Brunswick, NJ, revised March 1987.
7. Package insert. Hepatolite—kit for the preparation of technetium Tc [99m] Disofenin. DuPont, Billerica, MA, June 1989.

7

Genitourinary System

Mary F. Hauser
Douglas A. Collins

Dynamic Renal Scan

Summary Information

Radiopharmaceutical

Adult doses: 10 mCi (370 MBq) ^{99m}Tc mercapto-acetyl-glycylglycyl-glycine (MAG3)

Pediatric doses: Adjusted according to the patient's weight (see Appendix A-3).

Contraindications Radiographic contrast agents may interfere with kidney function. If contrast studies have been performed, the renal scan should be deferred for 24 hours. If the patient has undergone renal angiography or angioplasty, the study should be deferred for 3 days, if clinically feasible.[1]

Dose/Scan Interval Imaging begins immediately after the injection.

Views Obtained

Native kidneys: Posterior view of lower back. Ensure that the kidneys and bladder are in the field of view (if deconvolution analysis is required, positioning is higher with the heart included in the field of view; at the end of the study, a view of the bladder should be obtained). Occasionally, it may be helpful to inject a 200-μCi (7.4 MBq) ^{99m}Tc MAG3 dose to aid in positioning, before commencing the renal scan.

Transplant kidneys: Anterior view of pelvis.

Indications

^{99m}Tc MAG3 renal scintigraphy is used to assess renal function, particularly in renal failure, renovascular hypertension, and after renal transplantation. It is also used to evaluate urinary drainage from the kidneys and collecting systems.[2,3]

Principle

^{99m}Tc MAG3 is a technetium-labeled compound with many of the functional properties of iodohippurate.[4,5] After IV injection, it is highly protein-bound and excreted primarily by tubular secretion, with no retention in normal kidney parenchyma. Renogram curves for MAG3 are essentially the same as for iodohippurate, with the advantage of superior image quality and decreased radiation exposure to the patient.

Patient Preparation

Good hydration is required for all renal studies (urine flow rate of more than 1 ml/min).[6] Patients should void immediately before the scan. The specific gravity of the urine should be measured and should be 1.015 or less. Hydration status should be noted on the renal scan information sheet shown in Figure 7-1. If hydration is not satisfactory, the patient should drink 300–500 ml of water or juice, and the hydration status should be checked again after 20–30 minutes. *Note:* If the patient has an indwelling urinary catheter, check with the nuclear medicine physician about whether it should be clamped for the duration of the study.

GENITOURINARY : RENAL SCAN INFORMATION

Patient Name : _____

Clinic No. _____   Date : _____

HYDRATION STATUS

CONTRAST MEDIA :   o YES   o NO

PRE-TEST HYDRATION :   o YES   o PARTIAL   o NO

FIRST TRIAL   : SPECIFIC GRAVITY = _____

SECOND TRIAL : SPECIFIC GRAVITY = _____

Note : S.G. should be < 1.015 to start study
       If > 1.015, hydrate until S.G. at or < 1.015

BOLUS QUALITY

MAG-3 :   o GOOD   o SOME PROBLEM   o MAJOR PROBLEM

DTPA :   o GOOD   o SOME PROBLEM   o MAJOR PROBLEM

OTHER OBSERVATIONS

CATHETER :   o NO   o YES ------->   o CLAMPED   o DRAINING

OTHER REMARKS :

Technologist : _____

Figure 7-1. Renal scan information sheet.

Instrument Specifications

Gamma camera:	Any large field-of-view system can be used.
Collimators:	Low-energy, all-purpose collimator.
Energy setting:	140 keV, 15–20% energy window.
Analog formatter:	8 × 10 film, 70 mm (9-on-1) format.
Computer system:	Acquisition requirements—dynamic (64 × 64 matrix or 128 × 128), the latter is preferred for better region of interest (ROI) definition.
	Processing requirements—ROI analysis, curve generation and manipulation, deconvolution analysis (optional).

Imaging Procedure

For all studies, the patient should be positioned supine on the imaging table,[6] with the detector positioned posterior for native kidneys or anterior for transplant kidneys. The field of view should include the kidneys and bladder, unless deconvolution analysis is required, in which case the heart should be included in the field of view. ^{99m}Tc MAG3 should be injected via an antecubital vein.

Analog Formatter

Start the analog formatter when activity is first visualized in the descending aorta. Record the following:

1. Flow study (2 seconds per image for 9 images).
2. Acquire static images at 1, 5, 10, 15, and 20 minutes after injection, with 1,000 kct per image for the initial 1- and 5-minute images. The duration for the image acquired at 5 minutes should be used for subsequent images.
3. After the 20-minute image, acquire a static image (of the same duration) to include the bladder, if it was not included in the original field of view.
4. Postvoid image: If the renal collecting system appears to be dilated or if bladder outflow obstruction is a concern, acquire a static image (of the same duration) after the patient has voided.

Computer Acquisition

Start computer acquisition at the time the ^{99m}Tc MAG3 is injected. This is a 20-minute computer acquisition with the following acquisition variables:

1. Two-phase dynamic study in 128 × 128 word mode matrix. *Note:* A 64 × 64 matrix size is acceptable; however, a 128 × 128 matrix size permits more accurate definition of cortical and pelvic ROIs.
2. Phase 1 is 60 frames at 1 second per frame; phase 2 is 114 frames at 10 seconds per frame.

Computer Analysis

The following steps should be performed in renogram analysis:

1. Sum frames 61–66 (1–2 minutes), and draw ROIs around each kidney, as shown in Figure 7-2.

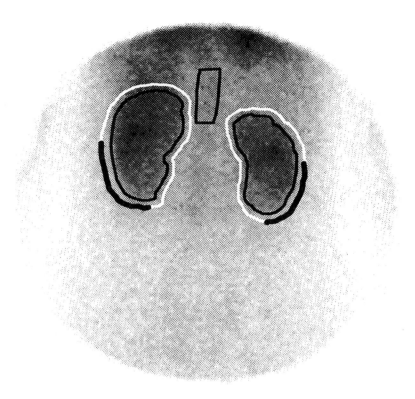

Figure 7-2. A 1–2- minute image showing placement of kidney, whole kidney background (white), cortical kidney background (black), and aortic ROIs.

2. Narrow (1–2-pixel-thick) background ROIs should be drawn around each kidney (see Fig. 7-2) but displaced 2–3-pixels from the edge of the kidney ROIs.
3. Record the size and counts within each ROI. Perform background (Bkg) correction to obtain the corrected kidney counts as follows:

$$\text{Kidney}_{corr} = \text{Kidney}_{raw} - \text{Bkg} \times (\text{Size}_{kidney}/\text{Size}_{bkg})$$

4. Determine differential renal function by expressing counts from each kidney as a percentage of total (right + left) kidney counts.
5. Draw an ROI over the descending aorta, as shown in Figure 7-2. Using all the preceding ROIs, generate time–activity curves from the phase 1 dynamic study (first 60 seconds). These curves are normalized to counts per pixel (rather than total counts) and can be used to assess relative renal perfusion (Fig. 7-3).
6. Sum frames 61–96 (1–7 minutes) to yield six 1-minute frames. Select the image that shows maximal renal pelvic activity. Draw ROIs around the pelvic and calyceal activity in each kidney, as shown in Figure 7-4. By subtracting the renal pelvic ROI from the entire renal ROI, the cortical renal ROI is derived, as shown in Figure 7-4. The cortical ROIs should not include any pelvic activity. The new background ROIs to correct the cortical kidney activity are derived by using the lower outer quadrant of the circumferential background ROIs (see Fig. 7-4).
7. Using all images (phase 1 and 2), generate time–activity curves from the cortical and background ROIs, and perform background correction, as described in step 3.

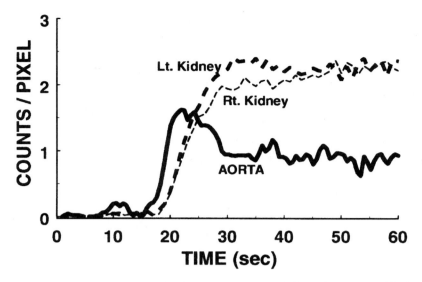

Figure 7-3. Time–activity curves normalized to counts per pixel, from the aorta and kidneys (background corrected) over the first 60 seconds postinjection.

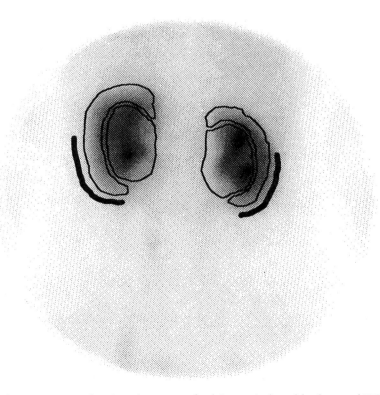

Figure 7-4. A 6-minute image showing placement of pelvic, cortical, and background ROIs. Cortical ROIs were derived by subtracting the pelvic ROIs from the whole-kidney ROIs shown in Figure 7-2.

8. From the (background-corrected) cortical kidney curves, two indices of renal function can be determined (Fig. 7-5):
   a. Time-to-peak counts (normal range, 1–4 minutes)
   b. Half-time ($t_{1/2}$) clearance (normal range, less than 10 minutes.[7]

9. If convolution/deconvolution software is available, then parenchymal mean transit time can be calculated by deconvolving the cortical kidney curves with the heart curve.[8,9] The validity of the deconvolution software should be checked with software phantoms.[10] *Note:* Many manufacturers provide comprehensive renal analysis software programs with their systems that eliminate the need for manual processing of the data. Full details of the renal analysis package, including references to the technique used, should be obtained.

Information on Film

Obtain a hard copy of all ROIs and both raw and background-corrected curves. On each analog and computer film, ensure that the following information is recorded:

1. Patient name and clinic/hospital number
2. Type of scan and radiopharmaceutical
3. Date and time of each image after injection
4. Orientation of each image (e.g., posterior) and appropriate labels for ROIs and curves

Interpretation

Normal kidneys demonstrate a rapid and symmetric perfusion, with a prompt increase in activity and symmetric prompt excretion, with peak times less than 4 minutes and

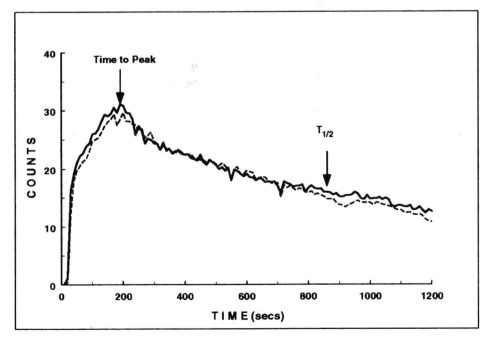

Figure 7-5. Left and right cortical kidney curves showing time to peak counts and $t_{1/2}$ clearance.

Table 7-1. Absorbed Radiation Dose Estimates in a 70-kg Adult
From 10 mCi (370 MBq) ^{99m}Tc MAG3

Tissue	Absorbed Radiation Dose	
	rad/10 mCi	mGy/370 MBq
Urinary bladder wall	4.80	48.0
Kidneys	0.14	1.4
Gallbladder wall	0.16	1.6
Small bowel	0.16	1.6
Upper large intestinal wall	0.19	1.9
Lower large intestinal wall	0.33	3.3
Liver	0.04	0.4
Ovaries	0.26	2.6
Testes	0.16	1.6
Red marrow	0.05	0.5
Total body	0.07	0.7

$t_{1/2}$ clearance times less than 10 minutes. Differential renal function should not differ by more than 10%.

Radiation Dosimetry

The estimated absorbed doses in organs and tissues of an average subject (70 kg) from the administration of 10 mCi (370 MBq) ^{99m}Tc MAG3 are shown in Table 7-1.[11]

References

1. Gates GF, Green GS. Transient reduction in renal function following arteriography: a radionuclide study. J Urol 1983; 129: 1107–1110.
2. Russell CD, Young D, Billingsley JD, Dubovsky EV. Technical procedures for use of the new kidney agent Technetium-99m MAG3. J Nucl Med Tech 1991; 19: 147–152.
3. Russell CD, Thorstad BL, Stutzman ME, et al. The kidney: imaging with Tc-99m mercaptoacetyl-triglycine, a technetium-labeled analog of iodohippurate. Radiology 1989; 172: 427–430.
4. Fritzberg AR, Kasina S, Eshima D, Johnson DL. Synthesis and biological evaluation of technetium-99m MAG3 as a hippuran replacement. J Nucl Med 1986; 27: 111–116.
5. Taylor A Jr, Eshima D, Fritzberg AR, Christian PE, Kasina S. Comparison of iodine-131 OIH and technetium-99m MAG3 renal imaging in volunteers. J Nucl Med 1986; 27: 795–803.
6. Cosgriff PS, Lawson RS, Nimmon CC. Towards standardization in gamma camera renography. Nucl Med Commun 1992; 13: 580–585.
7. Klingensmith WC III, Briggs DE, Smith WI. Technetium-99m-MAG3 renal studies: normal range and reproducibility of physiologic parameters as a function of age and sex. J Nucl Med 1994; 35: 1612–1617.
8. Britton KE, Nimmon CC, Whitfield HN, et al. The evaluation of obstructive nephropathy by means of parenchymal retention functions. In "Radionuclides in Nephrology," eds Hollenberg NK, Lange S, George Thieme, Stuttgart, Germany, 1980, pp 151–154.

9. Britton KE, Nawaz MK, Whitfield HN, et al. Obstructive nephropathy: comparison between parenchymal transit time index and frusemide diuresis. Br J Urol 1987; 59: 127–132.

10. Britton KE, Busemann Sokole E. Quality assurance in nuclear medicine software and "COST." Nucl Med Commun 1990; 11: 334–338.

11. Package insert. TechneScan MAG3 kit for the preparation of technetium Tc 99m mertiatide. Mallinckrodt Medical, St. Louis, 1992.

Dynamic Renal Scan With Furosemide

Summary Information

Radiopharmaceutical
Adult dose: 10 mCi (370 MBq) ^{99m}Tc MAG3.
Pediatric dose: The Pediatric Furosemide Renal Scan procedure should be used on all pediatric patients.

Contraindications Allergy to furosemide contraindicates its use. Radiographic contrast agents may interfere with kidney function. If contrast studies have been performed, the renal scan should be deferred for 24 hours. If the patient has undergone renal angiography or angioplasty, the study should be deferred for 3 days, if clinically feasible.[1]

Dose/Scan Interval Imaging begins immediately after the injection.

Views Obtained
Native kidneys: Posterior view of lower back. Ensure that the kidneys and bladder are in the field of view. Occasionally, it may be helpful to inject a 200-μCi (7.4 MBq) ^{99m}Tc MAG3 dose to aid in positioning before commencing the renal scan.
Transplant kidneys: Anterior view of the pelvis.

Indications

^{99m}Tc MAG3 renal scintigraphy with furosemide is used for the diagnosis of obstructive uropathy.[2]

Principle

^{99m}Tc MAG3 is cleared by the kidneys and may collect in the pelvic region because of a dilated collecting system. The use of a diuretic (furosemide) as an adjunct to the renal scan is helpful in distinguishing patients with obstruction from those without obstruction. In obstructed hydronephrosis, no washout of activity may occur, or a blunted response may occur after furosemide administration, whereas washout should be good in the nonobstructed system.[3]

Patient Preparation

Check that the patient is not allergic to furosemide. Good hydration is required for all renal studies. Patients should void immediately before the scan. The specific gravity of the urine should be measured and should be 1.015 or less. Hydration status should be noted on the renal scan information sheet shown in Figure 7-1. If hydration is not satisfactory, the patient should drink 300–500 ml of water or juice, and the hydration status should be checked again after 20–30 minutes.

An indwelling urinary catheter may be helpful in patients with outlet obstruction or obstruction of the ureterovesical junction. A catheter may also help avoid a false-positive test that is due to pressure from urine retained in the bladder. If present, an existing catheter should be unclamped.

Instrument Specifications

Gamma camera:	Any large field-of-view system can be used.
Collimators:	Low-energy, all-purpose collimator.
Energy setting:	140 keV, 15–20% energy window.
Analog formatter:	8 × 10 film, 70-mm (9-on-1) format.
Computer system:	Acquisition requirements—dynamic (64 × 64 matrix or 128 × 128), the latter is preferred for better ROI definition.) Processing requirements—ROI analysis and curve generation and manipulation.

Furosemide Administration

The furosemide dose is 0.5 mg/kg body weight, up to a maximum of 40 mg. Furosemide should be injected slowly over a 1–2 minute period. Be sure to flush the furosemide dose with saline. Furosemide is usually injected 10–20 minutes after the start of the study. The nuclear medicine physician will determine the optimal time for furosemide injection on the basis of visual inspection of the images.

Imaging Procedure—Prefurosemide

The patient should be positioned supine on the imaging table with the detector placed posteriorly for native kidneys or anteriorly for transplant kidneys. The field of view should include the kidneys and bladder. The ^{99m}Tc MAG3 should be injected in an antecubital vein, and analog and computer acquisitions performed as described later.

Analog Formatter

Start the analog formatter when activity is first visualized in the descending aorta. Record the following:

1. Flow study (2 seconds per image for 9 images).
2. Static images at 1 and 5 minutes after injection and subsequently at 5-minute intervals until furosemide injection is begun. Acquire 1,000 kct per image for the initial 1- and 5-minute images. Thereafter, all images should be acquired for a preset time equal to the time of the 5-minute image.

Computer Acquisition

Start computer acquisition at the time the ^{99m}Tc MAG3 is injected. This is a 30-minute computer acquisition, with the following acquisition variables:

1. A two-phase dynamic study in 128 × 128 word mode matrix (64 × 64 matrix is acceptable, but a larger matrix size permits better ROI definition).
2. Phase 1 is 60 frames at 1 second per frame; phase 2 is 87 frames at 20 seconds per frame.

Note: The analog formatter images and the phase-2 acquisition may be stopped any time before 30 minutes, depending on the accumulation of activity in the renal pelvic area. Consult with the nuclear medicine physician on the appropriate time to stop acquisition.

Imaging Procedure—Postfurosemide

Analog Formatter

Start the analog formatter at the time the furosemide is injected. Record static images at 1 and 5 minutes and subsequently at 5-minute intervals up to 30 minutes after the injection. Images should be acquired for a preset time equal to the time of the 5-minute prefurosemide image. Imaging may be stopped before 30 minutes if the images are visually diagnostic.

Computer Acquisition

Start computer acquisition at the time the furosemide is injected. This is a 10- to 30-minute computer acquisition. The study duration is at the discretion of the nuclear medicine physician and depends on the rate at which activity is cleared from the renal pelvic regions. The following acquisition variables should be used: a single-phase dynamic study in 128 × 128 word mode matrix, with 90 frames at 20 seconds per frame.

Computer Analysis

The following steps should be performed on the prefurosemide image data:

1. Sum frames 61–63 (1–2 minutes), and draw ROIs around each kidney, as shown in Figure 7-2.
2. Narrow (1–2-pixel-thick) background ROIs should be drawn around each kidney (see Fig. 7-2) but displaced 2–3 pixels from the edge of the kidney ROIs.
3. Record the number of pixels and counts within the ROIs. Perform background (Bkg) correction to obtain the corrected kidney count as follows:

$$\text{Kidney}_{corr} = \text{Kidney}_{raw} - \text{Bkg} \times (\text{Size}_{kidney}/\text{Size}_{bkg})$$

4. Determine differential renal function by expressing counts from each kidney as a percentage of total (right + left) kidney counts.
5. Draw an ROI over the descending aorta, as shown in Figure 7-2. Using all the preceding ROIs, generate time–activity curves from the phase-1 dynamic study (first 60 seconds). These curves are normalized to counts per pixel (rather than total counts) and can be used to assess relative renal perfusion (see Fig. 7-3).
6. Sum frames 61–78 (1–7 minutes) to yield six 1-minute images. Select the image that shows maximal renal pelvic activity. Draw ROIs around the pelvic and calyceal activity in each kidney, as shown in Figure 7-4. By subtracting the renal pelvic ROI from the entire renal ROI, the cortical renal ROI is derived, as shown in Figure 7-4. The cortical ROIs should not include any pelvic activity. The new background ROIs to correct the cortical kidney activity are derived by using the lower outer quadrant of the circumferential background ROI (see Fig. 7-4).

7. Using all images (phase 1 and 2), generate time–activity curves from the cortical and background ROIs and perform background correction, as described in step 3.
8. Depending on the duration of the prefurosemide acquisition, two indices of renal function (time-to-peak counts and $t_{1/2}$ clearance) can be determined from the (background-corrected) cortical kidney curves (see Fig. 7-5).

The following steps should be performed on the postfurosemide image data:

9. Using the pelvic ROIs shown in Figure 7-6, generate time–activity curves showing the washout of activity from the pelvic area after furosemide administration.
10. If the ureters are visualized, select an appropriate image (or a summed group of images). Draw ROIs over the left and right ureters, as shown in Figure 7-6. Generate time–activity curves of ureter activity after furosemide administration.

Note: Many manufacturers provide comprehensive renal analysis software programs with their systems that eliminate the need for manual processing of the data. Full details of the renal analysis package, including references to the technique used, should be obtained.

Information on Film

Obtain a hard copy of all ROIs and both raw and background-corrected curves. On each analog and computer film, ensure that the following information is recorded:

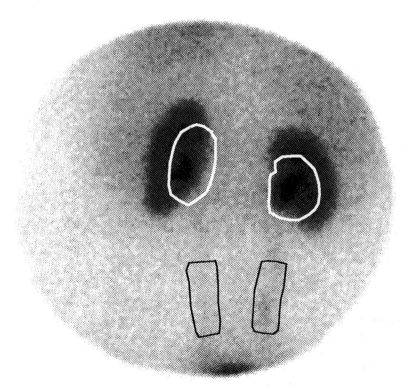

Figure 7-6. Postfurosemide image showing placement of pelvic and ureter ROIs.

1. Patient name and clinic/hospital number
2. Type of scan and radiopharmaceutical
3. Date and time of each image after injection and postfurosemide administration
4. Orientation of each image (e.g., posterior) and appropriate labels for ROIs and curves

Interpretation

1. Normal pattern: Kidneys show a prompt increase in activity, with spontaneous washout accelerated by diuresis (Fig. 7-7A). The ureters show a flat low level of activity, with a possible transient spike after furosemide injection.
2. Obstructed pattern: Kidneys show progressively increasing activity, with a flat response or further increase after furosemide injection (Fig. 7- 7B). The ureters may show a similar pattern (if the site of the obstruction is distal), with failure to decrease activity after furosemide.
3. Dilated nonobstructed pattern: Kidneys show progressively increasing activity that decreases after diuretic injection, with $t_{1/2}$ clearance less than 10 minutes (Fig. 7-7C). The ureters may show a pattern similar to that of the kidneys (although delayed in time), with gradual increase followed by washout after furosemide injection.
4. Blunted response: Kidneys show progressively increasing activity before furosemide injection, with a blunted response to furosemide ($t_{1/2}$ clearance of 10–20 minutes), which is indeterminate (Fig. 7-7D). It may represent a partial obstruction, a large reservoir effect, or an inability to mount an adequate diuretic response, possibly because of poor function. *Note:* A kidney with severely impaired function may be unable to respond to furosemide and thus give a false-positive pattern for obstruction.

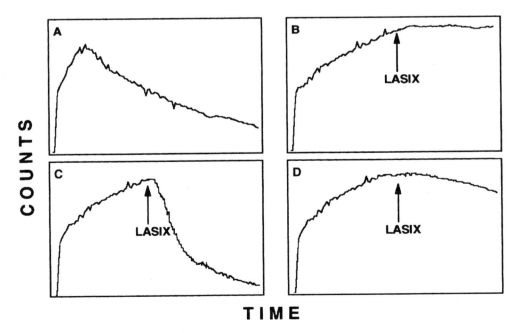

Figure 7-7. Cortical kidney activity. (**A**) Normal pattern. (**B**) Obstructed pattern. (**C**) Dilated nonobstructed pattern. (**D**) Equivocal/partially obstructed pattern.

Radiation Dosimetry

The estimated absorbed doses in organs and tissues of an average subject (70 kg) from the administration of 10 mCi (370 MBq) ^{99m}Tc MAG3 are shown in Table 7-1.[4]

References

1. Gates GF, Green GS. Transient reduction in renal function following arteriography: a radionuclide study. J Urol 1983; 129: 1107–1110.
2. Russell CD, Young D, Billingsley JD, Dubovsky EV. Technical procedures for use of the new kidney agent Technetium-99m MAG3. J Nucl Med Tech 1991; 19: 147–152.
3. O'Reilly PH, Britton KE, Nommon CC. Evaluation of urinary tract obstruction. In "Evaluation of Renal Function and Disease with Radionuclides," ed Blaufox MD. Karger, Basel, Switzerland, 1989, pp 116–129.
4. Package insert. TechneScan MAG3 kit for the preparation of technetium Tc 99m Mertiatide. Mallinckrodt Medical, St. Louis, 1992.

Dynamic Renal Scan
With Captopril

Summary Information

Radiopharmaceutical

Adult dose: 10 mCi (370 MBq) ^{99m}Tc MAG3.

Pediatric dose: Adjusted according to the patient's weight (see Appendix A-3).

Contraindications

1. Check for possible allergy to furosemide (Lasix).
2. Captopril can cause potentially dangerous hypotension in patients with high levels of renin or in patients who are dehydrated or salt-depleted or who recently have had dialysis.
3. Radiographic contrast agents may interfere with kidney function. If contrast studies have been performed, the renal scan should be deferred for 24 hours. If the patient has undergone renal angiography or angioplasty, the study should be deferred for 3 days.[1–3]

Dose/Scan Interval   Imaging begins immediately after the injection.

Views Obtained

Native kidneys: Posterior view of lower back. Ensure that the kidneys and bladder are in the field of view. Occasionally, it may be helpful to inject a 200-µCi (7.4 MBq) ^{99m}Tc MAG3 dose to aid in positioning before commencing the renal scan.

Transplant kidneys: Anterior view of the pelvis.

Indications

Dynamic renal scintigraphy with captopril is used in diagnosing renovascular hypertension and in assessing various therapeutic interventions.[3]

Principle

In patients with renin-dependent hypertension, angiotensin II, an octapeptide, acts to maintain renal function by increasing blood pressure in the kidneys. The production of angiotensin II can be inhibited with captopril, one of a family of drugs known as

Table 7-2. Angiotensin-Converting Enzyme Inhibitor[a]

Name of Drug		
Generic	Brand	Manufacturer
Captopril	Capoten	Bristol-Myers Squibb Co.
Captopril		
+ hydrochlorothiazide	Caposide	Bristol-Myers Squibb Co.
Fosinopril sodium	Monopril	Bristol-Myers Squibb Co.
Benazepril HCl	Lotensin	Ciba-Geigy Corp., Pharmaceuticals Division
Ramipril	Altace	Hoechst-Roussel Pharmaceuticals
Lisinopril	Zestril	ICI Pharmaceuticals, ICI Americas Inc.
Lisinopril		
+ hydrochlorothiazide	Zestoretic	ICI Pharmaceuticals, ICI Americas Inc.
Enalapril maleate	Vasotec	Merck Human Health Division
Enalapril maleate		
+ hydrochlorothiazide	Vaseretic	Merck Human Health Division
Lisinopril	Prinivil	Merck Human Health Division
Lisinopril		
+ hydrochlorothiazide	Prinzide	Merck Human Health Division
Quinapril HCl	Accupril	Parke-Davis, Division of Warner-Lambert Co.

[a]If the patient has taken any of these drugs within the last 3 days, inform the nuclear medicine physician who will decide on the appropriate course of action.

angiotensin-converting enzyme (ACE) inhibitors (Table 7-2). In the absence of angiotensin II, the function of the affected kidney is decreased. This reduction in function can then be detected with dynamic renal scintigraphy using ^{99m}Tc MAG3.[4–6] Furosemide is given during the MAG3 study to aid in washout of any activity that collects in the renal pelvic areas, thereby providing more accurate assessment of renal cortical clearance.[7]

Patient Preparation

Good hydration is required for all renal studies. Patients should void immediately before the scan. The specific gravity of the urine should be measured and should be 1.015 or less. Hydration status should be noted on the renal scan information sheet shown in Figure 7-1. If hydration is not satisfactory, the patient should drink 300–500 ml of water or juice, and the hydration status should be checked again after 20–30 minutes. *Note:* Patients should arrive at the nuclear medicine laboratory about 1.5 hours before the scheduled appointment so that hydration can be checked and the following pretest procedures can be completed.

Instrument Specifications

Gamma camera:	Any large field-of-view system can be used.
Collimator:	Low-energy, all-purpose collimator.
Energy setting:	140 keV, 15–20% energy window.

Analog formatter: 8 × 10 film, 70-mm (9-on-1) format.

Computer system: Acquisition requirements—dynamic (64 × 64 matrix or 128 × 128 matrix), the latter is preferred for more accurate ROI definition).

Processing requirements—ROI analysis and curve generation and manipulation.

Captopril and Furosemide Administration

After the patient arrives in the nuclear medicine laboratory, the following procedure should be used:[8]

GENITOURINARY : CAPTOPRIL RENOGRAM

Patient Name : _____

Clinic No. _____ Date : _____

PLEASE LIST YOUR CURRENT MEDICATIONS FOR BLOOD PRESSURE

1. _____
2. _____
3. _____
4. _____
5. _____
6. _____
7. _____
8. _____

ARE YOU TAKING ANY OF THE FOLLOWING SPECIFIC MEDICATIONS ?

CAPOTEN (Captopril)	○ yes ○ no	ZESTORETIC (Lisinopril)	○ yes ○ no
CAPOZIDE (Captopril)	○ yes ○ no	VASOTEC (Enalapril)	○ yes ○ no
MONOPRIL (Fosinopril)	○ yes ○ no	VASERETIC (Enalapril)	○ yes ○ no
LOTENSIN (Benazepil)	○ yes ○ no	PRINIVIL (Lisinopril)	○ yes ○ no
ALTACE (Ramipril)	○ yes ○ no	PRINZIDE (Lisinopril)	○ yes ○ no
ZESTRIL (Lisinopril)	○ yes ○ no	ACCUPRIL (Quinapril)	○ yes ○ no

If you answered YES to any of the above, please indicate   LAST DOSE : Time : _____   Date : _____

Are you taking any diuretic medications (e.g. Lasix, Diazide etc.)   ○ yes ○ no

---

Please return this form to the technologist, prior to undergoing the kidney scan.
Thank you for your co-operation.

....do not enter anything below this line...

For technologist use only

: _____
      Technologist

Pre-captopril BP : _____	Captopril given at : _____
Post-captopril BP : _____	Elapsed time : _____
Post-MAG3 BP : _____	Elapsed time : _____

Figure 7-8. Captopril renogram worksheet.

1. Ask the patient to complete the drug history portion of the captopril renogram form (Fig. 7-8) and return it to the technician. If the patient has taken an ACE inhibitor (listed in Table 7-2) within the last 3 days, check with the nuclear medicine physician before proceeding further.
2. Measure the blood pressure twice, and record the average of the two on the form.
3. Optional (for plasma renin determination)—Before administering captopril, draw 7 ml of blood into a 10-ml ethylenediamine tetraacetic acid (EDTA) anticoagulated tube for measurement of plasma renin. Obtain a second blood sample in the same manner 1 hour after captopril is administered.
4. Administer two crushed 12.5-mg tablets of captopril to the patient. Check and include the pharmacy slip indicating the 25-mg dose with the drug history form. For pediatric patients, consult with the referring physician for the appropriate dose of captopril.
5. The patient should be kept supine on a cart in the patient waiting area for 60 minutes, and the blood pressure should be measured every 15 minutes.
6. Ask the patient to void immediately before injection of the ^{99m}Tc MAG3.
7. Proceed with the ^{99m}Tc MAG3 study. When this is completed, measure the blood pressure again.
8. Inject furosemide 3–5 minutes after injecting ^{99m}Tc MAG3. The furosemide dose is 0.5 mg/kg body weight, up to a maximum of 40 mg. Furosemide should be injected slowly over a 1–2 minute period.

Imaging Procedure

Analog Formatter

Start the analog formatter when activity is first visualized in the descending aorta. Record the following:

1. Flow study (2 seconds per image for 9 images).
2. Static images at 1, 5, 10, 15, and 20 minutes after the injection, with 1,000 kct per image for the initial 1- and 5-minute images. The duration for the 5-minute image should then be used for subsequent images.

Computer Acquisition

Start computer acquisition when ^{99m}Tc MAG3 is injected. This is a 20-minute computer acquisition with the following acquisition variables:

1. Two-phase dynamic study in a 128 × 128 word mode matrix.
2. Phase 1 is 60 frames at 1 second per frame; phase 2 is 114 frames at 10 seconds per frame.

Computer Analysis

The following steps should be performed in renogram analysis:

1. Sum frames 61–66 (1–2 minutes), and draw ROIs around each kidney, as shown in Figure 7-2.
2. Narrow (1–2-pixel-thick) background ROIs should be drawn around each kidney (see Fig. 7-2) but displaced 2–3 pixels from the edge of the kidney ROIs.
3. Record the size and counts within the ROIs. Perform background (Bkg) correction to obtain the corrected kidney counts as follows:

$$\text{Kidney}_{corr} = \text{Kidney}_{raw} - \text{Bkg} \times (\text{Size}_{kidney}/\text{Size}_{bkg})$$

4. Determine differential renal function by expressing counts from each kidney as a percentage of total (right + left) kidney counts.

5. Draw an ROI over the descending aorta, as shown in Figure 7-2. Using all the preceding ROIs, generate time–activity curves from the phase-1 dynamic study (first 60 seconds). These curves are normalized to counts per pixel (rather than total counts) and can be used to assess relative renal perfusion (see Fig. 7-3).

6. Sum frames 61–96 (1–7 minutes) to yield six 1-minute frames. Select the image that shows maximal renal pelvic activity. Draw ROIs around activity in the pelvis and calyces of each kidney, as shown in Figure 7-4. The cortical renal ROI is derived by subtracting the renal pelvic ROI from the entire renal ROI, as shown in Figure 7-4. The cortical ROIs should not include any pelvic activity. The new background ROIs to correct the cortical kidney activity are derived by using the lower outer quadrant of the circumferential background ROI (see Fig. 7-4).

7. Using all images (phase 1 and 2), generate time–activity curves from the cortical and background ROIs and perform background correction, as described in step 3.

8. From the (background-corrected) cortical kidney curves, several indices of renal function can be determined[9] (see Fig. 7-5):
   a. Time-to-peak counts (normal range, 1–4 minutes)
   b. $t_{1/2}$ clearance (normal range, less than 10 minutes)
   c. Ratio of 20-minute counts to peak counts (normal range less than 30%)

Note: Many manufacturers provide comprehensive renal analysis software programs with their systems that eliminate the need for manual processing of the data. Full details of the renal analysis package, including references to the technique used, should be obtained.

Information on Film

Obtain a hard copy of all ROIs and both raw and background-corrected curves. On each analog and computer film, ensure that the following information is recorded:

1. Patient name and clinic/hospital number
2. Type of scan and radiopharmaceutical
3. Date and time of each image after the injection
4. Administered dose of captopril and furosemide
5. Orientation of each image (e.g., posterior) and appropriate labels for ROIs and curves

Interpretation

Because captopril acts by decreasing the glomerular filtration rate in renal artery stenosis, the clearance of tubular agents is decreased. Thus, the most sensitive finding is delayed clearance, as evident from visual assessment of the images or as manifested by prolonged parenchymal transit time, prolonged $t_{1/2}$, and a ratio of 20-minute counts to peak counts exceeding 30%. However, asymmetry of perfusion, flattening of the cortical activity curve, and delay in visualization of bladder activity may also be present. The test is most sensitive for unilateral renal artery stenosis. In bilateral disease, the more severely affected side is usually easier to detect. Bilaterally symmetric renal artery stenosis is hard to differentiate from other entities, but it is relatively uncommon.

If the results of the study are abnormal or equivocal, it may be helpful to perform a baseline study without captopril for comparison.

Additional Notes

If any reaction to captopril is observed, the attending nuclear medicine physician should be notified immediately. After interpretation, the drug form sheets should be filed with the patient's films for future reference.

Radiation Dosimetry

The estimated absorbed doses in organs and tissues of an average subject (70 kg) from the administration of 10 mCi (370 MBq) ^{99m}Tc MAG3 are shown in Table 7-1.[10]

References

1. Gates GF, Green GS. Transient reduction in renal function following arteriography: a radionuclide study. J Urol 1983;129: 1107–1110.
2. Wedeen RP, Blaufox MD. The normal radiorenogram. In "Evaluation of Renal Function and Disease With Radionuclides," ed Blaufox MD. Karger, Basel, Switzerland, 1989, pp 116–129.
3. Fine EJ, Britton KE, Nimmon CC. The scintirenogram in hypertensive disease. In "Evaluation of Renal Function and Disease With Radionuclides," ed Blaufox MD. Karger, Basel, Switzerland, 1989, pp 198–247.
4. Russell CD, Young D, Billingsley JD, Dubovsky EV. Technical procedures for use of the new kidney agent Technetium-99m MAG3. J Nucl Med Tech 1991; 19: 147–152.
5. Russell CD, Thorstad BL, Stutzman ME, et al. The kidney: imaging with Tc-99m mercaptoacetyltriglycine, a technetium-labeled analog of iodohippurate. Radiology 1989; 172: 427–430.
6. Tondeur M, Piepsz A, Dobbeleir A, Ham H. Technetium 99m mercaptoacetyltriglycine gamma camera clearance calculations: methodological problems. Eur J Nucl Med 1991; 18: 83–86.
7. Sfakianakis GN, Belles B, Vontorta K, et al. MAG3/Enalaprilat protocol for diagnosis of renovascular hypertension in a single visit. J Nucl Med 1993; 34: 249P.
8. Blaufox MD, Dubovsky EV, Hilson AJW, Taylor A Jr, de Zeeuw R. Report of the working party group on determining the radionuclide of choice. Am J Hypertension 1991; 4 Suppl: 747S–748S.
9. Klingensmith WC III, Briggs DE, Smith WI. Technetium-99m-MAG3 renal studies: normal range and reproducibility of physiologic parameters as a function of age and sex. J Nucl Med 1994; 35: 1612–1617.
10. Package insert. TechneScan MAG3 kit for the preparation of technetium Tc 99m mertiatide. Mallinckrodt Medical, St. Louis, 1992.

Dynamic Renal Scan With Glomerular Filtration Rate/ Effective Renal Plasma Flow

---

Summary Information

Radiopharmaceutical

Adult dose:
1 mCi (37 MBq) ^{99m}Tc DTPA.
10 mCi (370 MBq) ^{99m}Tc MAG3.
Exact doses should be recorded on the glomerular filtration rate/effective renal plasma flow (GFR/ERPF) worksheet (see Fig. 7-9).

Pediatric dose:
The pediatric furosemide (Lasix) renal scan procedure should be used on all pediatric patients.

Contraindications
Radiographic contrast agents may interfere with kidney function. If a contrast study has been performed, the renal scan should be deferred for 24 hours. If the patient has undergone renal angiography or angioplasty, the study should be deferred for 3 days, if clinically feasible.[1]

Dose/Scan Interval
Imaging begins immediately after the injection.

Views Obtained

Native kidneys:
Posterior view of lower back. Ensure that the kidneys and bladder are in the field of view.

Transplant kidneys:
Not usually done because of overlap with iliac vessels and the difficulty with background correction.

Indications

GFR and ERPF (or indices related to these variables) can be calculated from dynamic renal scintigraphy performed with ^{99m}Tc DTPA (diethylenetriamine pentaacetic acid) and ^{99m}Tc MAG3.[2,3] Both GFR and ERPF provide objective measurements of renal function and its change over serial studies. They also help determine whether renal disease is primarily tubular or glomerular.

Principle

GFR can be measured by determining the absolute amount of ^{99m}Tc DTPA in the kidneys at 2–3 minutes after injection and expressing this amount as a fraction of the injected dose.[2] Determination of the absolute amount in the kidneys requires knowledge of (1) the exact amount of activity injected, (2) correction for any residual activity in the syringe or in the patient's arm, (3) the conversion factor from counts in the kidneys to μCi (kBq) in the kidneys, and (4) kidney depth (to correct for attenuation by overlying tissue). A similar technique can be used to calculate ERPF from the ^{99m}Tc MAG3 uptake at 1–2 minutes after injection.[3]

Patient Preparation

If the GFR or ERPF (or both) is to be determined, no patient preparation is required. Good hydration is required if a dynamic renal scan is to be performed concomitantly. In such cases, the patients should void immediately before the scan. The specific gravity of the urine should be measured and should be 1.015 or less. The hydration status should be noted on the renal scan information sheet shown in Figure 7-1.

Instrument Specifications

Gamma camera:	Any large field-of-view system can be used.
Collimator:	Low-energy, all-purpose collimator.
Energy setting:	140 keV, 15–20% energy window.
Analog formatter:	8 × 10 film, 70-mm (9-on-1) format.
Computer system:	Acquisition requirements—dynamic (128 × 128 matrix). Processing requirements—ROI analysis and curve generation and manipulation.

Imaging Procedure

For all studies, the patient should be positioned supine on the imaging table, with the detector positioned posteriorly. The field of view should include the kidneys and bladder. Place a 21-gauge butterfly needle and tubing set in an antecubital vein. Inject the ^{99m}Tc DTPA, and flush the butterfly tubing with saline. After completion of the ^{99m}Tc DTPA study, inject the ^{99m}Tc MAG3, and again flush the butterfly tubing with saline. Remove the butterfly set, and discard it in the radioactive waste bin.

Note: If only GFR/ERPF measurement is required (i.e., no dynamic renal imaging), then the analog formatter and computer acquisition steps for ^{99m}Tc MAG3 are identical to those for ^{99m}Tc DTPA.

Dose Calibration—^{99m}Tc DTPA

1. Record the exact activity of ^{99m}Tc DTPA in the syringe (μCi/kBq) and the time of calibration.
2. Record the exact injection time.
3. Record the residual activity in the syringe (μCi/kBq).
4. Record the preceding times and activities on the GFR/ERPF worksheet (Fig. 7-9).

Analog Formatter—^{99m}Tc DTPA

Start the analog formatter at the time of the injection. Record static images for 6 minutes (1 minute per image).

GENITOURINARY : RENAL SCAN WITH GFR/ERPF

Patient Name : _____

Clinic No. _____   Date : _____

Height : _____ cm.   Weight : _____ kg

ESTIMATION OF KIDNEY DEPTH

Right Kidney Depth : _____ mm

Left Kidney Depth : _____ mm

Tc-99m DTPA	**Tc-99m MAG3**

Tc-99m DTPA Dose : _____ uCi   Tc-99m MAG3 Dose : _____ uCi

(corrected for injection site act.) :_____ uCi   (corrected for injection site act.) : _____ uCi

Calibration Time : _____   Calibration Time : _____

Injection Time : _____   Injection Time : _____

Residual syringe act. : _____ uCi   Residual syringe act. : _____ uCi

---

ACTIVITY AT INJECTION SITE

Injection site activity : _____ cts/min   % dose at injection site : _____ %

                = _____ uCi   Injected dose < 1% = ignore

Divide cts/min by system sensitivity factor to convert to uCi.   Injected dose > 1% and < 5% = subtract from calibrated dose act.

                                                              Injected dose > 5% = do not perform GFR / ERPF calculation.

GAMMA CAMERA : SENSITIVITY FACTOR

Gamma Camera : _____   Sensitivity Factor : _____ cts/min

Comments : _____

                     _____

Technologist : _____

Figure 7-9. Worksheet for GFR/ERPF calculation.

Computer Acquisition—^{99m}Tc DTPA

Start computer acquisition at the time ^{99m}Tc DTPA is injected. This is a 6-minute computer acquisition. Images are acquired into a 128×128 matrix at 15 seconds per frame.

Dose Calibration—^{99m}Tc MAG3

Repeat the same steps for measurement of the injected dose of ^{99m}Tc MAG3, as in steps 1–4 for ^{99m}Tc DTPA.

Analog Formatter—^{99m}Tc MAG3

Start the analog formatter when activity is first visualized in the descending aorta. Record the following:

1. Flow study (2 seconds per image for 9 images).
2. Static images at 1, 5, 10, 15, and 20 minutes after the injection, with 1,000 kct per image for the initial 1- and 5-minute images. The time duration for the 5-minute image should be used for subsequent images
3. Static image (of the same time duration) should include the bladder, if not seen on the images in steps 1 and 2.

Computer Acquisition—^{99m}Tc MAG3

Start computer acquisition at the time ^{99m}Tc MAG3 is injected. This is a 20-minute computer acquisition, with the following acquisition variables.

1. Two-phase dynamic study in 128 × 128 word mode matrix.
2. Phase 1 is 60 frames at 1 second per frame; phase 2 is 114 frames at 10 seconds per frame

Injection Site/Lateral Views

1. At the completion of the study, position the injection site under the gamma camera, as shown in Figure 7-10, and acquire a 1-minute acquisition on the gamma camera and on computer (256 × 256 word mode matrix). Under ROI analysis, draw a region around the injection site. Record the total counts. This is to check for residual activity at the site of injection.
2. Use the "counts to μCi/kBq" conversion factor (see "Measurement of System Sensitivity," following) to convert counts at the injection site to μCi or kBq. If the activity in the patient's arm is more than 5% of the ^{99m}Tc MAG3 dose, do NOT proceed with the

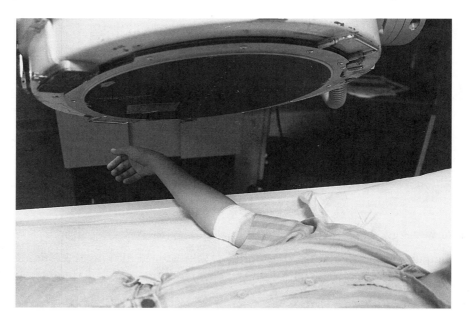

Figure 7-10. Injection site positioned under the gamma camera for measurement of residual activity. Detector has been moved away from the patient to illustrate the acquisition setup.

GFR/ERPF calculation. If the activity in the arm is less than 5%, subtract this amount from the administered ^{99m}Tc MAG3 dose to get the actual administered dose.

3. Because the detector is not moved between the ^{99m}Tc DTPA and ^{99m}Tc MAG3 studies, no image of the injection site is available for the ^{99m}Tc DTPA study. Therefore, it should be assumed that the percent administered dose at the injection site is the same for both radiopharmaceuticals and the appropriate adjustment made to the ^{99m}Tc DTPA administered dose.

4. With the patient still supine on the imaging table, orient the gamma camera to show a lateral view of the left kidney on the persistence screen, with a radioactive line source (^{57}Co) placed between the gamma camera and patient. Figure 7-11 shows a line source consisting of four point sources of ^{57}Co (5 µCi/185 kBq per source) attached to a vertical ruler. Adjust the height of the line source until the four ^{57}Co markers lie along the midline of the kidney. The image of the line source should then be acquired on computer in a 256 × 256 matrix. Record the ruler height in millimeters—this corresponds to the kidney depth. Repeat the process for the right kidney. *Note:* If lateral views are not available, a crude estimate of kidney depth in centimeters can be obtained with the following equations:[4]

$$\text{Right Kidney Depth} = 13.3 \, (\text{Weight/Height}) + 0.7$$
$$\text{Left Kidney Depth} = 13.2 \, (\text{Weight/Height}) + 0.7$$

where weight and height are expressed in kilograms and centimeters, respectively. *Note:* A correlation of calculated versus measured (ultrasonography) kidney depths has shown that the preceding equations provide a poor estimate of true kidney depth, with a correlation

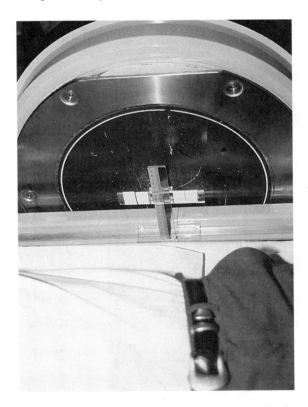

Figure 7-11. Line source and ruler for estimate of kidney depth. The ruler base should be positioned on the table surface. The patient should then be moved closer to the camera for best resolution.

coefficient less than 0.7.[5] Thus, whenever possible, a lateral scan or ultrasonographic estimate of kidney depth should be obtained.

Measurement of System Sensitivity

1. Draw 50–100 µCi (1.85–3.7 MBq) ^{99m}Tc into a syringe. The syringe should be assayed in a well calibrator, and the exact times at which the syringe activity was measured should be recorded. The gamma camera should be oriented with the head facing up, and the syringe should be placed on the collimator in the center of the field of view at a distance of 10 cm from the collimator surface, as shown in Figure 7-12.
2. A static image should be acquired on computer in a 128 × 128 word mode matrix for 2 minutes. The exact time of acquisition and the count rate should be recorded.
3. The syringe activity should be decay-corrected to the time of imaging. An ROI region should be drawn around the image of the syringe, and the total counts obtained should be divided by 2 to give ct/min and then divided by syringe activity to give ct/min per µCi (ct/min per kBq). This is the system sensitivity factor for converting kidney counts to activity.

Computer Analysis

The ^{99m}Tc MAG3 images should be analyzed as described in Procedure 7-1. For GFR/ERPF analysis, the following additional steps should be performed:

1. From the ^{99m}Tc DTPA study, sum frames 9–12 (2–3 minutes). Apply the total kidney ROIs and appropriate background ROIs drawn in the Dynamic Renal Scan analysis to

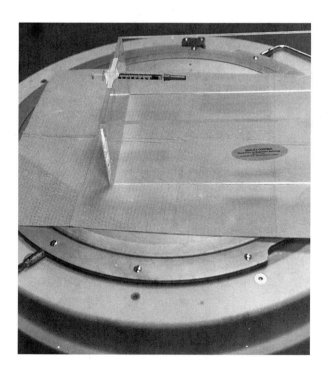

Figure 7-12. A syringe containing 50–100 µCi (1.85–3.7 MBq) ^{99m}Tc suspended 10 cm above the collimator surface for the measurement of system sensitivity.

the 2–3 minute ^{99m}Tc DTPA image. Compute the background-corrected counts for each kidney.

2. From the measured depth of each kidney, correct the counts for attenuation using the following equation:

$$\text{Counts}_{corr} = \text{Counts}_{measured} \times e^{0.12 \times \text{depth (cm)}}$$

An attenuation coefficient of 0.12 cm^{-1} (rather than 0.15 cm^{-1}) should be used to allow for the effects of scatter.[6]

3. Convert the depth-corrected counts to μCi (kBq) by dividing by the system sensitivity factor described previously. Kidney activity can then be divided by injected activity to obtain the percent injected dose in each kidney.

4. For ^{99m}Tc MAG3, repeat steps 1–3, using the 1–2 minute summed image (frames 61–66).

5. Each laboratory needs to generate an appropriate conversion table to convert percent uptake of ^{99m}Tc DTPA and ^{99m}Tc MAG3 to GFR and ERPF, respectively. This conversion will vary depending on choice of background ROI, attenuation correction factor, and estimate of kidney depth.

Information on Film

Obtain a hard copy of all ROIs and both raw and background-corrected curves. On each analog and computer film, ensure that the following information is recorded:

1. Patient name and clinic/hospital number
2. Type of scan and radiopharmaceutical
3. Date and time of each image after the injection
4. Orientation of each image (e.g., posterior) and appropriate labels for the ROIs and curves
5. Results of GFR and ERPF calculations, including percent injected dose in each kidney

Interpretation

Previous work by Gates[2] has shown a good correlation between the percent uptake of ^{99m}Tc DTPA in a kidney and its GFR as measured by creatinine clearance. The relationship is given by the equation

$$\text{GFR}_{creatinine} = (\% \text{ uptake } ^{99m}\text{Tc DTPA}) \times 9.75 - 6.20 \qquad R > 0.95$$

In our laboratory, the relationship between the percent uptake of ^{99m}Tc DTPA and GFR as measured by iothalamate clearance has been found to be

$$\text{GFR}_{iothalamate} = (\% \text{ uptake } ^{99m}\text{Tc DTPA}) \times 12.50 - 2.59 \qquad R > 0.88$$

For ^{99m}TC MAG3 studies in our laboratory, the relationship between ERPF and the percent uptake in the kidney is given by the equation

$$\text{ERPF} = (\% \text{ uptake } ^{99m}\text{Tc MAG3}) \times 31.15 + 41.88 \qquad R > 0.85$$

As can be appreciated from the difference in the results of Gates and our laboratory, the relationships between ^{99m}TC DTPA uptake and GFR, and ^{99m}Tc MAG3 uptake and ERPF, are technique dependent and need to be established for each laboratory.

Note: In vivo techniques such as those described are not as accurate as measurements made on serial blood samples.

Table 7-3. Absorbed Radiation Dose Estimates in a 70-kg Adult
From 1 mCi (37 MBq) ^{99m}Tc DTPA

Tissue	Radiation Absorbed Dose	
	rad/1mCi	mGy/37 MBq
Urinary bladder wall		
2-hr void	0.12	1.15
4.8-hr void	0.27	2.70
Kidneys	0.09	0.90
Ovaries		
2-hr void	0.011	0.11
4.8-hr void	0.016	0.16
Testes		
2-hr void	0.008	0.075
4.8-hr void	0.011	0.105
Total body	0.006	0.06

Radiation Dosimetry

The estimated absorbed doses in organs and tissues of an average subject (70 kg) from the administration of 10 mCi (370 MBq) ^{99m}Tc MAG3 and 1 mCi (37 MBq) ^{99m}Tc DTPA are shown in Tables 7-1 and 7-3, respectively.[7,8]

References

1. Gates GF, Green GS. Transient reduction in renal function following arteriography: a radionuclide study. J Urol 1983; 129: 1107–1110.
2. Gates GF. Glomerular filtration rate: estimation from fractional renal accumulation of ^{99m}Tc DTPA (stannous). Am J Roentgenol 1982; 138: 565–570.
3. Klingensmith WC III, Briggs DE, Smith WI. Technetium-99m-MAG3 renal studies: normal range and reproducibility of physiologic parameters as a function of age and sex. J Nucl Med 1994; 35: 1612–1617.
4. Tønnesen KH, Munck O, Hold T, Mogensen P, Wolf H. Influence on the radio-renogram of variation in skin to kidney distance and the clinical importance hereof. Read at International Symposium on Radionuclides in Nephrology, Berlin, Germany, April 1, 1974, cited by Schlegel JU, Hamway SA. Individual renal plasma flow determination in 2 minutes. J Urol 1976; 116: 282–285.
5. Gruenewald SM, Collins LT, Fawdry RM. Kidney depth measurement and its influence on quantitation of function from gamma camera renography. Clin Nucl Med 1985; 10: 398–401.
6. Harris CC, Greer KL, Jaszczak RJ, et al. Tc-99m attenuation coefficients in water-filled phantoms determined with gamma cameras. Med Phys 1984; 11: 681–685.
7. Package insert. TechneScan MAG3 kit for the preparation of technetium Tc 99m mertiatide. Mallinckrodt Medical, St Louis, 1992.
8. Package insert. MPI DTPA kit for the preparation of technetium Tc 99m pentetate injection. Medi-Physics Inc, Arlington Heights, IL, 1992.

Pediatric Furosemide Renal Scan

Summary Information

Radiopharmaceutical   The ^{99m}Tc MAG3 administered dose is 50 µCi/kg (1.85 MBq/kg), with a minimal dose of 1 mCi (37 MBq) and a maximal dose of 10 mCi (370 MBq).

Contraindications   If possible, the study should be delayed in children younger than 1 month old to allow for maturation of tubular function. However, an age of less than 1 month does not preclude a furosemide (Lasix) renal study if clinically indicated. Check for possible allergy to furosemide. Radiographic contrast agents or renal angiography/angioplasty may interfere with kidney function.[1] If a contrast study has been performed, the renal scan should be deferred for 24 hours.

Dose/Scan Interval   Imaging begins immediately after the injection.

Views Obtained

Native kidneys: Posterior view of lower back. Ensure that the kidneys and bladder are in the field of view. The proper magnification should be established before the study to include the midthorax at the top of the field of view to the upper thigh at the bottom of the field of view. This magnification should be performed at the camera console. Approximate magnification factors are given in Table 7-4 for a 40-cm circular field-of-view gamma camera.

Transplant kidneys: Anterior view of pelvis, with similar magnification as for native kidneys.

Indications

In pediatric patients, ^{99m}Tc MAG3 renal scintigraphy with furosemide is used to diagnose obstructive uropathy.[2]

Principle

^{99m}Tc MAG3 is cleared by the kidneys and may collect in the pelvic region because of a dilated collecting system. The use of a diuretic (furosemide) as an adjunct to the renal scan distinguishes patients with obstruction from those without obstruction who have delayed pelvic clearance that is due to a dilated collecting system. In obstructed uropathy, washout of activity does not occur after furosemide administration, whereas washout does occur in the nonobstructed system.[2,3] The procedure described next is based on the diuresis renography protocol recommended by the Pediatric Nuclear Medicine Club of the Society of Nuclear Medicine and the Society for Fetal Urology.[4]

Patient Preparation

1. Hydration: Intravenous fluids will be necessary for children up to 6–7 years old. Older children should be hydrated orally, and urine concentration monitored for specific gravity, as for adults. For children younger than 6–7 years, IV hydration should be set at 30 ml/hr per kg of 5% dextrose in 0.2% normal saline solution. This should be started 15 minutes before the renal scan and maintained for 30 minutes (i.e., a total of 15 ml/kg should be given over this period). After this, hydration should be reduced to 4.2 ml/hr per kg (0.07 ml/min per kg) for the rest of the study (minimal maintenance dose, not less than 3 ml/hr).
2. Catheterization: All children should be catheterized. The catheter should remain open throughout the renal study. The bladder should be emptied before the study, and urine should be collected in serial tubes every 10 minutes. Urine output should be recorded at 10-minute intervals for the entire study. If during the study it appears that the bladder is not emptying, urine should be removed at 10-minute intervals by syringe suction.
3. Sedation: Consult with the hospital/clinic pediatrician about the appropriate method of sedation.
4. Pediatric Furosemide Renogram Worksheet: All urine output, hydration rates, infused fluid volumes, and administered doses of furosemide and ^{99m}Tc MAG3 should be recorded on the Pediatric Furosemide Renogram Worksheet (Fig. 7-13). This worksheet should be retained and filed with the films.

Instrument Specifications

Gamma camera:	Any large field-of-view system can be used.
Collimator:	Low-energy, all-purpose collimator.
Energy setting:	140 keV, 15–20% energy window.
Analog formatter:	8 × 10 film, 70-mm (9-on-1) format.
Computer system:	Acquisition requirements—dynamic (64 × 64 matrix). Processing requirements—ROI analysis and curve generation and manipulation.

Furosemide Administration

The furosemide dose is 1.0 mg/kg body weight up to a maximum of 80 mg. Furosemide should be injected slowly over a 1–2 minute period. Be sure to flush the furosemide dose with saline. Furosemide is injected 20–30 minutes after the injection of ^{99m}Tc MAG3. Consult with the nuclear medicine physician to determine the optimum time for furosemide injection.

Imaging Procedure—Prefurosemide

Set the magnification factor to include the midthorax at the top of the field of view to the upper thigh at the bottom of the field of view. Appproximate magnification factors are given in Table 7-4 for a 40-cm circular field-of-view camera.

PEDIATRIC FUROSEMIDE RENOGRAM : WORKSHEET

Patient Name : _____

Clinic No. _____   Date : _____

Weight : _____   Age : _____

HYDRATION

Hydration rate = 30 ml/hr/kg
Maintenance Rate : 4.2 ml/hr/kg

IV Hydration Rate : _____ ml/min _____ ml/hr

IV Maintenance Rate : _____ ml/min _____ ml/hr

Tc-99m MAG3

Tc-99m MAG3 dose : 50 uCi/kg
Minimum = 1 mCi / Maximum = 10mCi

Tc-99m MAG3 Dose : _____ mCi

Volume MAG3 : _____ ml

Saline Flush Volume

_____ ml

FUROSEMIDE

Furosemide dose : 1 mg / kg
Maximum dose = 80 mg

Furosemide Dose : _____ mg

Volume Lasix : _____ ml

PROCEDURE TIMES

Start time = time of MAG3 injection
End time = end of post-furosemide study

Start Time : _____   End Time : _____

Total procedure time : _____ min.

URINARY OUTPUT

Empty bladder immediately prior to injection of Tc-99m MAG3.

Every 10 minutes, empty urine into serial tubes and record volume.

If bladder not emptying, remove urine by syringe suction every 10 minutes

Pre-Furosemide output   0-10 min : _____ ml

10-20 min : _____ ml

20-30 min : _____ ml
(only if delay between acq's)

Post-Furosemide output   0-10 min : _____ ml

10-20 min : _____ ml

20-30 min : _____ ml

TOTAL I.V. FLUIDS

Determine total volume that has been infused for the entire procedure

A. Initial IV volume in pump : _____ ml

B. End IV volume in pump : _____ ml

C. IV volume infused by pump (A-B) : _____ ml

TOTAL IV FLUID VOL. (Volume Furosemide + Volme MAG3 + Saline Flush + C) : _____ ml

Technologist : _____

Figure 7-13. Pediatric Furosemide Renogram Worksheet.

Analog Formatter

Start the analog formatter when the ^{99m}Tc MAG3 is injected. Record the following:

1. Flow study (3 seconds per image for 9 images).

Table 7-4. Image Magnification Factor as a Function of Patient Age

Age	Magnify
1–2 weeks	2.0
1 month	1.75
1 year	1.5
2 years	1.25
More than 2 years	None/1.25

Note: Children of this age can vary significantly in size. Please use these values only as a rough guide.

2. Static images at 1, 5, 10, 15, 20, 25, and 30 minutes after the injection. Total counts acquired on the 1- and 5-minute images should be based on patient age, as shown in Table 7-5.

Subsequent images should be acquired for a preset time equal to the time of the 5-minute image.

Computer Acquisition

Start computer acquisition when the ^{99m}Tc MAG3 is injected. This is a 30-minute computer acquisition with the following acquisition variables:

1. Two-phase dynamic study in 128 × 128 word mode matrix (64 × 64 matrix acceptable; however, the larger matrix permits more accurate ROI definition).
2. Phase 1 is 60 frames at 1 second per frame; phase 2 is 174 frames at 10 seconds per frame.

Imaging Procedure—Postfurosemide

The magnification factor should remain unchanged from that used in the prefurosemide imaging procedure.

Analog Formatter

Start the analog formatter when furosemide is injected. Record static images at 1, 5, 10, 15, 20, 25, and 30 minutes after the injection. *Note:* The time per image should be the same as the prefurosemide time per image.

Table 7-5. Total Counts Acquired as a Function of Patient Age

Age	kct per image
1–2 weeks	150
1 month	200
1 year	350
2 years	400
3–10 years	500–1,000
11–20 years	1,000

Computer Acquisition

Start computer acquisition when the furosemide is injected. This is a 30-minute computer acquisition with the following acquisition variables: single-phase dynamic study in a 128 × 128 word mode matrix, with 90 frames at 20 seconds per frame.

Note: The acquisition may be stopped at 20–30 minutes, depending on the visualization of activity in the renal pelvis and ureter. Consult with the nuclear medicine physician about the appropriate time to stop acquisition.

Computer Analysis

The following analysis should be performed on the prefurosemide image data:

1. Sum frames 61–66 (1–2 minutes), and draw ROIs around each kidney, as shown in Figure 7-2.
2. Narrow (1–2-pixel-thick) background ROIs should be drawn around each kidney (see Fig. 7-2) but displaced 2–3 pixels from the edge of the kidney ROIs.
3. Record the size and counts in the ROIs. Perform background (Bkg) correction to obtain the corrected kidney counts as follows:

$$Kidney_{corr} = Kidney_{raw} - Bkg \times (Size_{kidney} / Size_{bkg})$$

4. Determine differential renal function by expressing counts from each kidney as a percentage of total (right + left) kidney counts.
5. Draw an ROI over the descending aorta, as shown in Figure 7-2. Using all the preceding ROIs, generate time–activity curves from the phase-1 dynamic study (first 60 seconds). These curves are normalized to counts per pixel (rather than total counts) and can be used to assess relative renal perfusion (see Fig. 7-3). In the very small child, the flow study is usually suboptimal.
6. Sum frames 61–96 (1–7 minutes) to yield six 1-minute frames. Select the image that shows maximal renal pelvic activity. Draw ROIs around the pelvic and calyceal activity in each kidney, as shown in Figure 7-4. The cortical renal ROI is derived by subtracting the renal pelvic ROI from the entire renal ROI, as shown in Figure 7-4. The cortical ROIs should not include any pelvic activity. The new background ROIs to correct the cortical kidney activity are derived by using the lower outer quadrant of the circumferential background ROI (see Fig. 7-4).
7. Using all images (phase 1 and 2), generate time–activity curves from the cortical and background ROIs, and perform background correction, as described in step 3.
8. Depending on the duration of the prefurosemide acquisition, two indices of renal function (time-to-peak counts and $t_{1/2}$ clearance) can be determined from the (background-corrected) cortical kidney curves (see Fig. 7-5).

The following steps should be performed on the postfurosemide image data:

1. Using the pelvic ROIs shown in Figure 7-6, generate time–activity curves showing the washout of activity from the pelvic area after furosemide administration.
2. If the ureters are visualized, select an appropriate image (or a summed group of images). Draw ROIs over the left and right ureters, as shown in Figure 7-6. Generate time–activity curves of ureter activity after furosemide administration.

Note: Many manufacturers provide comprehensive renal analysis software programs with their systems that eliminate the need for manual processing of the data. Full details of the renal analysis package, including references to the technique used, should be obtained.

Information on film

Obtain a hard copy of all ROIs and both raw and background-corrected curves. On each analog and computer film, ensure that the following information is recorded:

1. Patient name and clinic/hospital number
2. Type of scan and radiopharmaceutical
3. Date and time of each image after injection and after furosemide administration
4. Orientation of each image (e.g., posterior), and appropriate labels for ROIs and curves

Interpretation

1. Normal pattern: Kidneys show a prompt increase in activity, with spontaneous washout accelerated by diuresis. In immature or poorly functioning kidneys, there may be reduced washout and an inadequate response to furosemide (Figs. 7-14 and 7-15).
2. Dilated nonobstructed pattern: Kidneys show progressively increasing activity, which decreases after diuretic injection (Figs. 7-14 and 7-15).
3. Obstructed pattern: Kidneys show progressively increasing activity with flat or blunted response or further increase after furosemide injection (Figs. 7-14 and 7-15). *Note:* A false-positive study may be seen with immaturity or poor function.

Radiation Dosimetry

The estimated absorbed doses in organs and tissues for an 8-day old, 1-year-old, 5-year-old, 10-year-old, and 15-year-old from the administration of ^{99m}Tc MAG3 are shown in Table 7-6.[5]

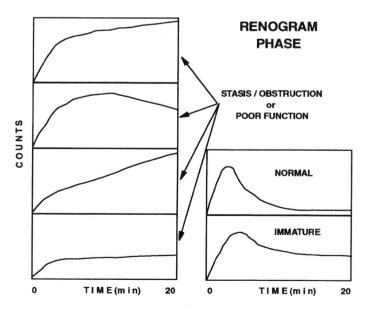

Figure 7-14. Renogram phase: examples of possible uptake and washout patterns for cortical kidney curves following MAG3 injection.

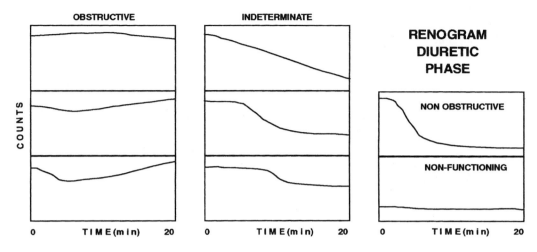

Figure 7-15. Diuretic phase: examples of possible washout patterns for MAG3 cortical kidney curves following furosemide injection.

Table 7-6. Absorbed Radiation Dose Estimates to Children Aged 8 Days to 15 Years, From ^{99m}Tc MAG3

Organ	8-day-old 3.4 kg 1 mCi/37 MBq rad/mGy	1-year-old 9.8 kg 1.96 mCi/73 MBq rad/mGy	5-year-old 19 kg 3.8 mCi/141 MBq rad/mGy	10-year-old 32 kg 6.4 mCi/237 MBq rad/mGy	15-year-old 57 kg 10 mCi/370 MBq rad/mGy
Urinary bladder wall	1.1/11.0	0.94/9.43	2.11/21.09	2.37/23.68	5.92/59.2
Kidneys	0.14/1.4	0.11/1.09	0.13/1.31	0.15/1.52	0.17/1.74
Gallbladder wall	0.27/2.7	0.25/2.47	0.16/1.55	0.17/1.66	0.20/1.96
Small bowel	0.052/0.52	0.05/0.54	0.12/1.20	0.14/1.40	0.20/2.04
Upper large intestinal wall	0.096/0.96	0.09/0.94	0.18/1.83	0.20/2.04	0.24/2.44
Lower large intestinal wall	0.170/1.70	0.16/1.60	0.23/2.25	0.24/2.37	0.41/4.07
Liver	0.032/0.32	0.03/0.30	0.04/0.39	0.04/0.43	0.05/0.48
Ovaries	0.058/0.58	0.06/0.62	0.13/1.32	0.15/1.54	0.33/3.33
Testes	0.051/0.51	0.05/0.53	0.11/1.08	0.12/1.18	0.24/2.37
Red marrow	0.016/0.16	0.02/0.16	0.03/0.28	0.04/0.36	0.06/0.63
Total body	0.024/0.24	0.02/0.22	0.04/0.37	0.04/0.40	0.08/0.81

References

1. Gates GF, Green GS. Transient reduction in renal function following arteriography: a radionuclide study. J Urol 1983; 129: 1107–1110.
2. O'Reilly PH, Britton KE, Nommon CC. Evaluation of urinary tract obstruction. In "Evaluation of Renal Function and Disease With Radionuclides," ed Blaufox MD. Karger, Basel, Switzerland, 1989, pp 116–129.
3. Russell CD, Young D, Billingsley JD, Dubovsky EV. Technical procedures for use of the new kidney agent technetium-99m MAG3. J Nucl Med Tech 1991; 19: 147–152.
4. Conway JJ, Maizels M. The "well tempered" diuretic renogram: a standard method to examine the asymptomatic neonate with hydronephrosis or hydroureteronephrosis. A report from combined meetings of The Society for Fetal Urology and members of The Pediatric Nuclear Medicine Council—The Society of Nuclear Medicine. J Nucl Med 1992; 33: 2047–2051.
5. Package insert. TechneScan MAG3 kit for the preparation of technetium Tc 99m mertiatide. Mallinckrodt Medical, St. Louis, 1992.

99mTc DMSA Renal Scan

Summary Information

Radiopharmaceutical

    Adult dose: 3 mCi (111 MBq) ^{99m}Tc DMSA (2,3-dimercaptosuccinic acid) injected intravenously.

    Pediatric dose: Adjusted according to the patient's weight (see Appendix A-3).

Contraindications   None.

Dose/Scan Interval   Imaging commences 3 hours after injection.

Views Obtained

    Planar imaging: Anterior and posterior views of the abdomen.

    SPECT imaging: Abdominal region, with the gamma camera centered on the kidneys.

Indications

^{99m}Tc DMSA can be used in the evaluation of acute pyelonephritis, for which it is considerably more sensitive than either an IV pyelogram or ultrasonography.[1] It provides information about renal tubular mass and can, thus, be used to determine the relative cortical function of each kidney as well as the size, shape, and number of kidneys.[2] It is also valuable in detecting renal masses, lacerations, contusions, abscesses, and inflammation and in evaluating renal pseudotumors.

Principle

After IV injection, ^{99m}Tc DMSA becomes tightly bound to plasma proteins and is extracted from the blood by the proximal renal tubules, thereby becoming localized in the renal cortex. Because DMSA is excreted only minimally, it is an excellent agent for displaying the renal cortex free of pelvocaliceal activity.[2,3]

Patient Preparation

None.

Instrument Specifications

Planar Imaging

    Gamma camera: Any large field-of-view system can be used.

    Collimator: Low-energy, all-purpose or low-energy, high-resolution collimator.

Energy setting:	140 keV, 15–20% energy window.
Analog formatter:	8 × 10 film, 70-mm (9-on-1) format.
Computer system:	Acquisition requirements—static (256 × 256 matrix).
	Processing requirements—ROI analysis.

SPECT Imaging

Gamma camera:	Single-, dual-, or triple-head SPECT system.
Collimator:	Low-energy, high-resolution collimator (single-head system).
	Low-energy, high- or ultrahigh-resolution collimator (dual- or triple-head systems).
Energy setting:	140 keV, 15–20% energy window.
Computer system:	Acquisition requirements—SPECT (128 × 128 matrix).
	Processing requirements—SPECT reconstruction software.

Imaging Procedure

1. About 3 hours after the injection, position the patient supine on the imaging table.
2. On an analog formatter, acquire posterior and anterior views of the kidneys, with 1,000 kct/view. Posterior oblique views may be of value in some cases. If little activity is visible on the anterior view, acquisition should be stopped after 5 minutes.
3. On computer, acquire posterior and anterior views of the kidneys (256 × 256 word mode matrix, 5 minutes per image).
4. In some patients, a SPECT acquisition may be required to better visualize renal anatomy. In such cases, the following acquisition variables should be used:

   Single-head system: Elliptical/body contour orbit, 128 × 128 word mode matrix, 120 views every 3° at 20 seconds per view (total acquisition time = 40 minutes).
   Dual- or triple-head systems: Elliptical/body contour orbit, 128 × 128 word mode matrix, 120 views every 3° at 30 seconds per view (total acquisition time is 20–30 minutes).

Computer Analysis

Planar Images

For calculating the percentage of functioning renal mass, draw ROIs around each kidney on both the anterior and posterior views. Background correction generally is not required. Obtain the geometric mean of counts for each kidney using the equation:

$$COUNTS_{GM} = (COUNTS_{ANT} \times COUNTS_{POST})^{0.5}$$

Sum the total geometric mean counts for both kidneys, and express each kidney as a percentage of total counts.

SPECT Images

The following steps should be followed:

1. Apply uniformity and center of rotation correction to the data (on newer systems, this may be done automatically).
2. If possible, prefilter the planar data before back-projection. The filter type and cutoff should be similar to those used for bone SPECT. Possible filters are Butterworth, order 10–12, cutoff at 0.4–0.6 Nyquist, and Metz filter with power of 3 and FWHM of 6–10 mm.

3. Reconstruct 1-pixel-thick transaxial slices. The back-projection filter may be a Ramp or Ramp-Butterworth with a cutoff at 0.6–0.8 Nyquist. Conventional sagittal and coronal slices should be generated.

Information on Film

On each analog and computer film, ensure that the following information is recorded:

1. Patient name and clinic/hospital number
2. Date and time of each image after injection
3. Type of scan and radiopharmaceutical
4. Orientation of each image (e.g., anterior, posterior)

Interpretation

The normal ^{99m}Tc DMSA renal scan shows homogeneous uptake throughout both renal cortices. The kidney margins may show some irregularity because of respiratory motion. The kidneys should be within 2 cm of each other in length and from 10 to 14 cm in overall length.

Acute pyelonephritis is characterized by varying degrees of decreased cortical uptake of ^{99m}Tc DMSA in single or multiple regions, predominantly located in the upper and lower poles of the kidneys. Generally, there is no apparent loss in kidney volume.[1] Renal tumors, cysts, infarcts, abscesses, and damage that is due to renal trauma such as rupture or intracapsular hematomas appear as cold defects in the renal parenchyma. These may not be distinguishable from each other on the scan. Diffuse renal disease may show patchy or diffusely decreased uptake of the radiopharmaceutical. Unilateral renal disease such as unilateral renal artery stenosis shows decreased size and/or decreased uptake on the involved side. Congenital defects such as ectopic kidneys show renal uptake in abnormal locations.

Radiation Dosimetry

The estimated absorbed doses in organs and tissues of an average subject (70 kg) from an IV injection of ^{99m}Tc DMSA are shown in Table 7-7.[4]

Table 7-7. Absorbed Radiation Dose Estimates in a 70-kg Adult From 3 mCi (111 MBq) ^{99m}Tc DMSA

Tissue	Absorbed Radiation Doses	
	rad/3 mCi	mGy/111 MBq
Bladder wall	0.42	4.2
Kidneys	3.78	37.8
Renal cortices	5.10	51.0
Liver	0.19	1.9
Bone marrow	0.13	1.3
Ovaries	0.08	0.8
Testes	0.04	0.4
Total body	0.09	0.9

References

1. Majd M, Rushton HG. Renal cortical scintigraphy in the diagnosis of acute pyelonephritis. Semin Nucl Med 1992; 22: 98–111.
2. Taylor A Jr. Quantitation of renal function with static imaging agents. Semin Nucl Med 1982; 12: 330–344.
3. Handmaker H. Nuclear renal imaging in acute pyelonephritis. Semin Nucl Med 1982; 12: 246–253.
4. Kit for the preparation of technetium Tc-99m succimer injections, product 4349. Medi-physics, Inc, Paramus, NJ, revised March 1989.

Voiding Cystography

Summary Information

Radiopharmaceutical   2 mCi (74 MBq) [99mTc] DTPA instilled into the bladder through a catheter for patients older than 1 year.
1 mCi (37 MBq) [99mTc] DTPA instilled into the bladder through a catheter for patients younger than 1 year.

Contraindications   None.

Dose/Scan Interval   Imaging begins immediately on injection of the [99mTc] DTPA and continues until the patient has voided completely.

Views Obtained
Filling phase: Posterior view of the bladder and ureters, with the patient supine.

Voiding phase: Posterior view of the bladder and ureters, with the patient upright and sitting on a urinal.

Indications

This procedure is useful for detecting vesicoureteral reflux and for follow-up examinations to determine the effects of time or therapy on reflux. The determination of whether a patient has vesicoureteral reflux is an important aspect of pediatric urology.[1,2]

Principle

[99mTc] DTPA is injected through a catheter into the bladder, and the bladder is slowly filled with saline until the patient has an urge to void. The patient's kidneys and ureters are monitored continuously during the filling, full bladder, and voiding phases to detect the amount of vesicoureteral reflux.[3]

Patient Preparation

Ask the patient to remove all clothing from the waist down and to put on a hospital gown. The technique requires catheterization of the bladder, which should be done by an experienced nurse. The patient should not void before this procedure, because urine samples may be required for assessing renal function and sterility testing. The following items are required for bladder catheterization:[2]

1. A 500-ml bag of sterile saline with an IV infusion set
2. One tubing clamp or 3-way stopcock

3. A sterile catheter kit—recommended catheter sizes are

Boys less than 1 year old—#5 or #8 infant feeding tube
Boys 1–3 years old—#8 Foley catheter
Girls less than 1 year old—#8 Foley catheter
Girls 1–3 years old—#10 Foley catheter
Girls more than 3 years old—#12 Foley catheter

4. Absorbent pads.
5. Urinal or commode.

When the catheter is in place, tape it so that the patient cannot easily push it out. When no more urine comes out of the catheter, attach it to the IV set and saline bag. Raise the saline bag 2–3 feet above the patient (if higher, the increased pressure may cause reflux).

Instrument Specifications

Gamma camera:	Any large field-of-view system can be used.
Collimator:	Low-energy, high-sensitivity or all-purpose collimator.
Energy setting:	140 keV, 15–20% energy window.
Analog formatter:	8 × 10 film, 70-mm (9-on-1) format.
Computer system:	Acquisition requirements—dynamic (64 × 64 matrix).
	Processing requirements—dynamic display of images.

Imaging Procedure

1. With sterile technique, insert the catheter through the urethra into the bladder. Connect the tubing clamp and sterile saline bag to the catheter.
2. Image the patient in a supine position in the posterior projection (the camera head is under the imaging table), as shown in Figure 7-16.[4] Use absorbent pads liberally under the patient.

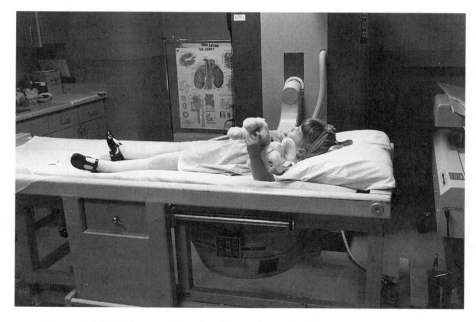

Figure 7-16. Patient position for filling phase of radionuclide cystography.

3. Immediately before the injection of ^{99m}Tc DTPA, start the computer acquisition (64 × 64 word mode matrix, 5 seconds per frame, 400 frames). Start the analog formatter after injection of the ^{99m}Tc DTPA, and acquire the first image for 250 kct. Note the acquisition time for the image, and set the formatter on continuous mode to acquire subsequent images for the same time.

4. Inject the ^{99m}Tc DTPA into the catheter, rinsing the syringe several times. Start the saline infusion to fill the patient's bladder. The degree of filling will vary from patient to patient; however, the expected capacity can be estimated with the following formula:[5]

$$\text{Expected bladder capacity (ml)} = (\text{Age in years} + 2) \times 29$$

Filling should continue until the bladder is full or until the patient is unable to tolerate the increased bladder pressure. Clamp the tube after filling is complete, and note the infused volume. Set the analog formatter to single mode, and allow it to complete the acquisition of the current image. Stop the computer acquisition.

5. In older children (more than 2 years), remove the catheter and sit these patients on the urinal with their backs to the gamma camera (Fig. 7-17). Younger children may not have adequate bladder control to wait until seated and should void supine. In these patients, place a bed pan under the patient to collect the urine. The gamma camera should be positioned to image the bladder and ureters.

6. Start the analog formatter, using the same setting as in step 3. Set up the computer acquisition as in step 3 and start computer. Instruct the patient to begin voiding. When the bladder is empty, stop the computer and analog formatter acquisitions and note the volume of urine voided.

7. Obtain a postvoiding image on computer (64 × 64 word mode) and on analog formatter for the time of the first image in step 3. *Note:* It is important not to confuse voided activity on the table, absorbent pads, clothes, or urinal with urethral reflux.

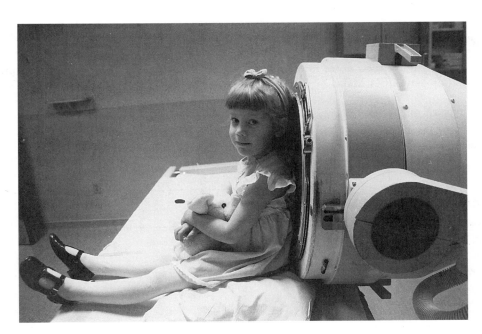

Figure 7-17. Patient position for voiding phase of radionuclide cystography.

Computer Analysis

Play back the dynamic computer studies using a window level optimized to show low-count regions. Note whether reflux occurs during the filling or voiding phase.

Information on Film

On analog and computer films, record the following information:

1. Patient name and clinic/hospital number
2. Date and time of each image after infusion of the ^{99m}Tc DTPA
3. Type of scan and radiopharmaceutical
4. Orientation and phase (e.g., filling phase) of each image
5. Volume instilled into the bladder and the volume voided

Interpretation

Any reflux is abnormal. This may occur during any phase of the study: at filling, after the bladder is full, or during voiding.[2]

Additional Notes

If there is a contraindication to catheterization, an indirect method based on the renal clearance of ^{99m}Tc DTPA can be used. This does not allow for detection of reflux during the filling phase, and it may be difficult to distinguish between reflux and activity descending from the kidney. The study should begin after most of the injected tracer has cleared the kidneys. With the indirect method, the patient is required to retain urine until accumulation of ^{99m}Tc DTPA in the bladder is sufficient. This indirect method may not work in patients with poor renal function.

Radiation Dosimetry

The estimated absorbed doses in organs and tissues of an average subject (70 kg) from an infusion of 2 mCi (74 MBq) ^{99m}Tc DTPA into the bladder are shown in Table 7-8. These

Table 7-8. Absorbed Radiation Dose Estimates in a 70-kg Adult
From an Infusion of 2 mCi (74 MBq) ^{99m}Tc DTPA Into the Bladder

Tissue	Absorbed Radiation Doses	
	rad/2 mCi	mGy/74 MBq
Bladder wall	0.331	3.31
Testes	0.009	0.09
Ovaries	0.015	0.15
Uterus	0.031	0.31
Total body	0.004	0.04

dose estimates were calculated using a maximal residence time of 1 hour and "S" values obtained from Kereiakes and Carey.[6]

References

1. Palmer EL, Scott JA, Strauss HW. Practical Nuclear Medicine. W.B. Saunders, Philadelphia, 1992, pp 264–266.
2. Taylor A Jr. Radionuclide imaging of the genitourinary tract. In "Clinical Practice of Nuclear Medicine," eds Taylor A Jr, Datz FL. Churchill Livingstone, New York, 1991, pp 119–152.
3. Brown ML. Cystography. In "Manual of Nuclear Medicine Procedures," 4th Edition, ed Carey JE, Klein RC, Keyes JW. CRC Press, Boca Raton, FL, 1983, pp 73–74.
4. Beschi RJ, Dubovsky EV, Kontzen FN, Scott JW, Billingsley JD. Genitourinary system. In "Nuclear Medicine: Technology and Techniques," 3rd Edition, eds Bernier DR, Christian PE, Langan JK. Mosby-Year Book, St. Louis, MO, 1994, pp 335–360.
5. Berger RM, Maizels M, Moran GC, Conway JJ, Firlit CF. Bladder capacity (ounces) equals age (years) plus 2 predicts normal bladder capacity and aids in diagnosis of abnormal voiding patterns. J Urol 1983; 129: 347–349.
6. Kereiakes JG, Carey KR. Biophysical effects of the medical use of technetium Tc-99m. AAPM Monograph No. 1, American Association of Physicists in Medicine, Cincinnati, 1976.

Determination of Residual Urine

Summary Information

Radiopharmaceutical
Adult dose: 2 mCi (74 MBq) ^{99m}Tc MAG3 injected intravenously.
Pediatric dose: Adjusted according to patient's weight (see Appendix A-3). *Note:* Larger doses may be used if this procedure is part of a renal study.

Contraindications   None.

Dose/Scan Interval   Imaging may commence 30–60 minutes after the injection.

Views Obtained   Obtain an anterior view of the bladder.

Indications

This procedure is indicated whenever there is a question of significant urine retention in the bladder after micturition. This may occur in patients with obstructive uropathy, neurogenic bladder dysfunction, and chronically overdistended bladder that is due to spinal cord injury or habitual suppression of the urge to void. Also, residual urine studies are used as a follow-up of patients after bladder retraining.[1] *Note:* In patients with poor renal function, this procedure may not be accurate, because there is a slow, continuous inflow of activity into the bladder, which corrupts the postvoiding bladder count.

Principle

This procedure can be performed with either ^{99m}Tc DTPA or ^{99m}Tc MAG3. However, ^{99m}Tc MAG3 is preferred because it accumulates more rapidly in the urinary bladder. Residual urine determinations can be quantitated by using a gamma camera and computer system, thus avoiding catheterization. The bladder is imaged both before and after voiding. The difference in counts together with the urine volume voided allows quantitation of the volume of residual urine in the bladder. Results from this procedure are comparable to those obtained with catheterization.[2]

Patient Preparation

The patient should be normally hydrated or slightly overhydrated and should void immediately before injection of ^{99m}Tc MAG3.

Instrument Specifications

Gamma camera: Any large field-of-view system can be used.
Collimator: Low-energy, all-purpose collimator.

Energy setting:	140 keV, 15–20% energy window.
Analog formatter:	8 × 10 film, 70-mm (9-on-1) format.
Computer system:	Acquisition requirements—static (256 × 256 matrix).
	Processing requirements—ROI analysis.

Imaging Procedure

1. Inject 2 mCi (74 MBq) ^{99m}Tc MAG3 intravenously. Up to 10 mCi (370 MBq) may be used if the test is performed in conjunction with a kidney scan.
2. Instruct the patient not to void and to return within 60 minutes (allows for the accumulation of ^{99m}Tc MAG3 in the bladder).
3. After the patient returns, image the patient in the supine position, with the gamma camera positioned anteriorly over the bladder area, and obtain a 5-minute image on analog formatter and on computer (256 × 256 word mode matrix).
4. Have the patient void into a graduated container, and save the urine. Give the patient adequate privacy for this collection.
5. Reposition the patient, and repeat step 3. This must be done quickly to reduce the error introduced by the accumulation of renal excretion between the prevoid and postvoid images.
6. Measure the volume of voided urine.

Computer Analysis

1. Select the prevoid image, and draw an ROI around the bladder and an adjacent background region, as shown in Figure 7-18. The background ROI should be located to the side of the bladder, excluding the ureters and femoral arteries.
2. Record the size and total counts in the ROIs on the worksheet for residual urine calculation (Fig. 7-19). Repeat this analysis for the postvoid image. The residual urine volume is then calculated from the following equation and should be recorded on the worksheet.

$$\text{Residual Urine Volume (ml)} = \frac{\text{Voided Urine Volume (ml)} \times \text{Background Corrected Postvoid ct}}{\text{Background Corrected Prevoid ct - Background Corrected Postvoid ct}}$$

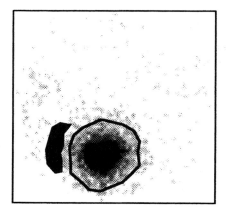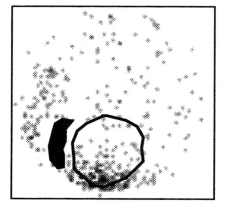

Figure 7-18. Anterior view of bladder showing placement of bladder and background ROIs.

RESIDUAL URINE : WORKSHEET

Patient Name : _____

Clinic No. _____   Date : _____

INJECTION / SCAN TIMES

TIME OF Tc-99m MAG3 INJECTION :   _____

TIME OF PRE-VOID SCAN :   _____

TIME OF POST-VOID SCAN :   _____

Was any urine lost between time of injection and pre-void scan ?   o **NO**   o **YES**

Comment :_____

RESIDUAL URINE CALCULATION

PRE-VOID IMAGE

    Bladder ROI :   Total Ct =   _____ (B1)   **Area (pixels) =**   _____ (B2)

    Background ROI: Total Ct =   _____ (A1)   **Area (pixels) =**   _____ (A2)

    Net full bladder counts : _____ (F) $\boxed{F = B1 - A1 \times (B2/A2)}$

POST-VOID IMAGE

    Bladder ROI :   Total Ct =   _____ (D1)   **Area (pixels) =**   _____ (D2)

    Background ROI: Total Ct =   _____ (C1)   **Area (pixels) =**   _____ (C2)

    Net empty bladder counts : _____ (E) $\boxed{E = D1 - C1 \times (D2/C2)}$

VOLUME OF URINE VOIDED (ml) :   _____ (V)

RESIDUAL URINE VOLUME (ml) :   _____ (RU) $\boxed{RU = V \times E / (F - E)}$

Technologist : _____

Figure 7-19. Residual urine worksheet.

Information on Film

On analog and computer films, record the following information:

1. Patient name and clinic/hospital number
2. Date and time of each image after injection

Table 7-9. Absorbed Radiation Dose Estimates in a 70-kg Adult
From 2 mCi (74 MBq) ^{99m}Tc MAG3

Tissue	Absorbed Radiation Doses	
	rad/2 mCi	mGy/74 MBq
Kidney	0.028	0.28
Bladder wall	0.960	9.60
Testes	0.032	0.32
Ovaries	0.052	0.52
Upper large intestinal wall	0.038	0.38
Lower large intestinal wall	0.066	0.66
Small intestine	0.032	0.32
Liver	0.007	0.07
Red marrow	0.010	0.10
Total body	0.013	0.13

3. Type of scan and radiopharmaceutical
4. Orientation of each image and whether prevoid or postvoid
5. Appropriate labels for ROIs

Interpretation

Residual urine volume should be less than 60 ml.

Radiation Dosimetry

The estimated absorbed doses in organs and tissues of an average subject (70 kg) from an IV injection of 2 mCi (74 MBq) ^{99m}Tc MAG3 are shown in Table 7-9.[3]

References

1. Brown ML. Residual urine determinations. In "Manual of Nuclear Medicine Procedures," 4th Edition, eds Carey JE, Klein RC, Keyes JW. CRC Press, Boca Raton, FL, 1983, pp 81–82.
2. Strauss BS, Blaufox MD. Estimation of residual urine and urine flow rates without ureteral catheterization. J Nucl Med 1970; 11: 81–84.
3. Kit for the preparation of technetium Tc-99m mertiatide, product 096. Mallinckrodt Medical, Inc, St. Louis, last revised November 1992.

Testicular Scan

Summary Information

Radiopharmaceuticals

Adult dose: 20 mCi (740 MBq) ^{99m}Tc sodium pertechnetate injected intravenously.

Pediatric dose: Adjusted according to the patient's weight (see Appendix A-3).

Contraindications None.

Dose/Scan Interval Imaging begins immediately after injection of the ^{99m}Tc sodium pertechnetate.

Views Obtained Obtain an anterior view of the pelvis (upper thigh to umbilicus).

Indications

The most useful application of testicular imaging is in differentiating epididymitis from testicular torsion as the cause of acute testicular pain.[1] The former condition requires conservative treatment, but the latter requires immediate surgical intervention if the testis is to be saved. Testicular torsion occurs when the testicle occludes its blood supply by twisting on the spermatic cord. Patients with a congenital abnormality called "bell-clapper" deformity (Fig. 7-20) may be predisposed to testicular torsion.[2] In patients with acute torsion, prompt detorsion is required for salvage of the testicle. The testicle can be saved in about 80% of patients if the operation is performed during the first 6 hours after the onset of symptoms. If surgery is delayed for 12 hours or more, the salvage rate decreases to 20% or less.[3,4]

Although chronic scrotal abnormalities such as hydrocele, spermatocele, tumor, abscess, traumatic hematoma, and chronic epididymitis may be detected with testicular imaging, ultrasonography is generally the method of choice for evaluating such lesions.[5]

Principle

Radionuclide angiography with ^{99m}Tc sodium pertechnetate is used to demonstrate the relative blood flow to the scrotal structures. Following this, static imaging is used to depict relative vascularity and nonspecific localization in areas of altered vascular permeability, such as sites of inflammation or vascular congestion.

Patient Preparation

Administer 30 ml of potassium perchlorate (200 mg) orally. Immediately before the scan, ask the patient to remove all clothing from the waist down and to put on a hospital gown.

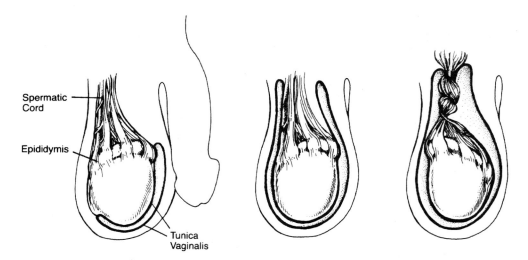

Figure 7-20. Scrotal anatomy. At left is the normal epididymis, spermatic cord, and tunica vaginalis. In a "bell-clapper" deformity, the tunica surrounds the testicle. At right is a testicular torsion. (From Palmer et al.,[2] with permission.)

Instrument Specifications

Adults

Gamma camera:	Any large field-of-view system can be used.
Collimator:	Low-energy, all-purpose collimator.
Zoom factor:	Use a zoom of approximately 2.0 for a 40-cm field-of-view gamma camera system.
Energy setting:	140 keV, 15–20% energy window.
Analog formatter:	8 × 10 film, 70-mm (9-on-1) format.
Computer system:	Acquisition requirements—dynamic (64 × 64 matrix), static (256 × 256 matrix).
	Processing requirements—cine display.

Small Children

Gamma camera:	Any large field-of-view system can be used.
Collimator:	Pin-hole collimator (6-mm aperture).
Zoom factor:	No zoom.
Analog formatter:	8 × 10 film, 70-mm (9-on-1) format.
Computer system:	Acquisition requirements—static (256 × 256 matrix).
	Processing requirements—none.

Note: A pin-hole collimator is required to achieve adequate magnification of the testes in small children.

Imaging Procedure

Adults

1. Position the patient supine on the imaging table with his legs apart.
2. Support the scrotum with a towel or adhesive tape sling to elevate and separate the testes to either side of the scrotum, as shown in Figure 7-21. The penis should be taped back to

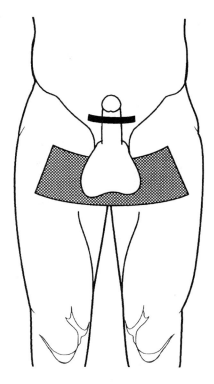

Figure 7-21. The setup for a testicular scan. The legs should be apart with the testes supported with a towel and the penis taped back.

the abdomen to eliminate potentially confusing overlying activity. It is important that the testes be symmetrically positioned and equally supported, because differences in their relative depth can give misleading results.

3. The gamma camera should be positioned with the base of the penis in the center of the field of view.
4. Inject 20 mCi (740 MBq) ^{99m}Tc sodium pertechnetate. Start the analog formatter (9 frames at 5 seconds per frame) after activity is visualized in the descending aorta. The computer should be started at the time of injection (60 frames at 5 seconds per frame, 64×64 word mode matrix).
5. Static views should be acquired at 1 and 5 minutes after injection for 1,000 kct on analog formatter and on computer (256×256 matrix).
6. If requested by the nuclear medicine physician, a lead shield may be placed under the scrotum, in a similar manner to the tape or towel sling, to eliminate soft tissue background activity from the thighs for the second static view. The lead shield should not be used for the flow study or the initial static view.
7. A marker view to outline the respective testes is often helpful (use a ^{57}Co line source).

Small Children

1. Follow steps 1–3 as for adults.
2. Inject the appropriate weight-adjusted dose of ^{99m}Tc sodium pertechnetate. No flow study is possible because of the low count rate with the pin-hole collimator.
3. Static views should be acquired at 1 and 5 minutes after injection for 500 kct on analog formatter and on computer (256×256 matrix).
4. Follow steps 6 and 7 as for adults.

Computer Analysis

The dynamic study should be played back to aid in determining perfusion to the testes.

Information on Film

On each analog and computer film, ensure that the following information is recorded:

1. Patient name and clinic/hospital number
2. Date and time of each image after injection
3. Type of scan and radiopharmaceutical
4. Orientation of each image (e.g., anterior)

Interpretation

Blood flow in the iliac and femoral vessels should be seen clearly during radionuclide angiography. On static imaging, normal testicular activity is symmetric and approximately equal to the thigh in intensity. In acute epididymitis, perfusion and tissue uptake on the affected side are increased. In acute testicular torsion, perfusion to the affected side is generally normal on the flow study. The static image reveals a cold defect at the location of the affected testis. Testicular abscess, missed torsion (more than 24 hours), and traumatic hematomas usually show a cool region surrounded by hyperemia. Hydroceles or spermatoceles are recognized as cool regions of characteristic shape and location. The appearance of testicular tumors varies.

Radiation Dosimetry

The estimated absorbed doses in organs and tissues of an average subject (70 kg) from an IV injection of 20 mCi (740 MBq) ^{99m}Tc sodium pertechnetate are shown in Table 7-10.[6]

Table 7-10. Absorbed Radiation Dose Estimates in a 70-kg Adult From 20 mCi (740 MBq) ^{99m}Tc Sodium Pertechnetate

Tissue	Absorbed Radiation Dose	
	rad/20 mCi	mGy/740 MBq
Bladder wall	1.06	10.6
Stomach wall	5.00	50.0
Upper large intestinal wall	1.37	13.7
Lower large intestinal wall	1.22	12.2
Red marrow	0.38	3.8
Testes	0.18	1.8
Ovaries	0.44	4.4
Thyroid	2.60	26.0
Brain	0.28	2.8
Total body	0.28	2.8

References

1. Holder LE, Melloul M, Chen D. Current status of radionuclide scrotal imaging. Semin Nucl Med 1981; 11: 232–249.
2. Palmer EL, Scott JA, Strauss HW. "Practical Nuclear Medicine." W.B. Saunders, Philadelphia, 1992, pp 267–273.
3. Allan WR, Brown RB. Torsion of the testis. A review of 58 cases. Br Med J 1966; 1: 1396–1397.
4. Skoglund RW, McRoberts JW, Ragde H. Torsion of the spermatic cord: a review of the literature and an analysis of 70 new cases. J Urol 1970; 104: 604–607.
5. Middleton WD, Siegel BA, Melson GL, Yates CK, Andriole GL. Acute scrotal disorders: prospective comparison of color Doppler US and testicular scintigraphy. Radiology 1990; 177: 177–181.
6. MIRD/Dose Estimate Report No. 8. Summary of current radiation dose estimates to normal humans from ^{99m}Tc as sodium pertechnetate. J Nucl Med 1976; 17: 74–77.

Infection–Bone

Lee A. Forstrom

^{111}In White Blood Cell Scan

Summary Information

Radiopharmaceutical

Adult dose:
300–500 µCi (11.1–18.5 MBq) ^{111}In-labeled white blood cells (WBCs) injected intravenously.

Pediatric dose:
Adjusted according to the patient's weight (see Appendix A-3). Where possible, ^{99m}Tc HMPAO-labeled white cells should be used, because of their lower radiation burden.

Note: Two types of ^{111}In WBC preparations are possible: a standard preparation and a purified granulocyte preparation. Check with the nuclear medicine physician to determine the appropriate WBC preparation for the patient. Whenever possible, the radiolabeled WBC preparation should be injected directly into a peripheral vein. If an IV catheter is used, the tubing should be flushed with normal saline before and after infusion of the dose. Avoid dextrose in water solutions, because they can cause the labeled cells to clump.

Standard Preparation
Used for osteomyelitis, septic arthritis, soft tissue infection, and fever of unknown origin.

Pure Granulocyte Preparation (Ficoll/Hypaque)
Used for prosthetic vascular graft infection and inflammatory bowel disease.

Contraindications
Severe leukopenia/granulocytopenia (less than 1×10^3 polymorphonuclear neutrophils per cubic millimeter).

Dose/Scan Interval
Imaging commences 24 hours after the injection, except in patients with inflammatory bowel disease, in whom imaging starts at 2–4 hours after the injection.

Views Obtained
Anterior and posterior whole-body images plus additional spot views, according to the area of interest specified on the examination request sheet or as requested by the nuclear medicine physician. Single photon emission computed tomography (SPECT) may occasionally be performed; however, unless a dual- or triple-head system is used, image quality may be compromised by poor counting statistics.

Indications

[111]In-labeled WBCs can be used to image various pathologic inflammatory conditions. Labeled WBCs have proved very useful in the evaluation of patients with fever of unknown origin and in the evaluation of osteomyelitis, inflammatory bowel disease, and prosthetic vascular graft infections.[1]

Principle

WBCs migrate into regions of inflammation or infection, particularly when the inflammation is acute. Radiolabeling techniques for WBCs include ^{111}In oxine, ^{111}In tropolone, and ^{99m}Tc HMPAO (hexamethyl propylene amine oxine). These labeling techniques adequately preserve WBC function to enable the radiolabeled cells to provide a pictorial representation of the inflammatory response.

Patient Preparation

None.

[111]In WBC Preparation

[111]In oxine is supplied as a sterile pyrogen-free isotonic aqueous solution of indium (^{111}In) oxine in a concentration of 1.0 mCi/ml (37 MBq/ml) at the time of calibration.

Equipment

The following items are required for the labeling process:

1. Two 60-ml syringes
2. 18 ml of anticoagulated citrate dextrose (ACD) solution (solution A as per USP National Formulary)
3. 32 ml of hetastarch solution
4. 6–12 ml of 12.6% ACD/saline (ACD mixed with 0.9% NaCl, v/v)
5. 600 μCi (22.2 MBq) [111]In oxine
6. Centrifuge
7. Sterile laminar flow hood
8. Test tube racks
9. Sterile test tubes
10. Sterile transfer pipettes
11. Ficoll/Hypaque gradients for Ficoll/Hypaque separation only

Standard Labeling Procedure

The entire separation procedure is performed in a sterile laminar flow hood using aseptic technique.

1. Collect 80 ml of whole blood into two 60-ml syringes, each containing 8–9 ml of ACD anticoagulant. Gently invert to mix.
2. Add 8 ml of hetastarch to each of four 50-ml conical tubes.
3. Add equal amounts of blood to each of the 50-ml conical tubes, and gently mix the contents with a sterile pipette. (Caution: avoid the formation of foam or bubbles.)
4. Cap the tubes and place them at a 45° angle in a rack for 25–35 minutes.

5. After sedimentation, remove the leukocyte-rich, platelet-rich plasma (with a sterile pipette), and put it into two 50-ml conical tubes. Avoid including erythrocytes in the suspension.

6. Centrifuge at 600 revolutions per minute (rpm) or $100 \times$ gravity (g) for 5 minutes to remove erythrocytes (Fig. 8-1, step 2). Take off the supernatant, put it into a 50-ml conical tube, and spin it at 800 rpm (150 g) for 8 minutes (Fig. 8-1, step 3). This produces a WBC pellet.

7. Take off the supernatant-platelet-rich plasma. Save 15 ml of supernatant in two conical tubes, and discard the rest. Spin at 4,000 rpm (3,200 g) for 10 minutes to get platelet-poor plasma. Save the platelet-poor plasma in a sterile capped tube for final resuspension of WBCs in step 11, later.

8. Wash the WBC pellet with 6 ml of 12.6% ACD/saline solution, and mix it slowly. Do not introduce air bubbles. Centrifuge it at 600 rpm (100 g) for 5 minutes. Take off the supernatant and discard it.

9. Add 600 µCi (22.2 MBq) ^{111}In oxine slowly, and assay it for initial radioactivity.

10. Incubate the WBCs for 20 minutes at room temperature. Centrifuge at 800 rpm (150 g) for 8 minutes. Take off the supernatant and discard it.

11. Add 7–8 ml of the platelet-poor plasma to the cell pellet and mix carefully to resuspend the WBCs. Draw the suspension into a labeled syringe and assay for final radioactivity.

12. Calculate labeling efficiency:

$$\frac{\text{Final Dose Activity}}{\text{Initial Activity}} \times 100 = \% \text{ Labeled Cells}$$

13. Discard all waste into radioactive waste bins.

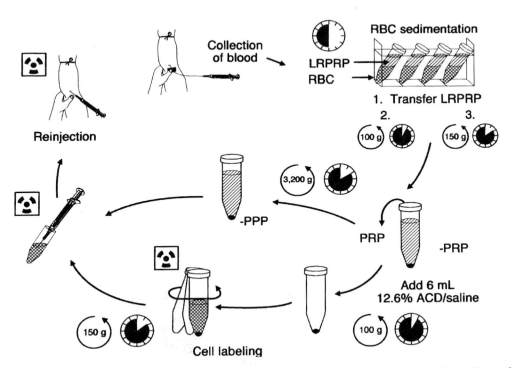

Figure 8-1. Schematic illustration depicting the various steps involved in the radiolabeling of WBCs. Refer to the text for a detailed description. LRPRP, leukocyte-rich platelet-rich plasma; PRP, platelet-rich plasma; PPP, platelet-poor plasma.

Ficoll/Hypaque Separation

1. Follow steps 1–5 in the standard labeling procedure.
2. Take off mixed WBC supernatant. Add equal amounts of the supernatant (approximately 3–5 ml) to sixteen 15-ml sterile conical tubes.
3. With a 12-ml syringe equipped with a long spinal needle, add 3 ml of Ficoll/Hypaque gradient I (1.08 g/ml) to the bottom of each tube. Add slowly, with great care.
4. Repeat step 3 with Ficoll/Hypaque gradient II (1.12 g/ml). Again, add with great care (Fig. 8-2).
5. Centrifuge at 2,300 rpm (1,200 *g*) for 13 minutes. Three layers separated by two bands of cells will be apparent in each tube (Fig. 8-2):
   a. Plasma (top layer)
   b. Monocytes, lymphocytes, and platelets (first band)
   c. Neutrophils (second band)
   d. Red blood cells (bottom)
6. Using sterile pipettes, very carefully remove the top layers and first band down to the neutrophil layer, and discard it.
7. Harvest neutrophil layer (no more than 1 ml), and save it in a 50-ml conical tube.
8. Add equal volumes of 12.6% ACD/saline to neutrophil aliquots, and centrifuge them at 1,300 rpm (300 *g*) for 6 minutes. Take off and discard the supernatant.
9. Wash again with 6 ml of 12.6% ACD/saline.
10. Finish by following steps 8–12 of the standard labeling procedure.
11. An aliquot (0.2 ml) of ^{111}In-labeled WBC suspension can be sent to a hematology laboratory to obtain a complete blood cell count and differential report.
12. Discard all waste into radioactive waste bins.

Notes: The labeled cells should be stored at room temperature. It is recommended that the labeled WBCs be used within 1 hour after preparation, if possible, and in no case more than 3 hours after preparation.

Use the "Policy for Patient Identification During Radiolabeled Blood Product Procedures," as described in Appendix A-2, to ensure correct patient identification and to minimize risk of mismatch.

Instrument Specifications

Gamma camera: Planar views—any large field-of-view system can be used. Whole-body views—dual-head rectangular field-of-view system preferred.

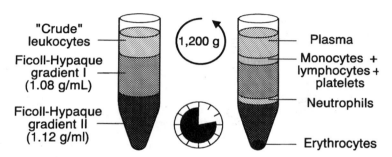

Figure 8-2. Schematic diagram of Ficoll/Hypaque gradients, before and after centrifugation.

SPECT—Single-, dual-, triple-head SPECT system.

Collimator:	Medium-energy collimators.
Energy setting:	174 and 247 keV, 20% energy window.
Analog formatter:	Spot views—8 × 10 film, 70-mm (9-on-1) format.
	Whole-body—11 × 14 film, 4-on-1 format.
Computer system:	Acquisition requirements—static (256 × 256 matrix), whole body (1,024 × 256 matrix), SPECT (64 × 64 matrix).
	Processing requirements—SPECT reconstruction software.

Imaging Procedure

Whole-Body Imaging

At 16–32 hours after injection, anterior and posterior whole-body images should be acquired on an analog formatter and on computer (1,024 × 256 word mode matrix) at a scan speed of 5 cm/min (approximately 40-minute scan time).

Planar Imaging

At 3 hours (inflammatory bowel disease) and 24 hours after injection, spot views of the abdomen should be acquired for 10 minutes per view. For low-count regions, e.g., the wrist, increase the imaging time to 15–20 minutes per view.

SPECT Imaging

When requested, SPECT studies should be acquired using the following acquisition variables:

Single-head system: 360° elliptical orbit, 64 × 64 word mode matrix, 60–64 views at 30–40 seconds per view. No zoom for 40-cm field-of-view system. Zoom of 1.2 for 50–60 cm field-of-view systems.

Dual-, triple-head system: 360° elliptical orbit, 64 × 64 word mode matrix, with a total of 120 views at 15–20 seconds per view. No zoom for 40-cm field-of-view system. Zoom of 1.2 for 50–60 cm field-of-view systems.

Computer Analysis

No analysis is required for planar images. For SPECT studies, the following steps should be followed:

1. Apply uniformity and center-of-rotation correction to the data (on newer systems, this may be done automatically).
2. If possible, prefilter the planar data. For a single-head system, possible filters include Butterworth, order 10, cutoff at 0.4–0.5 Nyquist and Hann filter with cutoff at 0.7–0.9 Nyquist. Dual- and triple-head systems can use sharper filters.
3. Reconstruct 1-pixel-thick transaxial slices. The back-projection filter may be a Ramp or Ramp-Butterworth with a cutoff at 0.6–0.8 Nyquist.

Information on Film

On each analog and computer film, ensure that the following information is recorded:

Table 8-1.   Absorbed Radiation Dose Estimates in a 70-kg Adult From 500 μCi (18.5 MBq)
[111]In-Labeled White Blood Cells

Tissue	[111]In rad/500 μCi	[111]In mGy/18.5 MBq	[114m]In/[114]In rad/1.25 μCi	[114m]In/[114]In mGy/46.3 kBq	Combined Dose rad	Combined Dose mGy
Spleen	13	130	7	70	20	200
Liver	1.9	19	0.71	7.1	2.66	26.6
Red marrow	1.3	13	0.69	6.9	1.99	19.9
Skeleton	0.364	3.6	0.085	0.85	0.45	4.5
Testes	0.01	0.1	0.004	0.04	0.014	0.14
Ovaries	0.19	1.9	0.006	0.06	0.2	2.00
Total Body	0.31	3.1	0.06	0.60	0.37	3.70

1. Patient name and clinic/hospital number
2. Type of scan and radiopharmaceutical preparation/dose used
3. Date and time after injection
4. Orientation of each image (e.g., anterior, posterior)

Interpretation

Activity is normally seen in the liver, spleen, and bone marrow. Images obtained at 0–4 hours after injection may show transient pulmonary distribution. Marrow activity is faintly visible throughout the skeleton, with uptake less in the distal extremities than in the central marrow. The most intense uptake occurs in the spleen.[2]

Accumulation of ^{111}In-labeled WBCs elsewhere in the body is abnormal. Inflammation and infection appear as focal regions of increased tracer uptake. No specific findings differentiate infection from nonseptic inflammation.

Radiation Dosimetry

The estimated absorbed doses in organs and tissues of an average subject (70 kg) from an IV injection of 500 μCi (18.5 MBq) ^{111}In-labeled WBCs are shown in Table 8-1.[3] [111]In may contain impurities of [114m]In and [114]In. Table 8-1 gives the additional radiation exposure that could result from 1.25 μCi (46.3 kBq) of [114m]In/[114]In in 1 mCi (37 MBq) [111]In at the time of calibration.

References

1. Froelich JW, Swanson D. Imaging of inflammatory processes with labeled cells. Semin Nucl Med 1984; 14: 128–140.
2. Palmer EL, Scott JA, Strauss HW. Non-organ-specific imaging: tumor and inflammation detection. In "Practical Nuclear Medicine." W.B. Saunders Co., Philadelphia, 1992, pp 343–364.
3. Indium In-111 oxyquinoline solution, Package insert. Amersham Corp. Code IN.15PA, last updated April 1986.

99mTc HMPAO
White Blood Cell Scan

Summary Information

Radiopharmaceutical

Adult dose: 5–10 mCi (185–370 MBq) 99mTc-(HMPAO)-labeled WBCs injected intravenously.

Pediatric dose: Adjusted according to the patient's weight (see Appendix A-3). *Note*: All preparation should be as described for ^{111}In WBCs in Procedure 8-1.

Contraindications None.

Dose/Scan Interval Imaging commences at 1–4 hours after the injection.

Views Obtained Anterior and posterior whole-body images plus additional spot views should be obtained according to the area of interest specified on the examination request sheet or as requested by the nuclear medicine physician. SPECT may occasionally be performed.

Indications

99mTc HMPAO-labeled WBCs can be used to image various pathologic inflammatory conditions. Labeled WBCs have proved useful in the evaluation of patients with fever of unknown origin and in the evaluation of osteomyelitis, inflammatory bowel disease, and prosthetic graft infections. In patients with inflammatory bowel disease, imaging should start at 1–3 hours after the injection, because normal intestinal excretion of 99mTc hexamethyl propylene amine oxine (HMPAO)-labeled WBCs becomes evident at about 4 hours.[1–3]

Principle

WBCs migrate into regions of inflammation or infection, particularly when the inflammation is acute. Radiolabeling techniques for WBCs include ^{111}In oxine, ^{111}In tropolone, and 99mTc hexamethyl propylene amine oxine (HMPAO). These labeling techniques adequately preserve WBC function to enable the radiolabeled cells to provide a pictorial representation of the inflammatory response.

Patient Preparation

None.

^{99m}Tc HMPAO-Labeled WBC Preparation

Equipment

The following items are required for the labeling process:

1. Two 60-ml syringes
2. 18 ml of ACD solution (solution A as per USP National Formulary)
3. 32 ml of hetastarch solution
4. 6–12 ml of 12.6% ACD/saline (ACD mixed with 0.9% NaCl, v/v)
5. 20 mCi (740 MBq) ^{99m}Tc HMPAO
6. Centrifuge
7. Sterile laminar flow hood
8. Test tube racks
9. Sterile test tubes
10. Sterile transfer pipettes

Labeling Procedure

The entire separation procedure is performed in a sterile laminar flow hood using aseptic technique.

1. Collect 80 ml of whole blood into two 60-ml syringes, each containing 8–9 ml of ACD anticoagulant. Gently invert to mix.
2. Add 8 ml of hetastarch to each of four 50-ml conical tubes.
3. Add equal amounts of blood to each of the 50-ml conical tubes, and gently mix the contents with a sterile pipette. (Caution: avoid the formation of foam or bubbles.)
4. Cap the tubes, and place them at a 45° angle in a rack for 25–35 minutes.
5. After sedimentation, remove the leukocyte-rich, platelet-rich plasma with a sterile pipette, and put it into two 50-ml conical tubes (see Fig. 8-1, step 1). Avoid including erythrocytes in the suspension.
6. Centrifuge at 600 rpm or 100 × gravity (*g*) for 5 minutes to remove erythrocytes (see Fig. 8-1, step 2). Take off the supernatant, and put it into a 50-ml conical tube, and spin it at 800 rpm (150 *g*) for 8 minutes (see Fig. 8-1, step 3). This produces a WBC pellet.
7. Take off the supernatant–platelet-rich plasma. Save 15 ml of supernatant in two conical tubes and discard the rest. Spin at 4,000 rpm (3,200 *g*) for 10 minutes to get platelet-poor plasma. Save the platelet-poor plasma in a sterile capped tube for final resuspension of WBCs in step 11, later.
8. Wash the WBC pellet with 6 ml of 12.6% ACD/saline solution, and mix it slowly. Do not introduce air bubbles. Centrifuge it at 600 rpm (100 *g*) for 5 minutes. Take off the supernatant, and discard it.
9. Slowly add approximately 20 mCi (740 MBq) of freshly prepared ^{99m}Tc HMPAO, and assay for initial radioactivity. *Note:* ^{99m}Tc HMPAO must be used within 30 minutes after preparation.
10. The tubes should be swirled gently. Incubate the WBCs for 20–25 minutes at room temperature, with occasional gentle swirling during incubation. Centrifuge at 800 rpm (150 *g*) for 8 minutes. Take off the supernatant, and discard it.
11. Add 5 ml of the platelet-poor plasma to the cell pellet, and mix it carefully to resuspend the WBCs. Assay the cell preparation for final radioactivity.
12. Calculate labeling efficiency:

$$\frac{\text{Final Dose Activity}}{\text{Initial Activity}} \times 100 = \% \text{ Labeled Cells}$$

13. Draw up 10 mCi (370 MBq) of the ^{99m}Tc HMPAO-labeled WBCs for reinjection.
14. Discard all waste into radioactive waste bins.

Notes: The labeled cells should be stored at room temperature. It is recommended that the labeled WBCs be used within 1 hour after preparation, if possible, and in no case more than 3 hours after preparation. Purified granulocytes, prepared as described for ^{111}In WBC (Procedure 8-1) can also be used for ^{99m}Tc HMPAO labeling.

Use the "Policy for Patient Identification During Radiolabeled Blood Product Procedures," as described in Appendix A-2, to ensure correct patient identification and to minimize risk of mismatch.

Instrument Specifications

Gamma camera:	Planar views—any large field-of-view system can be used. Whole-body views—dual-head rectangular field-of-view system. SPECT—single-, dual-, or triple-head SPECT system.
Collimator:	Low-energy, high-resolution collimator.
Energy setting:	140 keV, 20% energy window.
Analog formatter:	Spot views—8 × 10 film, 70-mm (9-on-1) format. Whole-body—11 × 14 film, 4-on-1 format.
Computer system:	Acquisition requirements—static (256 × 256 matrix), whole body (1,024 × 256 matrix), SPECT (128 × 128 matrix). Processing requirements—SPECT reconstruction software.

Imaging Procedure

Whole-Body Imaging

At 1–4 hours after injection, anterior and posterior whole-body images should be acquired on analog formatter and on computer (1,024 × 256 word mode matrix) at a scan speed of 5–10 cm/min (20–40 minute scan time).

Planar Local Views

At 1–4 hours after injection, spot views should be acquired for 5–10 minutes per view. For low-count regions, e.g., the wrist, increase imaging time to 10–15 minutes per view.

SPECT Imaging

When requested, SPECT studies should be acquired using the following acquisition variables:

Single-head system: 360° elliptical orbit, 128 × 128 word mode matrix, 60–64 views at 30–40 seconds per view. No zoom for 40-cm field-of-view system. Zoom of 1.2 for 50–60 cm field-of-view systems.

Dual- or triple-head system: 360° elliptical orbit, 128 × 128 word mode matrix, with a total of 120 views at 15–20 seconds per view. No zoom for 40-cm field-of-view system. Zoom of 1.2 for 50–60 cm field-of-view systems.

Computer Analysis

No analysis is required for planar or whole-body images. For SPECT studies, the following steps should be performed:

1. Apply uniformity and center-of-rotation correction to the data (on newer systems, this may be done automatically).
2. If possible, prefilter the planar data. Possible filters are Butterworth, order 10, cutoff at 0.4–0.5 Nyquist, and Hann filter with a cutoff at 0.8–0.9 Nyquist.
3. Reconstruct 1-pixel-thick transaxial slices. The back-projection filter may be a Ramp or Ramp-Butterworth with a cutoff at 0.6–0.8 Nyquist.

Information on Film

On each analog and computer film, ensure that the following information is recorded:

1. Patient name and clinic/hospital number
2. Type of scan and radiopharmaceutical preparation/dose used
3. Date and time after injection
4. Orientation of each image (e.g., anterior, posterior)

Table 8-2. Radiation Absorbed Dose Estimates in a 70-kg Adult From the Intravenous Injection of 10 mCi (370 MBq) ^{99m}Tc HMPAO-Labeled White Blood Cells

Tissue	Absorbed Radiation Dose	
	rad/10 mCi	mGy/370 MBq
Spleen	3.50	35.0
Liver	0.64	6.40
Upper large intestine	0.41	4.10
Lungs	0.39	3.90
Lower large intestine	0.30	3.00
Small intestine	0.26	2.60
Stomach	0.25	2.50
Urinary bladder	0.24	2.40
Bone surfaces	0.20	2.00
Ovaries	0.18	1.80
Red marrow	0.13	1.30
Blood	0.11	1.10
Thyroid	0.09	0.90
Breasts	0.09	0.90
Testes	0.08	0.80
Total body	0.15	1.50

Interpretation

Activity is normally seen in the liver, spleen, and bone marrow. Images obtained at more than 4 hours after injection may show intestinal excretion. Some activity will also be seen in the kidneys and urinary bladder. Bone marrow activity is faintly visible throughout the skeleton, with uptake less in the distal extremities than in the central marrow. The most intense uptake occurs in the spleen.[1,2]

Accumulation of [99mTc] HMPAO-labeled WBCs elsewhere in the body is abnormal. Inflammation and infection appear as focal regions of increased tracer uptake. There are no specific findings on a WBC scan that differentiate infection from nonseptic inflammation.

Additional Notes

Compared to [111In] WBCs, [99mTc] HMPAO-labeled WBCs provide lower patient radiation exposure and better image resolution. [99mTc] HMPAO-labeled WBCs have been especially useful in the evaluation of inflammatory bowel disease, where imaging at 1 and 3 hours after injection is recommended. [111In] WBCs may be preferable in the diagnosis of other forms of abdominal inflammations / infections or suspected chronic infections, including osteomyelitis.[4]

Radiation Dosimetry

The estimated absorbed doses in organs and tissues of an average subject from an IV injection of [99mTc] HMPAO WBCs are shown in Table 8-2.[1]

References

1. Brown ML, Hung JC, Vetter RJ, O'Connor MK, Chowdhury S, Forstrom LA. The radiation dosimetry and normal value study of [99mTc] HMPAO-labeled leukocytes. Invest Radiol 1994; 29: 443–447.
2. Peters AM, Roddie ME, Danpure HJ, et al. [99Tcm]-HMPAO labelled leucocytes: comparison with [111In]-tropolonate labelled granulocytes. Nucl Med Commun 1988; 9: 449–463.
3. Vorne M, Soini I, Lantto T, Paakkinen S. Technetium-99m HM-PAO-labeled leukocytes in detection of inflammatory lesions: comparison with gallium-67 citrate. J Nucl Med 1989; 30: 1332–1336.
4. Peters AM, Lavender JP. Imaging inflammation with radiolabelled white cells: [99mTc] HMPAO or [111In] (Editorial). Nucl Med Commun 1991; 12: 923–925.

^{67}Ga Gallium Scan

Summary Information

Radiopharmaceutical

    Adult doses: 5 mCi (185 MBq) ^{67}Ga citrate injected intravenously.

    Pediatric dose: Adjusted according to the patient's weight (see Appendix A-3).

Contraindications   None.

Dose/Scan Interval   Imaging commences 24 hours after the injection.

Views Obtained   Anterior and posterior whole-body images plus additional spot views or SPECT, according to the area of interest specified on the examination request sheet or as requested by the nuclear medicine physician.

Indications

^{67}Ga gallium citrate is useful in identifying sites of inflammation in conditions such as sarcoidosis, vertebral disk space infection, osteomyelitis, and pneumocystic pneumonia. Gallium imaging also serves as a screening procedure when occult abscess is suspected.[1]

Principle

After IV injection, ^{67}Ga gallium citrate rapidly binds to transferrin. It is distributed throughout the soft tissues and is concentrated particularly in the liver, spleen, bone, and bone marrow. It has significant renal and bowel excretion. In areas of intense inflammation, the uptake of ^{67}Ga is rapid. The mechanism of this localization is complex and thought to be due partly to the affinity of gallium (a transition metal) for ferritin, which mediates the incorporation of iron into bacteria.[2]

Patient Preparation

Laxatives or enemas given before scanning may help interpretation of abdominal activity by clearing normal gallium activity from the bowel. Instruct the patient in bowel cleansing if indicated by the nuclear medicine physician.

Instrument Specifications

    Gamma camera: Planar views—any large field-of-view system.

                             Whole-body views—dual-head large field-of-view rectangular system.

	SPECT—Single-, dual-, triple-head SPECT system.
Collimators:	Medium-energy collimator.
Energy setting:	93-keV, 184-keV, and 296-keV photopeaks, 20% energy windows.
Analog formatter:	Spot views—8 × 10 film, 70-mm (9-on-1) format.
	Whole-body views—10 × 14 film (4-on-1) format.
Computer system:	Acquisition requirements—static (256 × 256 matrix), whole body (1,024 × 256 matrix), SPECT (64 × 64 matrix).
	Processing requirements—SPECT reconstruction software.

Imaging Procedure

Whole-Body Imaging

At 24 hours after injection, place the patient supine on the imaging table, and acquire anterior and posterior whole-body images on analog formatter and on computer (1,024 × 256 word mode matrix) at a scan speed of 10 cm/min. Later views at 48 and 72 hours should be acquired at 5 cm/min.

Planar Imaging

At 24 hours after injection, anterior and posterior spot views of the abdomen should be acquired for 1,000 kct per view. Later views at 48 and 72 hours should be acquired for 1,000 kct per view or 5 minutes per view, whichever is shorter.

SPECT Imaging

When requested, SPECT studies should be acquired using the following acquisition variables:

Single-head system: 360° body-contouring orbit, 64 × 64 word mode matrix, 60–64 views at 30–40 seconds per view. No zoom for 40-cm field-of-view system. Zoom of 1.2 for 50–60-cm field-of-view systems.

Dual- or triple-head system: 360° body-contouring orbit, 64 × 64 word mode matrix, with a total of 120 views at 15 seconds per view. No zoom for 40-cm field-of-view system. Zoom of 1.2 for 50–60-cm field-of-view systems.

Computer Analysis

No analysis is required for planar images. For SPECT studies, the following steps should be performed:

1. Apply uniformity and center-of-rotation correction to the data (on newer systems, this may be done automatically).
2. If possible, prefilter the planar data. The suggested filter is Hann, with a cutoff at 0.8–0.9 Nyquist.
3. Reconstruct 1-pixel-thick transaxial slices. The back-projection filter may be a Ramp or Ramp-Butterworth with a cutoff at 0.6–0.8 Nyquist.

Information on Film

On each analog and computer film, ensure that the following information is recorded:

1. Patient name and clinic/hospital number
2. Type of scan and radiopharmaceutical dose injected
3. Date and time after injection
4. Orientation of each image (e.g., anterior, posterior)

Interpretation

Within the first 24 hours after administration, ^{67}Ga gallium citrate uptake can be seen in the kidneys and bladder, with occasional slight uptake in the large bowel. At 48–72 hours, renal excretion is nearly complete, and the kidneys may not be visualized. At 48 and 72 hours, significant bowel activity may be present (10–20% of the dose is excreted through the bowel) together with activity in the liver and spleen. With reduction in soft tissue activity, the uptake in bone is visible. Activity may also be visible in the breasts, particularly in patients with estrogen stimulation, and in the salivary and lacrimal glands, with faint uptake in the lungs. In children, activity may be seen in the epiphyseal plates and thymus.

Any area of focal uptake outside the areas described should be considered abnormal. Abnormal areas should be visualized better on later scans because of the reduction in soft tissue activity over time. If there is significant abdominal activity, bowel cleansing should be performed and the patient imaged again to determine the nature of the activity.

Radiation Dosimetry

The estimated absorbed radiation doses in a 70-kg adult from an IV injection of 5 mCi (185 MBq) ^{67}Ga gallium citrate are shown in Table 8-3.[3]

Table 8-3. Absorbed Radiation Dose Estimates in a 70-kg Adult
From Intravenous Administration of 5 mCi (185 MBq) ^{67}Ga Gallium Citrate

Tissue	Absorbed Radiation Doses	
	rad/5 mCi	mGy/185 MBq
Skeleton	2.20	22.0
Liver	2.30	23.0
Bone marrow	2.90	29.0
Spleen	2.65	26.5
Kidney	2.05	20.5
Ovaries	1.40	14.0
Testes	1.20	12.0
Stomach	1.10	11.0
Small intestine	1.80	18.0
Upper large intestine	2.80	28.0
Lower large intestine	4.50	45.0
Total body	1.30	13.0

References

1. Palmer EL, Scott JA, Strauss HW. "Practical Nuclear Medicine." W.B. Saunders Co., Philadelphia, 1992, pp 343–364.
2. Staab EV, McCartney WH. The role of gallium-67 in inflammatory disease. Semin Nucl Med 1978; 8: 219–234.
3. MIRD primer for absorbed dose calculations, Report No. 2, ed Loevinger R. Society of Nuclear Medicine, New York, 1988.

Bone Marrow Scan

Summary Information

Radiopharmaceutical

Adult dose: Standard scan—15 mCi (555 MBq) ^{99m}Tc sulfur colloid injected intravenously.

Combined ^{99m}Tc sulfur colloid/^{111}In-labeled WBC scan— 10 mCi (370 MBq) ^{99m}Tc sulfur colloid injected intravenously.

Pediatric dose: Adjusted according to the patient's weight (see Appendix A-3).

Contraindications None.

Dose/Scan Interval Imaging commences 45–60 minutes after the injection. *Note:* If blood pool activity persists, additional images may be required at 2–4 hours after the injection.

Views Obtained

Standard marrow scan: Anterior/posterior spot views of liver, anterior/posterior whole-body views.

Marrow/WBC scan: Spot view of the region of interest on the ^{111}In-labeled WBC scan.

Indications

The ^{99m}Tc sulfur colloid scan can be used to show the distribution of bone marrow throughout the body. Patients with chronic hemolytic anemia, stem-cell damage that is due to chemotherapy or radiotherapy, or with myeloproliferative disorders may show an altered distribution of marrow, with peripheral expansion. Some tumors, such as lymphomas and multiple myelomas, localize preferentially in bone marrow.[1] In these cases, the marrow scan may be more sensitive for their evaluation than the bone scan.

The marrow scan can also be used in conjunction with ^{111}In-labeled WBC scanning to help differentiate infection from a nonuniform marrow distribution pattern, because ^{111}In-labeled WBCs are normally seen in bone marrow.[2] This differentiation is most important in the femurs, hips, pelvis, shoulders, and humeri. Marrow scans may be helpful in the early diagnosis of avascular necrosis, as interruption of the blood supply to the femoral head decreases uptake in the marrow.

Principle

^{99m}Tc sulfur colloid localizes in the reticuloendothelial system and, thus, can be used to image the reticuloendothelial cells that populate the bone marrow. Hence, ^{99m}Tc sulfur colloid gives an indirect image of marrow function. It should be noted that in certain conditions and after radiotherapy, the distribution of the reticuloendothelial cells does not always reflect the distribution of the hematopoietic marrow. Absence of bone marrow uptake may be related to marrow depression following chemotherapy or radiotherapy or may be due to active necrosis in patients with aplastic anemia.

Patient Preparation

None.

Instrument Specifications

Gamma camera:	Any large field-of-view planar system can be used for spot views.
	A dual-head large field-of-view system is preferred for whole-body views.
Collimators:	Low-energy, high-resolution collimator.
	Medium-energy collimator is required if ^{111}In activity is present.
Energy setting:	140-keV peak, 15–20% energy window for ^{99m}Tc.
Analog formatter:	Spot views—70-mm (9-on-1) format, 8 × 10 film.
	Whole-body views—4-on-1 format, 10 × 14 film.
Additional items:	Velcro straps—40 cm long to prevent leg rotation.
	Lead shields—used to shield liver activity.
Computer system:	Minimum acquisition requirements—whole-body (1,024 × 256 matrix), static views (256 × 256 matrix).

Imaging Procedure

Standard Marrow Scan

1. At 45–60 minutes after injection, place the patient supine on the imaging table, and acquire anterior and posterior views of the liver (1,000 kct per view) on an analog formatter and on computer (256 × 256 matrix).
2. Place lead shields over the abdomen, both above and below the patient, as shown in Figure 8-3. This shields the gamma camera from activity in the liver and spleen and permits better visualization of the extremities.
3. Acquire anterior and posterior whole-body views at a scan speed of 10 cm/min on an analog formatter and on computer (1,024 × 256 matrix).
4. The nuclear medicine physician may request additional spot views of some regions of the body. If extramedullary hematopoiesis is suspected, acquire additional anterior and posterior spot views of the abdomen without a lead shield.

Marrow/White Blood Cell Scan

1. After completion of the ^{111}In-labeled WBC scan, the patient should be injected with 10 mCi (370 MBq) ^{99m}Tc sulfur colloid, and imaging should be started 45–60 minutes later.
2. Spot views of the abnormal regions seen on the ^{111}In-labeled WBC scan and corresponding contralateral regions should be acquired for 10 minutes per view on an analog formatter and on computer (256 × 256 matrix).

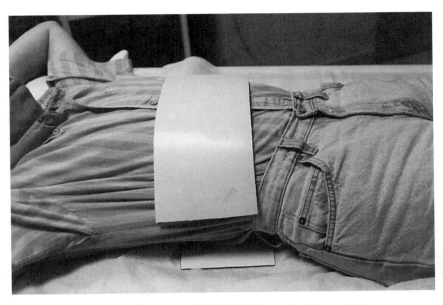

Figure 8-3. Placement of lead shields to reduce liver activity.

Computer Analysis

None.

Information on Film

On each analog or computer film, ensure that the following information is recorded:

1. Patient name and clinic/hospital number
2. Date and time of each image after injection
3. Type of scan and radiopharmaceutical dose administered
4. Orientation of each image (e.g., anterior, posterior)

Interpretation

Standard Scan

Normally 80–85% of the ^{99m}Tc sulfur colloid localizes in the liver, 10–15% in the spleen, and 1–5% in the bone marrow. A normal scan shows prominent uptake in the liver and spleen and uptake in the spine, pelvis, and sternum as well as in the proximal one-third of the femur and humerus. A marrow scan with absence of uptake in bone marrow (aplastic anemia), but with uptake in the liver and spleen, may be seen in patients with aplastic anemia or marrow replacement such as myelofibrosis. An abnormal scan with increased marrow activity as seen in early leukemia, chronic anemia, and polycythemia vera will show liver and spleen uptake and uptake in the distal long bones that is due to marrow expansion.

Marrow/White Blood Cell Scan

After joint replacement, bone surgery, or bone injury, many patients have uneven distribution of marrow. Hence, it may be difficult to ascertain whether ^{111}In-labeled WBC activity

Table 8-4. Absorbed Radiation Dose Estimates in a 70-kg Adult From the Intravenous Administration of 15 mCi (555 MBq) ^{99m}Tc Sulfur Colloid

Tissue	Absorbed Radiation Dose	
	rad/15 mCi	mGy/555 MBq
Liver	5.06	50.6
Spleen	3.19	31.9
Bone marrow	0.42	4.2
Testes	0.02	0.2
Ovaries	0.09	0.9
Total body	0.29	2.9

in a given region represents normal marrow or infection. Because ^{99m}Tc sulfur colloid localizes in marrow with little or no uptake in areas of infection or inflammation, a comparison of the colloid and WBC scans permits infection or inflammation to be differentiated from an abnormal marrow distribution.

Additional Notes

None.

Radiation Dosimetry

The estimated absorbed doses in organs and tissues of an average subject (70 kg) from an IV injection of 15 mCi (555 MBq) ^{99m}Tc sulfur colloid are shown in Table 8-4.[3]

References

1. Palmer EL, Scott JA, Strauss HW. "Practical Nuclear Medicine," W.B. Saunders Co., Philadelphia, 1992.
2. Schembri GP, Forstrom LA, Mullan BP, Hauser MF. The value of bone marrow scanning in the assessment of possible orthopedic infections (abstract). J Nucl Med 1992; 33: 840.
3. MIRD dose estimate report no. 3. Summary of current radiation dose estimates to humans with various liver conditions from technetium Tc-99m sulfur colloid. J Nucl Med 1975; 16: 108A–108B.

Bone Scan

Radiopharmaceutical

Adult dose: 20 mCi (740 MBq) ^{99m}Tc HDP (hydroxymethylene diphosphonate) or 20 mCi (740 MBq) ^{99m}Tc MDP (methylene diphosphonate) injected intravenously.

Pediatric dose: Adjusted according to the patient's weight (see Appendix A-3). *Note:* If upper extremity imaging is required, ensure that the injection is given in the contralateral normal arm.

Contraindications   None.

Dose/Scan Interval

Flow study: Imaging commences immediately after the injection.

Whole-body, spot views, SPECT: Imaging commences about 3 hours after the injection. A longer interval (4–5 hours) may be required for extremity imaging.

Views Obtained   The number of views depends on the indications for the examination.

Indications

In general, bone scintigraphy is considered a survey technique to evaluate patients with malignancy, diffuse musculoskeletal symptoms, abnormal laboratory results, and hereditary or metabolic disorders. The other major application is the evaluation of patients with suspected localized disease such as with focal pain or trauma or the assessment of abnormalities detected with other imaging modalities. Three-phase bone scintigraphy is helpful in areas of suspected trauma and musculoskeletal sepsis. The flow and early blood pool phases are positive in very active processes and may help in determining whether the abnormalities are recent.

Principle

It is not clear how ^{99m}Tc-labeled diphosphonates are incorporated into bone at the molecular level; however, it appears that regional blood flow, osteoblastic activity, and extraction efficiency are the major factors that influence uptake. In areas of increased osteogenic activity, active crystals of hydroxyapatite with large surface areas appear to be the most suitable sites for chemisorption of the diphosphonate ligands.[1]

Patient Preparation

The patient should drink 2–3 glasses of water between the time of injection and the scan. Have the patient void before scanning, and remove all metal objects from areas to be scanned.

Instrument Specifications

Gamma camera:	Planar views or flow study—any large field-of-view system can be used. Whole-body—dual-head large field-of-view system is preferred; any large field-of-view system can be used. Body SPECT—single-, dual-, or triple-head system with elliptical or body-contouring orbit.
Collimator:	Low-energy all-purpose collimator for flow studies and spot views of hands or feet. Pinhole collimator for local views of the hips. Low-energy high-resolution collimator for SPECT, whole-body, and spot views of body.
Energy setting:	140 keV, 15–20% energy window
Analog formatter:	8 × 10 film, 70-mm (9-on-1) format for spot views. 8 × 10 or 11 × 14 film for whole-body images.
Additional items:	Velcro strap— 40 cm long to prevent leg rotation. Sandbag—for restraint of feet or hands during spot views.
Computer system:	Minimum acquisition requirements—whole body (1,024 × 256 matrix), static (256 × 256 matrix), dynamic (64 × 64 matrix), SPECT (128 × 128 matrix). Processing requirements— SPECT reconstruction software.

Imaging Procedure

Flow Study/Immediate Views

1. Position the patient supine on the imaging table, and position the gamma camera so that the appropriate region of the body is in the field of view.
2. For flow phase study of the upper limbs, do not use a tourniquet. If a tourniquet is used for IV needle placement, release it and wait 5 minutes before injecting the ^{99m}Tc HDP or ^{99m}Tc MDP bolus.
3. When activity begins to appear in the field of view, acquire a dynamic study on analog formatter (9 frames at 3 seconds per frame for the trunk and 5 seconds per frame for the extremities) and on computer (64 × 64 word mode matrix, 30 frames at 3 seconds per frame). Immediate views should be acquired on an analog formatter for 200–1,500 kct per view (about 200 kct for hands and wrists, 600 kct for knees, and 1,000–1,500 kct for abdominal and thoracic regions). All immediate views should be acquired on computer (256 × 256 matrix, 2 minutes per view).

Whole-Body Views

1. At 3 hours after injection, position the patient supine on the whole-body imaging table. Adjust the upper detector to minimize the distance between the patient and collimator (Fig. 8-4). If the patient has discomfort lying on the back, place a pillow under the knees to reduce the discomfort. Place a Velcro strap around the feet to prevent rotation of the legs during acquisition (Fig. 8-5).
2. Acquire a 10-second static view over the chest to determine the appropriate intensity setting for the analog formatter. Acquire anterior and posterior whole-body images at a scan speed of 10 cm/min on an analog formatter and on computer (1,024 × 256 matrix).

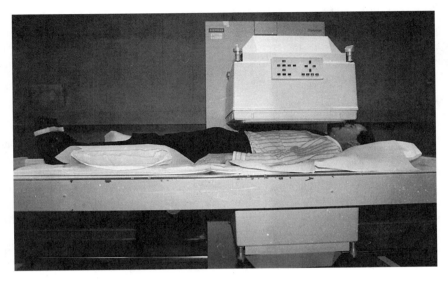

Figure 8-4. Patient setup for whole-body scan acquisition. Note close proximity of upper detector to patient and use of pillow under knees.

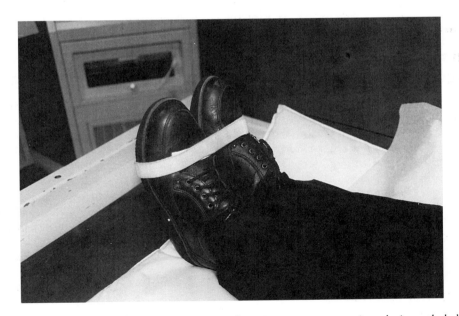

Figure 8-5. Foot strap around shoes to prevent leg movement or rotation during whole-body acquisition.

3. After the detector head passes the abdomen, reposition its height for proximity to the lower extremities.

Spot Views—Trunk

The number of counts per image depends on the region being imaged; however, as a general rule, for a large field-of-view system, 1,000 kct should be acquired over the thoracic spine, with other images being acquired for a similar time per image. All images should be acquired on an analog formatter and on computer (256 × 256 matrix).

Spot Views—Extremities

1. Images of the hands, wrists, feet, and ankles should be acquired for 400–800 kct per view using a low-energy, all-purpose collimator.[2] Images should be acquired on an analog formatter and on computer (256 × 256 matrix). The correct patient setup for extremity imaging is shown in Figures 8-6 and 8-7. Note the use of small sandbags to assist in keeping the extremities still during the scan period (Figs. 8-6B and 8-7). For dorsal views of the hands, the hands should be placed on a tabletop or flat surface and the gamma camera should be oriented to face down. The collimator face can be lowered to slightly touch the hands between the collimator and tabletop.
2. If early phase images were acquired, then at a minimum, acquire spot views of these regions for comparison.

Pinhole Views—Hip

Pinhole images of the hip should be acquired using a pinhole collimator with a 6-mm aperture (Fig. 8-8). Images should be acquired for 200–250 kct for the abnormal hip, with the same time per image being used for the contralateral hip. Images should be acquired on an analog formatter and on computer (256 × 256 matrix).

SPECT Study

SPECT acquisition variables will depend on the number of detector heads on the system.

1. For a single-head system, acquire 60–64 views over 360° into a 128 × 128 word mode matrix at 30–40 seconds per view using a high-resolution collimator and appropriate body contouring to minimize patient-to-collimator distance.
   Note: For studies of the lumbar or thoracic spine only, acquire 60–64 views over 180° from 90° right lateral to posterior to 90° left lateral. If possible, the patient should be prone on the imaging table.
2. For a dual-head or triple-head system, acquire as in step 1, with the time per frame decreased to 20 seconds per view. *Note:* The time per frame should be increased to 30–40 seconds for large patients (men greater than 100 kg, women greater than 80 kg) or if an ultrahigh-resolution collimator is used (collimator sensitivity less than 150 ct/min per μCi).
3. Check that all loose clothing and straps are tucked away, because they may interfere with a body-contouring orbit.

Computer Analysis

No analysis is required for whole-body or spot views. For SPECT studies, the following steps should be performed:

1. Apply uniformity and center-of-rotation correction to the data (on newer systems, this may be done automatically).
2. If possible, prefilter the planar data. A suggested filter is a Butterworth, order 10–12, cutoff at 0.4–0.5 Nyquist. Increase the cutoff frequency for dual- or triple-head systems.

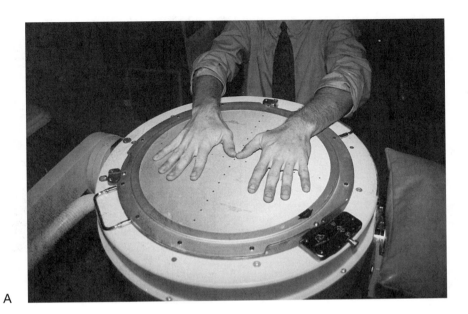

A

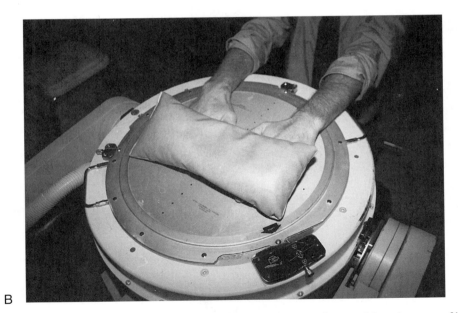

B

Figure 8-6. (A) Patient setup for scan of hands and wrists. (B) Sandbag positioned on top of hands to reduce motion artifacts.

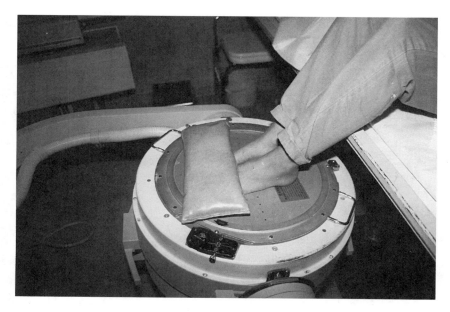

Figure 8-7. Patient setup for scan of feet (plantar view).

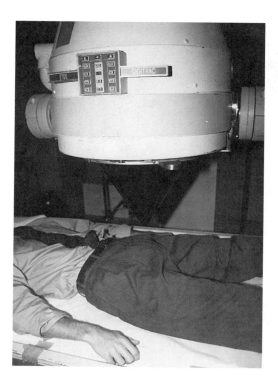

Figure 8-8. Patient and gamma camera setup for pinhole view of the left hip.

3. Reconstruct 1-pixel-thick transaxial slices. The back-projection filter may be a Ramp or Ramp-Butterworth with a cutoff at 0.6–0.8 Nyquist.

Information on Film

On each analog and computer film, ensure that the following information is recorded:

1. Patient name and clinic/hospital number
2. Date, type of scan, and radiopharmaceutical dose administered
3. Time of each image after injection
4. Orientation of each image (e.g., anterior, posterior)

Interpretation

Normal skeletal structures are usually visualized clearly, and activity is seen in the kidneys and bladder. Most skeletal abnormalities are focal areas of increased uptake. Focal cold areas may reflect absence of bone blood supply or bone destruction/resection.

Additional Notes

None.

Radiation Dosimetry

The estimated absorbed doses in organs and tissues of an average subject (70 kg) from an IV injection of 20 mCi (740 MBq) ^{99m}Tc MDP or ^{99m}Tc HDP are shown in Table 8-5.[3,4] *Note:* Dosimetry of ^{99m}Tc HDP is similar to that of ^{99m}Tc MDP.

Table 8-5. Absorbed Radiation Dose Estimates in a 70-kg Adult Following the Intravenous Administration of 20 mCi (740 MBq) ^{99m}Tc-HDP or ^{99m}Tc-MDP

Tissue	Absorbed Radiation Doses (^{99m}Tc-HDP or ^{99m}Tc-MDP)	
	rad/20 mCi	mGy/740 MBq
Bone total	0.70	7.0
Red marrow	0.56–0.96	5.6–9.6
Kidneys	0.44–0.80	4.4–8.0
Liver	0.06	0.6
Bladder wall		
2-hr void	2.60	26.0
4.8-hr void	6.20	62.0
Ovaries		
2-hr void	0.24	2.4
4.8-hr void	0.34	3.4
Testes		
2-hr void	0.16	1.6
4.8-hr void	0.22	2.2
Total body	0.13–0.25	1.3–2.5

References

1. Frances MD, Tofe AJ, Benedic JJ. Imaging the skeletal system. In "Radiopharmaceuticals II," ed Sorenson JA. Society of Nuclear Medicine, New York, 1974, pp 603–614.
2. O'Connor MK, Brown ML, Hung JC, Hayostek RJ. The art of bone scintigraphy—technical aspects. J Nucl Med 1991; 32: 2332–2341.
3. Technetium ^{99m}Tc Medronate Kit. Squibb Diagnostics. Princeton, NJ. Last revision January 1992.
4. Kit for the preparation of Technetium ^{99m}Tc Oxidronate, product # 099. Mallinckrodt, Inc,. St. Louis. Last revision June 1991.

Joint Scan

Summary Information

Radiopharmaceutical
   Adult dose: 20 mCi (740 MBq) [99mTc] pertechnetate injected intravenously.
  Pediatric dose: Adjusted according to the patient's weight (see Appendix A-3).

Contraindications None.

Dose/Scan Interval Imaging can commence immediately after the injection.

Views Obtained The following views are acquired:
   1. Anterior and posterior whole-body views
   2. Lateral views of the knees and ankles
   3. Plantar views of the feet
   4. Palmar views of the hands and wrists

Indications

[99mTc] pertechnetate can be used to document the severity and extent of inflammatory joint disease (synovitis). In some joints, synovitis can readily be ascertained by clinical examination. In certain situations, however, [99mTc] pertechnetate imaging is a useful adjunctive procedure in determining the severity and extent of the inflammation.[1]

Principle

Synovitis is characterized by increased vascular capacity, increased blood flow, and interstitial edema. Shortly after injection of [99mTc] pertechnetate, about 90% of the radiopharmaceutical becomes bound to serum albumin. This complex appears at the site of the inflamed joint because of the increased blood flow and extravasation into thickened and edematous interstitium. Although some uptake is present in periarticular bone, pertechnetate concentrates primarily in the inflamed synovium.[2]

Patient Preparation

   Adult dose: Orally administer 200 mg of $KClO_4$ (potassium perchlorate) 30 minutes before the injection, to block [99mTc] uptake in the thyroid gland.
  Pediatric dose: Oral $KClO_4$ dose-adjusted based on the patient's weight.

Instrument Specifications

   Gamma camera: Any large field-of-view planar system can be used for spot views.

455

	A dual-head large field-of-view system is preferred for whole-body views.
Collimators:	Low-energy, all-purpose collimator for views of the hands, wrists, or feet.
	Low-energy, high-resolution collimator for all other joints and for whole-body views.
Energy setting:	140-keV peak, 15–20% energy window for ^{99m}Tc.
Analog formatter:	Spot views—70-mm (9-on-1) format, 8 × 10 film.
	Whole-body views— 4-on-1 format, 10 × 14 film.
Additional items:	Velcro strap—40 cm long to prevent rotation of legs.
	Sandbag—for restraining the feet or hands during spot views.
Computer system:	Minimum acquisition requirements—static (256 × 256 matrix), whole body (1,024 × 256 matrix).
	Processing requirements—none.

Imaging Procedure

1. Immediately after the injection, position the patient supine on the imaging table, and acquire anterior and posterior whole-body views at a scan speed of 10 cm/min on an analog formatter and on computer (1,024 × 256 matrix).
2. For the left knee, position the patient on the patient's right side with the knees bent and the left knee forward of the right, as shown in Figure 8-9.
3. Acquire a left lateral view of the knees for 500 kct on an analog formatter and on computer (256 × 256 matrix). Note the acquisition time. Acquire a right lateral view and all other views for the same time.
4. Lateral views of the ankles should be acquired with the patient in the same position as for the lateral views of the knees.
5. Plantar views of the feet and palmar views of the hands and wrists should be acquired as shown in Figures 8-6 and 8-7. Note the use of a small sandbag to assist in keeping the extremities immobile during the scan period.

Computer Analysis

None.

Information on Film

On each analog or computer film, ensure that the following information is recorded:

1. Patient name and clinic/hospital number
2. Type of scan and radiopharmaceutical dose administered
3. Date and time after injection
4. Orientation of each image (e.g., anterior, posterior)

Interpretation

Normally, joint uptake of ^{99m}Tc is symmetric, diffuse, and homogeneous, and does not exceed the background activity in the soft tissue. In the shoulder, the dominant side may show slight increased uptake of tracer. Focal areas of increased activity and asymmetry between comparable joints are abnormal. Joints may be scintigraphically positive before radiographic or clinical evidence of synovitis appears.

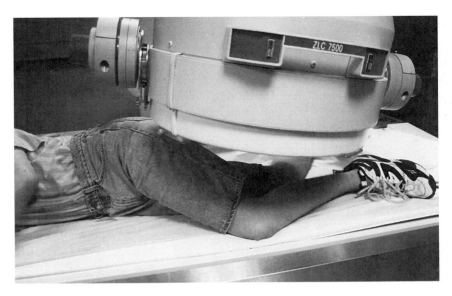

Figure 8-9. Patient setup for left lateral view of the knees. Detector has been moved away from the patient so that the orientation of the knees can be seen.

Additional Notes

None.

Radiation Dosimetry

The estimated absorbed doses in organs and tissues of an average subject (70 kg) from an IV injection of 20 mCi (740 MBq) ^{99m}Tc sodium pertechnetate are shown in Table 8-6.[3]

Table 8-6. Absorbed Radiation Dose Estimates in a 70-kg Adult From the Intravenous Administration of 20 mCi (740 MBq) ^{99m}Tc Sodium Pertechnetate

	Radiation Absorbed Dose	
Tissue	rad/20 mCi	mGy/740 MBq
Bladder wall	1.06	10.6
Stomach wall	5.00	50.0
Upper large intestinal wall	1.37	13.7
Lower large intestinal wall	1.22	12.2
Red marrow	0.38	3.8
Testes	0.18	1.8
Ovaries	0.44	4.4
Thyroid	2.60	26.0
Brain	0.28	2.8
Total body	0.28	2.8

References

1. Greyson ND. Radionuclide bone and joint imaging in rheumatology. Bull Rheum Dis 1979–1980; 30: 1034–1038.
2. Rosenspire KL, Blau M, Kennedy AC, et al. Assessment and interpretation of radiopharmaceutical joint imaging in an animal model of arthritis. Arthritis Rheum 1981; 24: 711–716.
3. MIRD dose estimate report no. 8. Summary of current radiation dose estimates to normal humans from ^{99m}Tc as sodium pertechnetate. J Nucl Med 1976; 17: 74–77.

9

Respiratory System

Douglas A. Collins
Mary F. Hauser

^{133}Xe Lung Ventilation Scan

Summary Information

Radiopharmaceutical
  Adult dose: 15–30 mCi (555–1,110 MBq) ^{133}Xe gas inhalation.
  Pediatric dose: Adjusted according to the patient's weight (see Appendix A-3).

Contraindications None.

Dose/Scan Interval Imaging commences immediately after inhalation of the xenon gas. With ^{133}Xe, the ventilation study must precede the ^{99m}Tc perfusion scan.

Views Obtained Posterior views for first breath, equilibrium, and washout. If possible, left posterior oblique (LPO) and right posterior oblique (RPO) views should be obtained between the first breath and equilibrium images and again after the washout phase.

Indications

Lung ventilation scans are used in conjunction with lung perfusion scans in the differential diagnosis of pulmonary embolism versus chronic obstructive pulmonary disease (COPD) or other lung disorders.

Principle

Pulmonary embolism usually has little or no effect on lung ventilation. In the absence of other disease, functional images of lung ventilation with xenon gas typically show no abnormality. Thus, the ventilation/perfusion (V/Q) scan shows pulmonary emboli as segmental zones of reduced or absent pulmonary perfusion associated with normal ventilation. The gas used for a ventilation study must diffuse easily, must not be absorbed significantly by the lungs, and must have a low density. Isotopes of xenon, ^{133}Xe, and ^{127}Xe meet these criteria. This gas has adequate imaging properties, and typically, less than 15% of it is absorbed by the body.

Patient Preparation

The procedure should be explained fully to the patient before starting the scan. This test requires the cooperation of the patient.

461

Instrument Specifications

Gamma camera:	Any large field-of-view system can be used. A ring gantry will permit easy acquisition of LPO and RPO views, as will acquisition in an upright position.
Collimators:	Low-energy all-purpose collimator for ^{133}Xe.
Energy setting:	20% energy window around the 80-keV photopeak.
Analog formatter:	8×10 film, 70-mm (9-on-1) format.
Additional items:	Closed ventilation machine with output to a xenon trap or to a room exhaust system. The room should have a negative pressure relative to connecting rooms or corridors. This is obtained by setting the air flow in the room exhaust system higher than that in the room supply system. This will permit removal of any xenon released accidentally.
Computer system:	Acquisition requirements—static (256×256 matrix). Processing requirements—region of interest (ROI) analysis if quantitation is required.

Imaging Procedure

Please remember that patients will be frightened when they are placed on a closed breathing system.

1. The operator should be thoroughly familiar with the operation of the closed ventilation system.
2. On the ventilation machine, check the absorbers. White soda-lime is normally used to absorb carbon dioxide from the patient's breath. This often needs to be replaced after each study. Moisture is removed from the system with anhydrous $CaSO_4$, which usually is supplied in the form of blue pellets. These pellets should be replaced when their color changes from blue to pink.
3. Attach the oxygen tank to the machine, and adjust the oxygen regulator to give the recommended pressure and flow rate (6–8 liters/min). Fill the rebreathing reservoir in the ventilation machine with oxygen.
4. Check that the outflow from the ventilation machine is connected to either a xenon trap or a room exhaust system.
5. Position the patient supine on the imaging table, with the gamma camera posteriorly. Alternatively, if the patient is able to cooperate, position the patient upright on a stool, with the gamma camera posteriorly. Use a transmission source (^{57}Co sheet source or ^{133}Xe vial) to determine the exact location of the lung fields. If necessary, place a lead apron over the patient's chest to shield the breathing hose from the field of view.
6. With the system set so that the patient can breath room air (bypassing the system), attach the face mask, as shown in Figures 9-1 and 9-2. Check that the fit is tight to avoid leakage of xenon gas into the room.
7. Do a dry run with no radioactive xenon to ensure that the patient comprehends what it is like to breath on a closed breathing system and can comply with your instructions.
8. *First breath phase:*
   a. With the gamma camera positioned posteriorly, set up the computer acquisition (dynamic acquisition, 256×256 matrix, 20 images at 5 seconds per image). Set the analog formatter to acquire 300–400-kct first breath image (9-on-1 format). With the

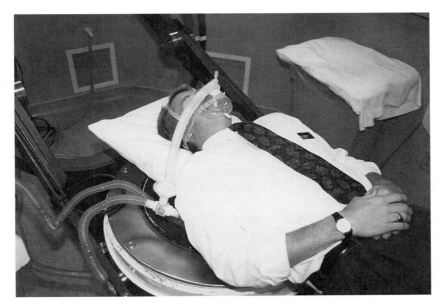

Figure 9-1. Setup for ^{133}Xe lung ventilation scan. Detector is positioned posteriorly.

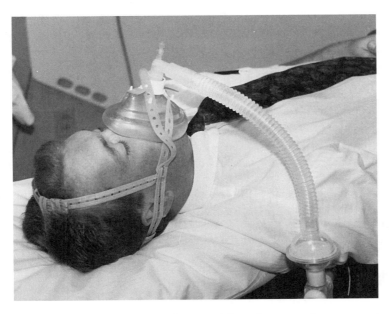

Figure 9-2. Position of face mask. Check for a good fit with no gaps between mask and face.

injection of ^{133}Xe, start the computer and analog formatter. It may be necessary to manually stop acquisition on both the analog formatter and computer, if the patient cannot hold first breath for a time long enough to acquire 300 kct.

b. Set up the ventilation machine for the first breath phase. Inject xenon gas into the system (usually into the tubing close to the face mask to maximize uptake into the lungs) as the patient begins to take a deep breath.

c. The patient should hold his or her breath for as long as possible and should signal the technologist when he or she can no longer hold it. At the patient's signal or at 300 kct (whichever comes first), stop the first breath acquisition and proceed to the equilibrium phase.

9. *Equilibrium phase:* After the first breath, when the patient resumes normal breathing, adjust the system so that the patient is breathing on a closed system. Take an "equilibrium" image after about 1–2 minutes of normal breathing. The equilibrium image should be acquired on computer and analog formatter for 300–400 kct. *Note:* If the detector head is mounted on a ring gantry or if the patient is sitting, acquire right and left posterior oblique views immediately after the first breath. Oblique views should be acquired on computer and analog formatter for up to 200 kct per view. After the oblique views, reposition the gamma camera and acquire a posterior view, as described.

10. *Washout phase:*

a. For washout images, set the analog formatter to acquire five 1-minute images in a 9-on-1 format. On the computer, set up a dynamic acquisition (64 × 64 matrix, 20 images at 15 seconds per image).

b. After the equilibrium image, switch the machine to the washout mode and start the computer and analog formatter. In this mode, the patient should be breathing in room air but be breathing out through the machine.

c. After washout is complete, remove the patient from the system. Follow the manufacturer's instructions for purging the system of any radioactive gas that remains in it.

Note: Monitor the trap effluent at regular intervals to ensure that the trap is functioning correctly and that no xenon is being released into the room.

Computer Analysis

No analysis of the computer data is required for conventional lung ventilation scans; however, these images may serve as the primary images if the analog images are unsatisfactory. Quantitative analysis of regional uptake in the lungs may be helpful in certain patients (e.g., lung transplant patients or patients undergoing resection for lung carcinoma). For these patients, select the first breath study, and sum the images that span the first breath time period. Draw rectangular ROIs around each lung (ROIs of the same size must be used for each lung), and subdivide these ROIs into three regions: apical, middle, and basal lung regions. Compute the ratio of left-to-right lung activity, as shown in Figure 9-3. Obtain a hard copy of the ROIs and results.

Information on Film

On each analog and computer film, ensure that the following information is recorded:

1. Patient name and clinic/hospital number
2. Date, type of scan, and radiopharmaceutical

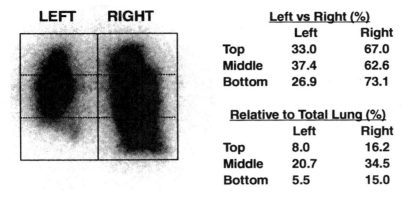

Figure 9-3. Example of quantitative analysis of regional ^{133}Xe lung ventilation.

3. Time of each image after injection
4. Orientation and phase (e.g., anterior/posterior, washout, first breath) of each image

Interpretation

In normal subjects, the distribution of the xenon should be uniform throughout both lungs with a rapid washout, with the lungs being cleared by 3 minutes (half-time of less than 1 minute). Lung ventilation scanning is an integral part of the scanning procedure for detecting pulmonary embolism. This is because several common causes of ventilatory abnormalities secondarily cause regional perfusion abnormalities. These include asthma, chronic bronchitis, COPD, bulla, and old inflammatory processes such as tuberculosis. Pulmonary emboli are the most common cause of an abnormal lung perfusion scan with a normal lung ventilation scan. The lung ventilation scan adds considerable specificity to lung perfusion scanning. Ventilation scanning does not resolve all the difficulties with lung perfusion scanning, because pulmonary edema, interstitial lung disease, and lymphatic obstruction may affect lung perfusion without affecting lung ventilation. A chest radiograph is necessary in evaluating these other causes of positive findings on lung perfusion scans and in excluding other causes of pleuritic chest pain (i.e., pneumothorax and pneumonic infiltrates).[1]

See the interpretative criteria in Procedure 9-4, "^{99m}Tc Macroaggregated Albumin Lung Perfusion Scan."

Additional Notes

The patient should be constantly reassured that all is routine and going well; this will give the patient more confidence and lead to a more successful study.

Radiation Dosimetry

The estimated radiation doses in organs and tissue of an average subject (70 kg) from inhalation of 20 mCi (740 MBq) of gaseous ^{133}Xe are shown in Table 9-1.[2]

Note: The data assume 5 minutes of rebreathing, activity delivered into a spirometer with a 10-liter capacity.

Table 9-1. Absorbed Radiation Dose Estimates in a 70-kg Adult
After Inhalation of 20 mCi (740 MBq) [133]Xe

Tissue	Absorbed Radiation Dose	
	rad/20 mCi	mGy/740 MBq
Lungs	0.14	1.4
Red marrow	0.02	0.2
Ovaries	0.02	0.2
Testes	0.02	0.2
Brain	0.001	0.01
Total body	0.002	0.02

References

1. Palmer EL, Scott JA, Strauss HW. In "Practical Nuclear Medicine." W.B. Saunders Co., Philadelphia, 1992, pp 185–240.
2. Lonnyer R et al., eds. MIRD primer for absorbed dose calculations. Society of Nuclear Medicine, New York, 1988.

^{99m}Tc DTPA Lung Aerosol Scan

Summary Information

Radiopharmaceutical

Adult dose: 0.5–1.0 mCi (18.5–37 MBq) ^{99m}Tc-DTPA when performed before the perfusion study.

Pediatric dose: Adjusted according to the patient's weight (see Appendix A-3).

Note: The ratio of ^{99m}Tc macroaggregated albumin (MAA) to ^{99m}Tc DTPA should be 5:1 or greater to ensure adequate image quality in the perfusion study.[1]

Contraindications None.

Dose/Scan Interval Imaging commences immediately after inhalation of the ^{99m}Tc DTPA aerosol.

Views Obtained Obtain eight views of the lungs: posterior, anterior, right and left lateral, right and left anterior oblique, and right and left posterior oblique.

Indications

Lung aerosol scans are used in conjunction with lung perfusion scans in the differential diagnosis of pulmonary embolism versus COPD or other lung disorders. Aerosol imaging can also be used to assess changes in alveolar-capillary permeability, which may be altered in patients with interstitial lung disease or inflammation of the lungs.[2,3]

Principle

Pulmonary embolism usually has little or no effect on lung ventilation. In the absence of other disease, functional images of lung ventilation using a radioactive gas or aerosol typically show no abnormality. Thus, the V/Q scan shows pulmonary emboli as segmental zones of reduced or absent pulmonary perfusion associated with normal ventilation. The radioaerosol particles used for a ventilation study must be uniform in size and less than 2 μm in diameter to travel distally into the alveoli.[4] After inhalation, ^{99m}Tc DTPA (diethylenetriamine pentaacetic acid) aerosol particles are deposited in the lungs by sedimentation and gravitational impaction.[5] They then diffuse across the alveolar capillary membrane with a half-time of more than 1 hour in normal subjects, although this clearance is greatly accelerated in subjects who smoke (half-time about 30–40 minutes).[6]

Patient Preparation

Immediately before the study, ask the patient to drink a small glass of water. This helps to clear excess saliva from the mouth, and it reduces the oral accumulation of ^{99m}Tc DTPA.

The procedure should be fully explained to the patient before starting the test. This test requires the cooperation of the patient. Rehearse the breathing procedure with the patient to ensure optimal patient cooperation. Ensure that the mouthpiece is positioned correctly (flange between the teeth and gums) and that the nose clip is in place, as shown in Figure 9-4.

Instrument Specifications

Gamma camera:	Any large field-of-view system can be used.
Collimators:	Low-energy, all-purpose collimator.
Energy setting:	20% energy window around the 140-keV photopeak.
Analog formatter:	8 × 10 film, 70-mm (9-on-1) format.
Additional items:	Aerosol generator (nebulizer) and oxygen supply. Filter system to trap expired radioactivity in the exhaled air.
Computer system:	Acquisition requirements—static (256 × 256 matrix). Processing requirements—ROI analysis if lung quantitation is required.

Imaging Procedure

1. Before commencing, the technologist should be thoroughly familiar with the operation of the radioaerosol delivery unit.
2. Position the patient supine on the imaging table, with the detector positioned posteriorly.
3. Slowly introduce 40 mCi (1,480 MBq) ^{99m}Tc DTPA in a volume of 3–4 ml into the nebulizer.

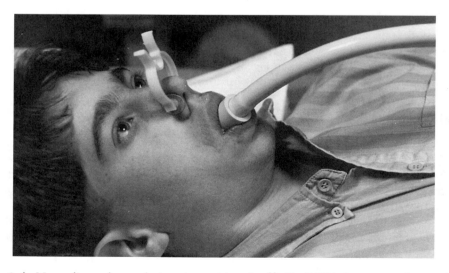

Figure 9-4. Nose clip and mouthpiece in position for ^{99m}Tc DTPA lung aerosol scan. Ensure mouthpiece is positioned between the gums and teeth to minimize leakage.

4. Fit the patient with the mouthpiece and nose clamp (see Fig. 9-4), and instruct him or her to breathe at a normal rate.
5. Attach the oxygen supply to the aerosol delivery system, and adjust the oxygen regulator to give a flow rate of at least 12 liters/min.
6. The patient should breathe on the system for 2–3 minutes or until the count rate has reached about 2–3 kct per second.
7. Turn off the oxygen flow to the nebulizer.
8. Remove the nose clip and mouthpiece, and wipe off any saliva that may be around the patient's mouth. The patient should also expel any saliva into a disposable tissue to reduce gastric accumulation of the ^{99m}Tc DTPA.
9. Dispose of the contaminated tissue, nebulizer, tubing, and mouthpiece in a plastic bag and place it in the radioactive waste bin.
10. On the analog formatter and computer (256×256 word mode matrix), acquire images for 400 kct per image. The following images should be acquired: posterior, anterior, right and left lateral, right and left anterior oblique, and right and left posterior oblique.

Computer Analysis

No analysis is required for conventional lung ventilation images. Quantitative analysis of regional uptake in the lungs may be helpful in certain patients (e.g., lung transplant patients or patients undergoing resection for lung carcinoma). For these patients, select the anterior and posterior views. Draw rectangular ROIs around each lung (ROIs of the same size must be used for each lung), and subdivide these ROIs into three regions: apical, middle, and basal lung regions. Calculate the geometric mean of counts for each lung region. For example, the geometric mean for the right basal region = (anterior right basal region $\times$ posterior right basal region)$^{0.5}$. Compute the ratio of left-to-right lung activity, as shown in Figure 9-3. Obtain hard copy of the ROIs and results.

Information on Film

On each analog and computer film, ensure that the following information is recorded:

1. Patient name and clinic/hospital number
2. Date, type of scan, and radiopharmaceutical
3. Orientation (e.g., anterior/posterior) of each image

Interpretation

Aerosol imaging often shows central airway deposition, even in normal subjects. In patients with lung disease, excessive central deposition of the ^{99m}Tc DTPA may result in inadequate activity reaching the lung periphery, thereby making interpretation difficult. Activity may also be seen in the esophagus and stomach because of swallowed activity. Lung ventilation scanning is an integral part of the scanning procedure for detecting pulmonary embolism. This is because several common causes of ventilation abnormalities secondarily cause regional perfusion abnormalities. These include asthma, chronic bronchitis, COPD, bulla, and old inflammatory processes such as tuberculosis. Pulmonary emboli are the most common cause of an abnormal lung perfusion scan with a normal lung ventilation scan. The lung ventilation scan adds specificity to lung perfusion scanning. Ventila-

Table 9-2. Absorbed Radiation Dose Estimates in a 70-kg Adult
After Inhalation of 1 mCi (37 MBq) ^{99m}Tc DTPA[a]

Tissue	Absorbed Radiation Dose	
	rad/1 mCi	mGy/37 MBq
Trachea	0.30	3.00
Lungs	0.080	0.80
Red marrow	0.004	0.41
Kidneys	0.010	0.01
Ovaries	0.006	0.06
Testes	0.004	0.04
Bladder wall	0.093	0.93
Total body	0.005	0.05

[a]Assumes 2–4 hr voiding schedule and patient in a supine position.

tion scanning does not resolve all of the difficulties with lung perfusion scanning, because pulmonary edema, interstitial lung disease, and lymphatic obstruction may affect lung perfusion without affecting lung ventilation. A chest radiograph is useful and necessary in evaluating these other causes of positive lung perfusion scans and in excluding other causes of pleuritic chest pain (i.e., pneumothorax and pneumonic infiltrates).[1]

See the interpretative criteria in Procedure 9-4, "^{99m}Tc Macroaggregated Albumin Lung Perfusion Scan."

Additional Notes

Aerosol studies are more prone to technical problems than those using either ^{99m}Tc pertechnegas or ^{133}Xe. Variables such as the tube diameter and length, air flow, and design of the nebulizer all affect the pattern of aerosol deposition in the lungs.

Radiation Dosimetry

The estimated radiation doses in organs and tissue of an average subject (70 kg) from the inhalation of 1 mCi (37 MBq) ^{99m}Tc DTPA are shown in Table 9-2.[7]

References

1. Palmer EL, Scott JA, Strauss HW. "Practical Nuclear Medicine." W.B. Saunders Co., Philadelphia, 1992, pp 185–240.
2. Coates G, O'Brodovich H. Measurement of pulmonary epithelial permeability with ^{99m}Tc-DTPA aerosol. Semin Nucl Med 1986; 16: 275–284.
3. Staub NC, Hyde RW, Crandell E. NHLBI workshop summary. Workshop on techniques to evaluate lung alveolar-microvascular injury. Am Rev Respir Dis 1990; 141: 1071–1077.
4. Miki M, Isawa T, Teshima T, Anazawa Y, Motomiya M. Difference in inhaled aerosol deposition patterns in the lungs due to three different sized aerosols. Nucl Med Commun 1992; 13: 553–562.

5. Heyder J. Mechanism of aerosol particle deposition. Chest 1981; 80(Suppl. 6): 820–823.

6. Coates G, Dolovich M, Koehler D, Newhouse MT. Ventilation scanning with technetium labeled aerosols: DTPA or sulfur colloid? Clin Nucl Med 1985; 10: 835–838.

7. Atkins HL, Weber DA, Susskind H, Thomas SR. MIRD dose estimate report no. 16: radiation absorbed dose from technetium-99m diethylenetriaminepentacetic acid aerosol. J Nucl Med 1992; 33: 1717–1719.

^{99m}Tc Pertechnegas Ventilation Scan

Summary Information

Radiopharmaceutical

Adult dose: 1–2 mCi (37–74 MBq) ^{99m}Tc pertechnegas.

Pediatric dose: No pediatric dose has been established.

Note: In the United States, the pertechnegas generator is not an approved device; hence, a signed consent form must be obtained before the study.

Contraindications None.

Dose/Scan Interval Imaging commences immediately after inhalation of the ^{99m}Tc pertechnegas.

Views Obtained Obtain eight views of the lungs in the following orientation and order: posterior, left posterior oblique, right posterior oblique, right lateral, right anterior oblique, anterior, left anterior oblique, and left lateral.

Indications

Lung ventilation scans are used in conjunction with lung perfusion scans in the differential diagnosis of pulmonary embolism versus COPD or other lung disorders.

Principle

Pulmonary embolism usually has little or no effect on lung ventilation. In the absence of other disease, functional images of lung ventilation using a radioactive gas typically show no abnormality. Thus, the V/Q scan shows pulmonary emboli as segmental zones of reduced or absent pulmonary perfusion associated with normal ventilation. The gas used for a ventilation study must diffuse easily, must not be absorbed significantly by the lungs, and must have a low density. ^{99m}Tc pertechnegas is a gaseous form of ^{99m}Tc sodium pertechnetate that diffuses into the lungs, depositing rapidly on the surfaces of the alveoli.[1] Pertechnegas crosses the alveolar-capillary membrane and leaves the lungs through the pulmonary circulation.[2] The biologic half-life of pertechnegas in the lungs ranges from 2 to 20 minutes. This rapid clearance limits the time available for acquisition of the ventilation images, but it has the advantages of allowing assessment of lung permeability (through

473

measurement of global or regional lung clearance times) and minimizing the superposition of residual activity from the ventilation scan on the lung perfusion images.[2,3]

Patient Preparation

The procedure should be explained fully to the patient before starting. In the United States, this is not currently an approved procedure. Hence, approval by the institutional review board and informed signed consent must be obtained. This test requires the cooperation of the patient. *Note:* Airway resistance is very low with the pertechnegas procedure, and in patients with severely compromised lung function, this test generally is tolerated better than a ^{133}Xe ventilation scan.

Instrument Specifications

Gamma camera:	Any large field-of-view system can be used.
Collimators:	Low-energy, all-purpose collimators.
Energy setting:	15–20% energy window around the 140-keV photopeak of ^{99m}Tc.
Analog formatter:	8 × 10 film, 70-mm (9-on-1) format.
Computer system:	Acquisition requirements—static (256 × 256 matrix).
Additional items:	Pertechnegas generator (Tetley Manufacturing, Ltd., Sydney, Australia), cylinder of argon gas, and disposable patient administration set.

Pertechnegas Generator Procedure

1. Draw 0.1 ml or less of 10–20 mCi (370–740 MBq) ^{99m}Tc sodium pertechnetate into a 1-ml syringe.
2. If the required activity cannot be obtained in a volume of 0.1 ml or less, draw up activity into additional syringes until the required activity is obtained. These will be added to the carbon crucible during multiple evaporation steps to obtain the required ^{99m}Tc concentration in the crucible. *Note:* The patient dose is not determined by the activity in the crucible, but rather by the number of breaths taken. The greater the activity in the crucible, the fewer breaths the patient must take in order to achieve the required activity in the lungs.
3. Connect the gas outlet from the argon cylinder to the back of the generator (Fig. 9-5). Open the regulator on the argon cylinder (clockwise) until the gauge needle is in the green area.
4. Check that the generator is plugged into a 220-volt outlet. Turn on the main switch on the back panel (Fig. 9-5). The system will automatically go through a 3-minute purge cycle to remove any remaining pertechnegas from the system.
5. Wet the graphite crucible with 2–3 drops of absolute alcohol or ethanol, removing excess alcohol. This step should only be done once—do not repeat it if multiple drying steps are required. *Note:* The crucible is very fragile, handle it carefully.
6. Press the "OPEN" button to open the drawer of the generator. Remove the old crucible and discard in the radioactive waste. *Note:* Gloves should be worn because the internal components may be radioactive.
7. Pick up the crucible with forceps (Fig. 9-6), and carefully place it between the two electrodes, as shown in Figure 9-7. To place the crucible, retract the right electrode by pressing the lever located on the left side under the platform (Fig. 9-8) and carefully position the crucible before releasing the lever.

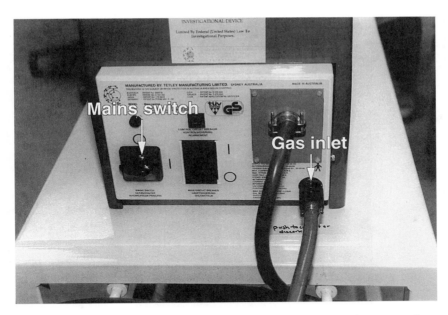

Figure 9-5. Back of pertechnegas generator showing gas inlet and main switch.

8. When in place, gently rotate the crucible to ensure good contact. Add up to 0.1 ml of ^{99m}Tc pertechnetate to the crucible. Measure the residual activity in syringe.
9. Close the drawer by simultaneously pressing the "CLOSE" button and depressing the drawer interlock knob (Fig. 9-9).

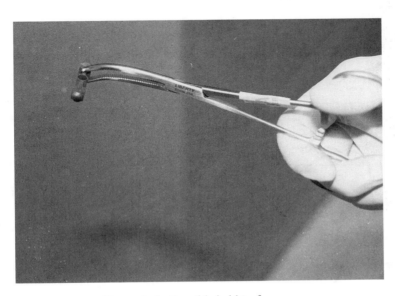

Figure 9-6. Crucible held in forceps.

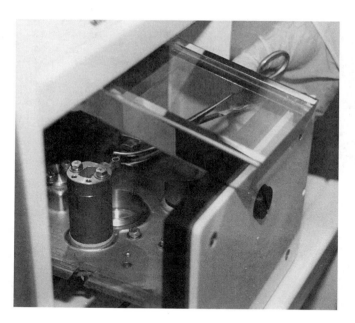

Figure 9-7. Crucible in position between electrodes.

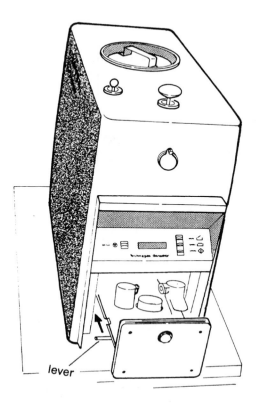

Figure 9-8. Diagram of generator showing position of lever for electrodes. (Courtesy of Tetley Manufacturing Ltd.)

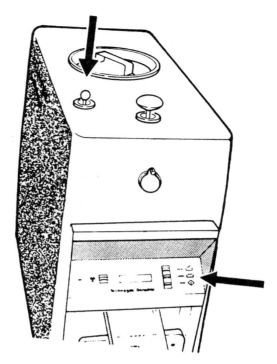

Figure 9-9. To close drawer, simultaneously press CLOSE button (right arrow) and depress drawer interlock knob (top arrow). (Courtesy of Tetley Manufacturing Ltd.)

10. Press the "START" button and the generator will heat the crucible to 70°C and begin a 6-minute cycle to evaporate the ^{99m}Tc eluate in the crucible with the argon/oxygen gas mixture. The gas flow should be 8–12 liters per minute.

11. If it is necessary to add more activity to the crucible, then at the end of the cycle, press the "CANCEL" button twice within 2 seconds. This permits the drawer to be opened and more ^{99m}Tc to be added (do not re-wet the crucible with alcohol). The evaporation cycle can then be run again.

12. The dried ^{99m}pertechnetate in the carbon crucible can be left at this stage as long as there is enough ^{99m}Tc activity to complete the patient study.

13. The final stage of the pertechnegas generation requires a short burn of 20 seconds at 2,500°C. Before performing this burn, perform all the required patient setup described below.

Patient Setup

1. Position the patient supine on the imaging table.
2. Move the table until the detector is positioned posteriorly with the lungs in the field of view. *Note:* It is not necessary at this stage to bring the detector in close to the patient).
3. Familiarize the patient with the patient administration set, which contains the face mask (or mouthpiece and noseclip), tubing, and filter unit. Do a dry run with the patient administration set so the patient understands what it will feel like.
4. Instruct the patient that he or she will be required to take a number of deep breaths and to hold each one for 3–5 seconds if possible.

Imaging Procedure

1. Before performing the pertechnegas study, set up a static acquisition on the analog formatter (9-on-1 format) and on computer (256 × 256 matrix) to terminate at 400 kct or 3 minutes, whichever comes first.
2. Press the "START" button on the generator to initialize the burn phase. This phase takes only 20 seconds.
3. When the burn is completed (display reads "DISCONNECT THE MAINS PLEASE"), shut off the argon gas, disconnect the gas hose, and open the gas regulator to release remaining gas.
4. Unplug the generator and wrap the electrical cord around the cart handle.
5. Wheel the unit to the patient positioned on the imaging table. The countdown timer will indicate the useful life of the gas in the generator (the useful life is 20 minutes from the time of burn).
6. Connect the end of the patient administration set to the generator, and position the face mask (or mouthpiece and nose clip) on the patient, as shown in Figure 9-10.
7. Adjust the detector head to give the minimum patient-to-collimator separation, with the detector oriented for a posterior image of the lungs.
8. When the patient is ready, first press the "START" button to open the patient delivery valve, then depress the patient delivery knob, as shown in Figure 9-11.
9. Ask the patient to take in a deep breath and to hold it for 3–5 seconds. Note the count rate on the gamma camera/computer system.
10. Repeat steps 8 and 9 until a count rate is obtained, consistent with a dose of 1 mCi ^{99m}Tc in the lungs (approximately 3 kcps for a single-head system with a low energy all-purpose collimator).

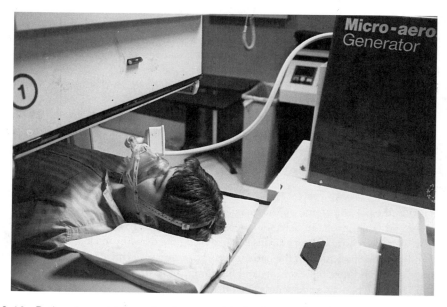

Figure 9-10. Patient in position under detector with the face mask, tubing, and filter unit in place. The tubing is connected to the generator via the front port.

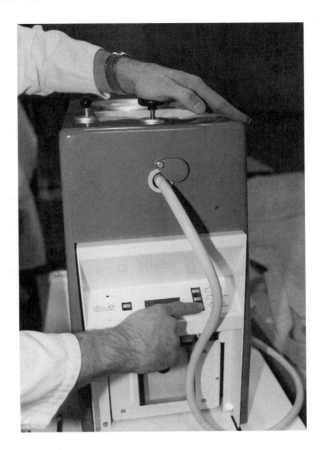

Figure 9-11. To release gas, (**A**) depress start button and then (**B**) depress top knob.

11. When this count rate is achieved, release the patient delivery knob. Have the patient breathe up to 10 more breaths to clear any remaining gas from the tubing. If possible, the patient administration set should be left on the patient until the completion of image acquisition.

12. Acquire all images on the analog formatter and on the computer, as described in step 1.

13. Acquire images in the following order: POST, LPO, RPO, RT LAT, RAO, ANT, LAO, LT LAT. A final posterior view may be obtained to determine the residual count rate in the lungs at the completion of the study.

14. If the count rate drops below 1 kcps, repeat steps 8–11 until a count rate of approximately 3 kcps is again achieved.

15. After acquisition, press the "CANCEL" button twice to shut down the system. Disconnect the patient administration set. Place it in a plastic bag, and discard it in the radioactive waste bin.

16. Return the generator to its original location, and plug in the power supply.

17. If a lung perfusion scan is to be performed following this procedure, the count rate from residual ^{99m}Tc pertechnegas in the lungs should be less that 2 kcps prior to the administration of the ^{99m}Tc perfusion agent. This is to ensure a 5-1 count ratio of the perfusion agent to the pertechnegas, assuming an administered dose of 4 mCi (148 MBq) for the perfusion agent.

Computer Analysis

No analysis of the computer data is required for conventional lung pertechnegas scans.

Information on Film

On each film, ensure that the following information is recorded:

1. Patient name and clinic/hospital number
2. Type of scan and radiopharmaceutical
3. Date and time after administration
4. Orientation of each image (e.g., anterior, posterior)

Interpretation

The interpretation of ^{99m}Tc pertechnegas lung ventilation scans is similar to that of ^{133}Xe lung ventilation scans, with the additional advantage of views in multiple projections that can be compared directly with the views obtained from perfusion imaging. The lung ventilation scan adds specificity to lung perfusion scanning. Ventilation scanning does not resolve all the difficulties with lung perfusion scanning, because pulmonary edema, interstitial lung disease, and lymphatic obstruction may affect lung perfusion without affecting lung ventilation. A chest radiograph is necessary in evaluating these other causes of positive lung perfusion scans and in excluding other causes of pleuritic chest pain (i.e., pneumothorax and pneumonic chest pain).[4]

See the interpretative criteria in Procedure 9-4, "^{99m}Tc Macroaggregated Albumin Lung Perfusion Scan."

Additional Notes

The patient should be reassured constantly that all is routine and going well, because this will give the patient more confidence and lead to a more successful study.

Table 9-3. Absorbed Radiation Dose Estimates to a 70-kg Adult From the Inhalation of 1 mCi (37 MBq) ^{99m}Tc Pertechnegas

Tissue	Absorbed Radiation Dose	
	rad/mCi	mGy/37 MBq
Bladder wall	0.053	0.53
Stomach wall	0.250	2.50
Upper large intestine wall	0.069	0.69
Lower large intestine wall	0.061	0.61
Red marrow	0.019	0.19
Testes	0.009	0.09
Ovaries	0.022	0.22
Thyroid	0.130	1.30
Brain	0.014	0.14
Total body	0.014	0.14

Radiation Dosimetry

The estimated radiation doses in organs and tissue of an average subject (70 kg) from inhalation of 1 mCi (37 MBq) of ^{99m}Tc pertechnegas are shown in Table 9-3.[5] Dosimetry is based on the assumption that the pertechnegas is absorbed into the body as sodium pertechnetate.

References

1. Bellen JC, Penglis S, Tsopelas C. Radiochemical characterization of modified Technegas. Nucl Med Biol 1993; 20: 715–717.
2. Monaghan P, Provan I, Murray C, et al. An improved radionuclide technique for the detection of altered pulmonary permeability. J Nucl Med 1991; 32: 1945–1949.
3. Ashburn WL, Belezzuoli EV, Dillon WA, et al. Technetium-99m labeled micro aerosol "Pertechnegas." A new agent for ventilation imaging in suspected pulmonary emboli. Clin Nucl Med 1993; 18: 1045–1052.
4. Palmer EL, Scott JA, Strauss HW. "Practical Nuclear Medicine." W.B. Saunders Co., Philadelphia, 1992, pp 185–240.
5. Lonnyer R et al., eds. MIRD primer for absorbed dose calculations. Society of Nuclear Medicine, New York, 1988.

$99mTc$ Macroaggregated Albumin Lung Perfusion Scan

Summary Information

Radiopharmaceutical

Adult dose: 4 mCi (148 MBq) ^{99m}Tc MAA.

Pediatric dose: Adjusted according to the patient's weight (see Appendix A-3).

Dose preparation: The vial of MAA contains approximately 8,000,000 particles. The vial should be reconstituted to 8 ml, giving a concentration of 1,000,000 particles per milliliter. The recommended number of particles per dose is 200,000–1,200,000, with an optimal number of 600,000.[1]

There are situations in which a smaller number of particles are indicated (see relative contraindications 1, 3, and 4, following). In adults, a minimum of about 50,000–75,000 particles is necessary to produce a diagnostic quality image. In children, the number of particles should be decreased to 10,000–50,000 in neonates and about 100,000 in children less than 8 years of age.

Contraindications There are several relative contraindications to the use of ^{99m}Tc MAA:

1. ^{99m}Tc MAA should be used with caution in patients with severe pulmonary hypertension, because of their compromised vascular bed. The scan can be performed, but the number of particles of ^{99m}Tc MAA in the dose may need to be decreased.

2. ^{99m}Tc MAA should not be administered to patients with a known hypersensitivity to products containing human serum albumin.

3. In patients with known right-to-left shunt, the MAA may bypass the lungs and become trapped in other organs, and hence a smaller number of particles may be indicated.

Continues

<table>
<tr><td colspan="2" align="center">**Summary Information** *(Continued)*</td></tr>
<tr><td></td><td>4. In children and patients with severely impaired pulmonary blood flow, fewer labeled particles should be administered (see preceding discussion).</td></tr>
<tr><td>**Dose/Scan Interval**</td><td>Imaging commences at 5 minutes after the injection.</td></tr>
<tr><td>**Views Obtained**</td><td>Eight views should be obtained: anterior, posterior, right and left lateral, right and left anterior oblique, and right and left posterior oblique. Additional views may be requested by the nuclear medicine physician.</td></tr>
</table>

Indications

Lung perfusion scintigraphy demonstrates blood flow to the lungs. The most common clinical indications for lung imaging include the following:

1. Evaluation of pulmonary emboli, which can include initial screening to rule out pulmonary embolism and follow-up to evaluate the response to therapy.
2. Evaluation of COPD, such as emphysema.
3. Evaluation of regional lung perfusion.

Principle

^{99m}Tc-labeled particles of MAA typically range in size from 10 to 40 µm. Within 1–5 minutes after injection, more than 90% of these particles become trapped in the arterioles and capillaries of the lung. The distribution of these particles in the lungs is a function of regional pulmonary blood flow. In a normal subject, these particles usually block about 1/1,000th of the lung's arterioles and capillaries. The MAA particles are fragile, gradually fragment, and leave the pulmonary arterial bed with a biologic half-time of 2–9 hours.[1]

Patient Preparation

All patients should have a chest radiograph within 24 hours before the lung scan. In patients with suspected pulmonary emboli, a lung ventilation scan should be performed before the perfusion scan.

Instrument Specifications

Gamma camera:	Any large field-of-view system can be used.
Collimator:	Low-energy all-purpose collimator.
Energy setting:	15–20% energy window around the 140-keV photopeak of ^{99m}Tc.
Analog formatter:	8 × 10 film, 70-mm (9-on-1) format.
Computer system:	Acquisition requirements—static (256 × 256 matrix). Processing requirements—ROI analysis.

Imaging Procedure

1. ^{99m}Tc MAA should always be injected slowly (over 15 seconds) with the patient supine. To ensure good mixing of the MAA particles, the syringe should be agitated just before the injection. If blood is drawn into the syringe, any unnecessary delay before injection may lead to clot formation. Do not back flush the syringe.
2. Preferably, the patient should be imaged in the upright position. However, the position of the patient needs to be the same as for the lung ventilation scan (upright or supine).
3. On the analog formatter and computer (256 × 256 word mode matrix), acquire the anterior and posterior images for 1,000 kct. The right lateral view should be acquired for 1,000 kct and the left lateral acquired for the same time. Acquisition should be conducted similarly for the right and left anterior and the right and left posterior oblique views.

Computer Analysis

No computer analysis is required for conventional lung perfusion scans for pulmonary emboli. For patients undergoing partial pneumonectomy, quantitation of right-versus-left or superior-versus-inferior activity may be required. For these patients, select the anterior and posterior views. Draw rectangular ROIs around each lung (ROIs of the same size must be used for each lung), and subdivide these ROIs into three regions—apical, middle, and basal lung regions. Calculate the geometric mean of counts for each lung region. For example, the geometric mean for the right basal region = (anterior right basal region × posterior right basal region)$^{0.5}$. Compute the ratio of left-to-right lung activity, as shown in Figure 9-3. Obtain a hard copy of the ROIs and results.

Information on Film

On each analog film, ensure that the following information is recorded:

1. Patient name and clinic/hospital number
2. Type of scan and radiopharmaceutical
3. Date and time of each image after injection
4. Orientation of each image (e.g., anterior, posterior)

Interpretation

Areas of decreased pulmonary arterial perfusion appear as areas of decreased tracer localization (perfusion defects). However, these defects can be caused by many things. Points in favor of pulmonary embolism on the scan include defects that are clearly segmental in distribution, multiple defects, and defects without corresponding abnormalities on chest radiographs. Interpretation of the lung V/Q scans should be done using a modified version of the criteria developed for the prospective investigation of pulmonary diagnosis (PIOPED) study.[2,3] The relevant terminology for different lung segments and the interpretive criteria are given in the additional notes.

Additional Notes

The typical incidence and size of pulmonary emboli are given in Tables 9-4 and 9-5. Interpretative criteria for high, intermediate, low, and very low probability of pulmonary emboli, as well as for normal scans, are also given in "Interpretative Criteria" using the modified PIOPED criteria.[2,3]

Table 9-4. Typical Incidence of Embolus by Scan Probability

Probability	Incidence, %
High	88
Intermediate	30
Low	13
Very low	5
Normal	0

Interpretative Criteria

The following are the categories and criteria for the interpretation of a V/Q scan.[2,3]

High Probability

1. Two or more large segmental equivalent perfusion defects (or the arithmetic equivalent in moderate, or large plus moderate perfusion defects, with two moderate defects equal to one large defect) without matching ventilation or chest radiographic abnormalities in those areas.
2. Two or more large perfusion defects associated with chest radiographic abnormalities, with the perfusion defects being substantially larger than either matching ventilation or chest radiographic abnormalities.

Intermediate Probability

1. One moderate but less than 2 large perfusion defects (or the arithmetic equivalent in moderate or large plus moderate perfusion defects, with two moderate defects equal to one large defect), without matching ventilation or chest radiographic abnormalities in those areas.
2. Perfusion defects with matched ventilation abnormalities and equally sized chest radiographic abnormalities in the lower lung zone.
3. Difficult to categorize as low or high or falling between the criteria for low and high.

Low Probability

1. Any perfusion defect regardless of the ventilation scan, which is substantially smaller than the chest radiographic abnormality in the same area.

Table 9-5. Defect Size as Percent of Lung Segment

Size	% of Lung Segment
Large	>75
Moderate	>25 and <75
Small	<25

Table 9-6. Absorbed Radiation Dose Estimates in a 70-kg Adult From Intravenous Administration of 4 mCi (148 MBq) ^{99m}Tc Macroaggregated Albumin

	Absorbed Radiation Dose	
Tissue	rad/4 mCi	mGy/148 MBq
Liver	0.07	0.72
Lungs	0.88	8.80
Spleen	0.07	0.68
Kidneys	0.04	0.44
Bladder wall		
2-hr void	0.12	1.20
4.8-hr void	0.22	2.20
Ovaries		
2-hr void	0.03	0.30
4.8-hr void	0.03	0.34
Testes		
2-hr void	0.02	0.24
4.8-hr void	0.03	0.26
Total body	0.06	0.60

2. Perfusion defects with matched ventilation abnormalities and equally-sized chest radiographic abnormalities in the upper or middle lung zone.
3. Perfusion defects (even externsive) that are matched by ventilation abnormalities, provided that the areas with the defects are normal on chest radiographs and that there are some normal areas of perfusion in the lung.
4. Any number of small perfusion defects with normal chest radiographic findings.
5. Nonsegmental perfusion defects (e.g., pleural effusion; fluid in a fissure; cardiomegaly; enlarged aorta, hila, and mediastinum; and elevated diaphragm).

Very Low Probability

Mild irregularity is present on perfusion imaging without segmental or subsegmental defects and normal chest radiographic findings.

Normal

No perfusion defects are present.

Radiation Dosimetry

The estimated absorbed doses in organs and tissues of an average subject (70 kg) from intravenous injection of 4 mCi (148 MBq) 99mTc MAA are shown in Table 9-6.4

References

1. Newman RD, Sostman HD, Gottschalk A. Current status of ventilation-perfusion imaging. Semin Nucl Med 1980; 10: 198–217.
2. Ralph DD. Pulmonary embolism. The implications of prospective investigation of pulmonary embolism diagnosis. Radiol Clin North Am 1994; 32: 679–687.
3. Worsley DF, Alan A. Comprehensive analysis of the results of the PIOPED study. J Nucl Med 1995; 36: 2380–2387.
4. Technescan MAA. Kit for the preparation of Technetium Tc-99m albumin aggregated, package insert. Mallinckrodt Medical, St. Louis. Last revision June 1988.

10

Tumor Imaging Procedures

Gregory A. Wiseman

Lymphoscintigraphy for Melanoma/Breast Cancer

Summary Information

Radiopharmaceutical

Adult Dose: 300–500 µCi (11.1–18.5 MBq) of ^{99m}Tc antimony colloid in a volume of 0.1 ml per injection site. If ^{99m}Tc antimony colloid is not available, filtered ^{99m}Tc sulfur colloid can be used (see following section entitled "Radiopharmaceutical Preparation").

Pediatric Dose: None established.

Melanoma The site and method of injection depend on the clinical situation. Typically, 3–6 injections are given. Each 0.1-ml volume is injected intradermally around the periphery of the lesion or surgical site. This gives an administered dose of approximately 1–3 mCi (37–111 MBq) of radiolabeled colloidal particles per lesion or site. Each injection should be administered using a 1-ml insulin syringe with a 28-gauge needle, using a separate syringe and needle for each injection.

Breast Carcinoma As described for melanoma, 3–6 injections are given. Each 0.1-ml volume is injected subcutaneously around the suspected tumor. This gives an administered dose of approximately 1–3 mCi (37–111 MBq) of radiolabeled colloidal particles per tumor. Each injection should be administered using a 1-ml insulin syringe with a 28-gauge needle for superficial lesions or a 27-gauge (1.25 inches long) needle for deeper lesions. A separate syringe and needle should be used for each injection.

Contraindications None.

Dose/Scan Interval ^{99m}Tc antimony colloid or filtered ^{99m}Tc sulfur colloid—the imaging should commence 15 minutes after the injection.

Views Obtained For malignant melanoma, acquire planar views such that the collimator is orthogonal to the skin surface. Additional oblique, anterior, or posterior views of the sentinel lymph nodes will be required.

For breast lesions, acquire anterior and lateral views of the breasts and axillae.

Indications

Many tumors metastasize through lymphatic channels. Defining the anatomy of nodes that drain a primary tumor site helps guide surgical and radiation treatment for certain tumor types. Contrast lymphangiography, magnetic resonance imaging (MRI), and computed tomography (CT) are the standard methods to evaluate the status of the lymph nodes. In cases in which the channels are relatively inaccessible to routine lymphangiographic methods (generally the trunk), radionuclide lymphoscintigraphy has been of value. This method has been used primarily in patients with truncal melanomas and prostate and breast cancer to map the routes of lymphatic drainage and to permit more effective surgical or radiation treatment of draining regional lymph nodes. It has also been used occasionally in patients in whom lymphangiography is difficult to perform because of lymphedema.[1]

Principle

Colloidal particles injected intradermally or subcutaneously adjacent to a lesion or biopsy site demonstrate a drainage pattern similar to that of the lesion.[2,3] Colloidal particles in the 10–50 nm range appear to be the most effective for this application. The colloidal particles drain into the sentinel lymph node, where they are trapped by phagocytic activity. This aids in the identification of the lymph nodes most likely to be sites of metastatic deposits from the tumor.

Radiopharmaceutical Preparation

If ^{99m}Tc antimony colloid is not available, the following procedure can be used to generate colloidal particles of less than 100 nm in size.

1. Draw up 1 ml of ^{99m}Tc sulfur colloid (25–30 mCi/925–1,110 MBq) into a lead-shielded 3-ml syringe.
2. Carefully remove the needle of the ^{99m}Tc sulfur colloid syringe, and aseptically attach the syringe to the female inlet of a sterile 0.1 μm filter (Millex-VV, Millipore Corp., Bedford, MA).
3. Attach a fresh 23-gauge needle to the male outlet end of the filter. Push the 1 ml of solution through the filter into a 5-ml sterile vial. This will give approximately 15 mCi (555 MBq) in 0.9 ml.
4. Add 2 ml of sterile saline to the vial to give a final concentration of approximately 5 mCi/ml (185 MBq/ml).
5. For each injection site, inject 0.1 ml of the filtered ^{99m}Tc sulfur colloid subcutaneously using a 1-ml insulin syringe with a 28-gauge needle. This will give a dose of 400–500 μCi (14.8–18.5 MBq) ^{99m}Tc per injection.

Patient Preparation

The procedure should be explained fully to the patient. The patient should remove all clothing from the injection site and, if necessary, change into a hospital gown. The injection itself may be associated with a stinging sensation lasting 5–10 seconds. The injection will be performed by the nuclear medicine physician after skin preparation with povidone-iodine swabs (providing the patient is not allergic to povidone-iodine).

Instrument Specifications

Gamma camera:	Any large field-of-view system may be used.
Collimator:	Low-energy, all-purpose or low-energy, high-resolution collimator.

Energy setting: 140 keV, 20% energy window.
Analog formatter: 8 × 10 film, 70-mm (9-on-1) format.
Computer system: Acquisition requirements—static (256 × 256 word mode matrix).
Processing requirements—none.

Imaging Procedure

Breast Cancer

1. The patient should be positioned supine on the imaging table with the arms extended over the head.
2. At 15 minutes after the injection, acquire an anterior view of the injection site.
3. All images should be acquired on an analog formatter and computer (256 × 256 word mode matrix) for 5 minutes per image.
4. Repeat step 2 every 15–30 minutes for 2 hours or until the sentinel lymph nodes are visualized.
5. When the sentinel nodes have been visualized, acquire additional lateral and oblique views of the node. If nodal uptake is proximal to the injection site, it may be necessary to shield the injection site with a lead apron.
6. It is important to mark appropriate anatomic landmarks to aid in identifying the draining lymph nodes on film. For this purpose, acquire additional images with ^{57}Co or ^{99m}Tc point source markers placed over the anatomic sites.
7. If requested, locate the lymph nodes that show uptake of the radiocolloid using a small ^{57}Co marker, and mark the overlying region of the patient's skin with an indelible ink marker.
8. For a patient receiving the injection immediately before an operation, an intraoperative probe can be used to detect lesion drainage into the axillary lymph nodes.

Malignant Melanoma

1. Depending on the injection site, the patient should be positioned supine or prone on the imaging table. Position the gamma camera over the injection site.
2. At 15 minutes after the injection, acquire an image of the injection site on the analog formatter and computer (256 × 256 word mode matrix) for 5 minutes per image.
3. Repeat step 2 every 15–30 minutes for 2 hours. In addition, check regionally around the injection site (this may require moving the patient or detector) to ensure that any uptake in the sentinel lymph nodes is detected.
4. When the sentinel nodes have been visualized, acquire additional lateral and oblique views of the node. If nodal uptake is proximal to the injection site, it may be necessary to shield the injection site with a lead apron.
5. With a small ^{57}Co marker, locate the lymph nodes that show uptake of the radiocolloid, and mark the overlying region of the patient's skin with an indelible ink marker.
6. Appropriate anatomic landmarks should be identified on the film with ^{57}Co or ^{99m}Tc point source markers.

Information on Film

On each analog and computer film, ensure that the following information is recorded:

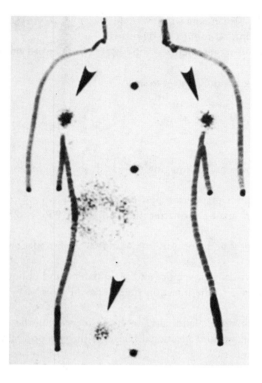

Figure 10-1. Anterior view of the abdomen showing the drainage from a melanoma on the left side of the abdomen to both axillae and the left inguinal (arrow) lymph nodes. The injection site is covered with a thin lead shield. (From Bennett and Lago,[1] with permission.)

1. Patient name and clinic/hospital number
2. Date and time of each image after injection
3. Type of scan and radiopharmaceutical
4. Orientation of each image (e.g., anterior, posterior)
5. Injection sites and location of anatomic markers

Interpretation

Lymphoscintigraphy permits identification of the sentinel nodes responsible for drainage from the lesion or biopsy site. The drainage from the injection site to the lymph nodes depends on the exact site of injection and on changes to the lymph drainage pattern caused by surgical treatment or lymphadenectomy. An example of drainage from a melanoma in the left abdomen to the left inguinal and both axillae lymph nodes is shown in Figure 10-1.

Radiation Dosimetry

Dosimetry for filtered ^{99m}Tc sulfur colloid and for ^{99m}Tc antimony trisulfide colloid are similar because the distribution of the activity, metabolism, and excretion is the same. The estimated absorbed doses in organs and tissues of an average subject (70 kg) from an injection of 2 mCi (74 MBq) of ^{99m}Tc antimony trisulfide colloid are shown in Table 10-1.[4]

Table 10-1. Absorbed Radiation Dose Estimates in a 70-kg Adult From Injection of 2 mCi (74 MBq) of ^{99m}Tc Antimony Colloid[a]

| | Absorbed Radiation Doses | | | |
| | Scenario 1[b] | | Scenario 2[c] | |
Tissue	rad/2 mCi	mGy/74 MBq	rad/2 mCi	mGy/74 MBq
Urinary bladder wall	0.00	0.00	2.80	28.0
Bone (total)	0.00	0.02	0.02	0.16
Liver	0.80	8.00	0.00	0.00
Ovaries	0.01	0.08	0.12	1.20
Testes	0.00	0.01	0.08	0.80
Red marrow	0.00	0.03	0.04	0.40
Uterus	0.01	0.08	0.28	2.80
Blood	0.04	0.40	0.00	0.03
Total body	0.04	0.40	0.00	0.03

[a]Estimated dose to the skin at the injection site (assuming all activity remains at injection site): 66 rad/2 mCi (660 mGy/74 MBq). Estimated dose to lymph node (assuming uptake of 0.4% per node, with no clearance of activity from node): 40 rad/2 mCi (400 mGy/74 MBq).
[b]Scenario 1, the entire dose is in the liver.
[c]Scenario 2, the entire dose is in the bladder.

References

1. Bennett LR, Lago G. Cutaneous lymphoscintigraphy in malignant melanoma. Semin Nucl Med 1983; 13: 61–69.
2. Krag DN, Weaver DL, Alex JC, Fairbank JT. Surgical resection and radiolocalization of the sentinel lymph node in breast cancer using a gamma probe. Surg Oncol 1993; 2: 335–339.
3. Alex JC, Weaver DL, Fairbank JT, Rankin BS, Krag DN. Gamma-probe-guided lymph node localization in malignant melanoma. Surg Oncol 1993; 2: 303–308.
4. Technetium Tc-99m antimony trisulfide colloid kit. Package insert, Cadema Medical Products, Middletown, NY, October 1984.

^{67}Ga Gallium Tumor Scan

Summary Information

Radiopharmaceutical

Adult dose: 10 mCi (370 MBq) gallium citrate (^{67}Ga) injected intravenously.

Pediatric dose: Adjusted according to the patient's weight (see Appendix A-3).

Contraindications None.

Dose/Scan Interval Imaging starts at 48 hours after the injection and may be required for up to 10 days after the injection.

Views Obtained Anterior and posterior whole-body images are obtained as well as additional spot views or single photon emission computed tomography (SPECT), according to the area of interest as specified on the examination request sheet or as requested by the nuclear medicine physician.

Indications

Gallium citrate is useful in assessing the extent of involvement in malignancies such as Hodgkin's disease, non-Hodgkin's lymphoma, hepatoma, lung cancer, and melanoma.[1] Gallium citrate is most often used in patients with non-Hodgkin's lymphoma or Hodgkin's disease to determine the effectiveness of therapy.[2]

Principle

The mechanism of gallium citrate localization in tumors is not fully understood; however, it appears that the initial step involves protein binding to transferrin. The ^{67}Ga transferrin complex most likely binds to specific transferrin receptor sites on the surface or within the tumor.[3,4] Gallium uptake appears to be an in vivo measurement of tumor differentiation; hence, it may be used as a prognostic indicator in predicting response to therapy and overall survival rate in patients with lymphomas.

Patient Preparation

Laxatives or enemas given before scanning may help interpretation of abdominal activity by clearing normal gallium activity from the bowel. Instruct the patient in bowel cleansing if indicated by the nuclear medicine physician. If bowel cleansing is required, instruct the patient to drink one bottle of magnesium citrate on the night before the imaging study.

Instrument Specifications

Gamma camera:	Planar views—any large field-of-view system may be used. Whole-body views—dual-head large field-of-view rectangular system. SPECT—single-, dual-, or triple-head SPECT system.
Collimator:	Medium-energy collimator.
Energy setting:	20% energy windows around the three main photopeaks at 93, 184, and 296 keV.
Analog formatter:	Spot views—8 × 10 film, 70-mm (9-on-1) format. Whole-body views—10 × 14 film (4-on-1 format).
Computer system:	Acquisition requirements—static (256 × 256 matrix), whole body (1,024 × 256 matrix), SPECT (64 × 64 matrix). Processing requirements—SPECT reconstruction software.

Imaging Procedure

Whole-Body Imaging

At 48 and 72–96 hours after injection, acquire anterior and posterior whole-body images on an analog formatter and on computer (1,024 × 256 word mode matrix) at a scan speed of 5 cm/min.

Planar Imaging

At 48 and 72–96 hours, acquire anterior and posterior spot views of the abdomen for 1,000 kct per view or 5 minutes per view, whichever is shorter. Views of the chest should exclude the liver and spleen, or these organs should be shielded with a lead apron. Abdominal views should include the liver and spleen but may be improved by imaging with these organs shielded or excluded from the field of view.

SPECT Imaging

When requested, SPECT studies should be acquired using the following acquisition variables:

1. Single-head system: 360° body-contouring orbit, 64 × 64 word mode matrix, 60–64 views at 30–40 seconds per view. No zoom for 40-cm field-of-view system. Zoom of 1.2–1.5 for 50–60 cm field-of-view systems.
2. Dual- or triple-head systems: 360° body-contouring orbit, 64 × 64 word mode matrix, with a total of 120 views at 15 seconds per view. No zoom for 40-cm field-of-view system. Zoom of 1.2–1.5 for 50–60-cm field-of-view systems.

Computer Analysis

No analysis is required for planar or whole-body images. For SPECT studies, perform the following steps:

1. Apply uniformity and center-of-rotation correction to the data (on newer systems, this may be done automatically).
2. If possible, prefilter the planar data (possible filters are Butterworth, order 10, cutoff at 0.5 Nyquist, and Hann filter, cutoff at 0.8–0.9 Nyquist).
3. Reconstruct 1-pixel-thick transaxial slices. The back-projection filter may be a Ramp or Ramp-Butterworth with a cutoff at 0.6–0.8 Nyquist.

Information on Film

On each analog and computer film, ensure that the following information is recorded:

1. Patient name and clinic/hospital number
2. Type of scan and radiopharmaceutical
3. Date and time after injection
4. Orientation of each image (e.g., anterior, posterior)

Interpretation

At 48 hours after injection, renal clearance of gallium citrate should be complete and soft tissue activity should be low. However, significant bowel activity may still be present (10–20% of the dose is excreted through the bowel) together with activity in bone, liver, and spleen. Activity may also be present in the salivary and lacrimal glands and in breast tissue, with faint activity in the lungs. In children, activity may be seen in the epiphyseal plates and thymus.

Any area of focal uptake outside the areas described should be considered abnormal. These focal areas may be visualized better on the 72-hour and later scans, because of the decrease in soft tissue activity over time. If there is significant abdominal activity, bowel cleansing should be performed and the patient imaged again to determine the nature of the activity. Recent or concurrent chemotherapy or radiation therapy may alter both the normal and tumor uptake of gallium citrate.[5,6] *Note:* Children and, occasionally, adults may have "thymic rebound" with ^{67}Ga uptake in the thymus unrelated to tumor involvement.[7] This generally occurs in the early months after chemotherapy, and SPECT imaging is particularly helpful in distinguishing between thymic and mediastinal uptake of [67]Ga.

Radiation Dosimetry

The estimated absorbed radiation doses in organs and tissues of an average subject (70 kg) from an IV injection of 10 mCi (370 MBq) of gallium citrate are shown in Table 10-2.[8]

Table 10-2. Absorbed Radiation Dose Estimates in a 70-kg Adult From Intravenous Injection of 10 mCi (370 MBq) of (^{67}Ga) Gallium Citrate

Tissue	Absorbed Radiation Doses	
	rad/10 mCi	mGy/370 MBq
Skeleton	4.40	44.0
Liver	4.60	46.0
Bone marrow	5.80	58.0
Spleen	4.30	43.0
Kidney	4.10	41.0
Ovaries	2.80	28.0
Testes	2.40	24.0
Stomach	2.20	22.0
Small intestine	3.60	36.0
Upper large intestine	5.60	56.0
Lower large intestine	9.00	90.0
Total body	2.60	26.0

References

1. Palmer EL, Scott JA, Strauss HW. "Practical Nuclear Medicine," W.B. Saunders Co., Philadelphia, 1992, pp 343–364.

2. Kaplan WD, Jochelson MS, Herman TS, et al. Gallium-67 imaging: a predictor of residual tumor viability and clinical outcome in patients with diffuse large-cell lymphoma. J Clin Oncol 1990; 8: 1966–1970.

3. Feremans W, Bujan W, Neve P, Delville J-P, Schandene L. CD71 phenotype and the value of gallium imaging in lymphomas. Am J Hematol 1991; 36: 215–216.

4. Bekerman C, Hoffer PB, Bitran JD. The role of gallium-67 in the clinical evaluation of cancer. Semin Nucl Med 1985; 15: 72–103.

5. Bekerman C, Pavel DG, Bitran J, Ryo UY, Pinsky S. The effects of inadvertent administration of antineoplastic agents prior to Ga-67 injection: concise communication. J Nucl Med 1984; 25: 430–435.

6. Wylie BR, Southee AE, Joshua DE, et al. Gallium scanning in the management of mediastinal Hodgkin's disease. Eur J Haematol 1989; 42: 344–347.

7. Peylan-Ramu N, Haddy TB, Jones E, et al. High frequency of benign mediastinal uptake of gallium-67 after completion of chemotherapy in children with high-grade non-Hodgkin's lymphoma. J Clin Oncol 1989; 7: 1800–1806.

8. Loevinger R, ed. MIRD primer for absorbed dose calculations, report no. 2. Society of Nuclear Medicine, New York, 1988.

99mTc Sestamibi Breast Scan

Summary Information

Radiopharmaceutical

Adult dose: 30 mCi (1,110 MBq) of 99mTc sestamibi injected intravenously. Inject in the arm opposite the suspected breast lesion. Whenever possible, injections should be made in a lower extremity vein, because even a small amount of extravasation may lead to lymph node uptake.

Pediatric dose: Not applicable.

Contraindications None.

Dose/Scan Interval Imaging begins 5 minutes after the injection.

Views Obtained Lateral views of each breast and an anterior view of the breasts and axillae.

Indications

99mTc sestamibi imaging of the breast has been reported to have a high sensitivity (greater than 95%) and a high negative predictive value (96%) but a lower specificity (about 50%) for the detection of malignant breast lesions.[1-3] It is primarily indicated as a complementary imaging test to mammography in patients with indeterminate mammographic findings or findings suggestive of a malignant breast lesion. Recent reports have attested to the potential clinical usefulness of this agent in patients with suspected breast cancer.[1,2]

Principle

99mTc sestamibi accumulates in various malignant tumors (e.g., lung cancer, lymphoma, peripheral soft tissue, and bone sarcomas). Currently, it is the agent of choice for the detection of parathyroid adenomas. Sestamibi is thought to diffuse into tumors because of their high negative membrane potential and/or by mitochondrial metabolism. Other possible mechanisms include transport or retention by a 170-kD p-glycoprotein that is an integral plasma membrane lipoprotein encoded by the human multidrug-resistant gene.[4,5]

Patient Preparation

The patient should remove all clothing and jewelry above the waist and put on a hospital gown open at the front. An in-dwelling intravenous catheter or butterfly infusion set, in the arm opposite to the breast with the lesion, should be used to avoid infiltration of the 99mTc sestamibi. For patients with lesions in both breasts, the injection should be given in

501

a lower extremity vein. The patient may be more comfortable if the study is performed by a female technologist.

Note: According to the previous reports, image quality varies depending on the time in the patient's menstrual cycle. In premenopausal women, the best image quality is obtained during the middle 2 weeks of the menstrual cycle.[6]

Instrument Specifications

Gamma camera:	Any large field-of-view system may be used.
Imaging table:	Modified SPECT tabletop with cutouts for breasts (Fig. 10-2). Alternatively, a raised board with cutouts for the breast is required. This should be placed on top of a conventional imaging table. The cutout should permit the breast to be suspended and allow the detector to be positioned close to the lateral wall of the breast.
Collimator:	Low-energy, high-resolution collimator.
Energy setting:	140-keV, 10% energy window (a narrow window is recommended to reduce scatter and to improve lesion detectability).
Analog formatter:	8 × 10 film, 70-mm (9-on-1) format.
Computer system:	Acquisition requirements—static (256 × 256 matrix). Processing requirements—none.

Imaging Procedure

1. Inject 30 mCi (1,110 MBq) of ^{99m}Tc sestamibi intravenously and wait 5 minutes. (*Note:* If a long period, greater than 40 minutes, elapses between injection and imaging, the study may not be diagnostic because of the washout of the sestamibi from the tumor.)
2. The injection should be in the arm opposite to the breast with the suspected lesion or, if possible, into a lower extremity vein to avoid artifacts that are due to retention of activity in the veins proximal to the injection site.
3. Place the patient prone on the modified SPECT imaging table, with one arm above her head, the shoulder flat against the table, and the head turned to the side opposite the breast

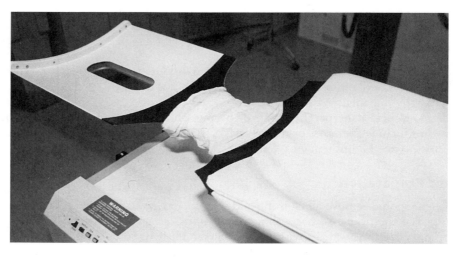

Figure 10-2. Modified tomographic imaging table with cutouts for prone breast imaging.

to be imaged. Position the patient so that the breast to be imaged is suspended freely through the cutout in the table, as in Figure 10-3.

4. Always image first the breast with the suspected lesion. *Note:* In patients who are undergoing biopsy of both breasts, the nuclear medicine physician will determine which breast should be imaged first.

5. Position the gamma camera laterally, and magnify the region around the breast using a 1.5–1.75 zoom. Check that the breast and chest wall are in the field of view, as in Figure 10-4.

6. Acquire a 10-minute static image on an analog formatter (4-on-1 format) and on computer (256 × 256 word mode matrix).

7. Repeat step 6 for the other breast.

8. Next, position the patient supine on the imaging table, with her hands behind her head. Acquire an anterior 10-minute static image of the breast and chest on an analog formatter (4-on-1 format) and on computer (256 × 256 word mode matrix).

9. Place ^{57}Co or ^{99m}Tc markers on each nipple, and acquire a second view of the breasts and chest for 5 minutes on an analog formatter and on computer (256 × 256 word mode matrix).

10. Delayed imaging may be requested at 1–2 hours after the injection. For delayed images, repeat steps 3–9.

Additional Notes

For deep lesions close to the chest wall, rotate the detector head to obtain 30° right or left posterior oblique projections.

Computer Analysis

No analysis is required. Whenever possible, images should be reviewed on a computer screen, because adjustment of image contrast may improve lesion detection.

Information on Film

On each analog and computer film, ensure that the following information is recorded:

1. Patient name and clinic/hospital number
2. Type of scan and radiopharmaceutical
3. Date and time of each image after the injection
4. Orientation of each image

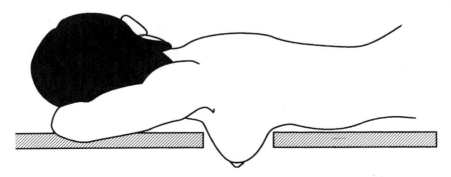

Figure 10-3. Schematic diagram showing the position of the patient on the tomographic table for imaging of the left breast. The breast should be freely suspended.

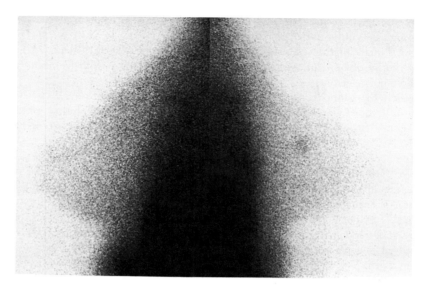

Figure 10-4. Images of the left and right breasts, illustrating the correct zoom to include chest wall and breast. A small tumor is visible in the right breast.

Table 10-3. Absorbed Radiation Dose Estimates for a 70-kg Adult at Rest (After Injection of 30 mCi [1,110 MBq] of ^{99m}Tc Sestamibi)

Tissue	Absorbed Radiation Dose	
	rad/30 mCi	mGy/1,110 MBq
Heart wall	0.5	5.1
Liver	0.6	5.8
Kidneys	2.0	20.0
Testes	0.3	3.4
Ovaries	1.5	15.5
Breasts	0.2	2.0
Thyroid	0.7	7.0
Stomach wall	0.6	6.1
Gallbladder wall	2.0	20.0
Small intestine	3.0	30.0
Upper large intestinal wall	5.6	55.5
Lower large intestinal wall	4.0	40.0
Urinary bladder wall	2.0	20.0
Total body	0.5	4.8

Interpretation

Normal breasts show a low uniform diffuse uptake, with occasional increased uptake in the region of the nipples. Bilateral patchy diffuse uptake may be seen during the first and fourth weeks of a woman's menstrual cycle.[6] Focal uptake is indicative of a malignant lesion, although false-positive uptake may be seen in epithelial hyperplasia. The findings of the sestamibi scan should be correlated with those found on mammography. Note that lesions located medially may be more difficult to visualize because of attenuation from the breast on lateral views.

Radiation Dosimetry

The estimated absorbed doses in organs and tissues of an average subject (70 kg) from the administration of 30 mCi (1,110 MBq) ^{99m}Tc sestamibi are presented in Table 10-3.[7]

References

1. Waxman A, Ashok G, Kooba A, et al. The use of Tc-99m methoxy isobutyl isonitrile (MIBI) in evaluation of patients with primary carcinoma of the breast: comparison with Tl-201 (abstract). J Nucl Med 1993; 34: 139P.
2. Khalkhali J, Mena I, Jouanne E, et al. Tc-99m sestamibi prone breast imaging in patients with suspicion of breast cancer (abstract). J Nucl Med 1993; 34: 140P.
3. Campeau RJ, Kronemer KA, Sutherland CM. Concordant uptake of Tc-99m sestamibi and Tl-201 in unsuspected breast tumor. Clin Nucl Med 1992; 17: 936–937.
4. Piwnica-Worms D, Chiu ML, Croop JM, Kronauge JF. Enhancement of Tc-99m sestamibi accumulation in multidrug resistant (MDR) cells by cytotoxic drugs and MDR reversing agents (abstract). J Nucl Med 1993; 34: 140P.
5. Piwnica-Worms D, Croop JM, Kramer RA, Kronauge JF. Tc-99m-sestamibi in a transport substrate recognized by the multidrug resistance P-glycoprotein (abstract). Proc Annu Meet Am Assoc Cancer Res 1993; 34: 309.
6. Diggles L, Mena I, Khalkhali I. Bilateral increased uptake of Tc-99m sestamibi in scintimammography: its correlation with the menstrual cycle (abstract). J Nucl Med Tech 1994; 22: 111.
7. Stabin M. Oak Ridge Associated University, Package insert for Cardiolite (Tc-99m sestamibi), DuPont, July 1990.

^{111}In OncoScint Scan

Summary Information

Radiopharmaceutical

Adult doses: 5 mCi (185 MBq) of ^{111}In OncoScint (satumomab pendetide) injected intravenously over a 5-minute period.

Pediatric dose: Not applicable. The safety and efficacy of this agent have not been established in children.

Contraindications ^{111}In OncoScint is not approved by the FDA for use in patients who have previously received this agent. The study should not be performed in patients with known hypersensitivity to other products of murine origin.

Dose/Scan Interval Imaging starts 72 hours after the injection and may be requested up to 5 days after injection.

Views Obtained Anterior and posterior spot views are obtained of the chest, liver and spleen, and pelvic regions. Usually, SPECT imaging of some of these regions will be requested by the nuclear medicine physician.

Indications

^{111}In OncoScint is indicated in patients with colorectal[1] or ovarian cancer.[2] A multicenter study of patients with colorectal cancer showed that ^{111}In OncoScint had a sensitivity of 69% and a specificity of 77%. It proved to be superior to CT in the detection of pelvic and extrahepatic abdominal tumors but inferior to CT in the detection of liver metastases. In patients with ovarian cancer, it had a higher sensitivity than CT (59% vs. 30%) but a lower specificity. OncoScint cannot reliably distinguish between benign and malignant primary ovarian tumors and is not recommended for the evaluation of patients with suspected primary ovarian cancer.

Principle

OncoScint is a conjugate produced from a murine monoclonal antibody directed against the glycoprotein TAG-7 antigen associated with various adenocarcinomas, including colorectal and ovarian carcinoma. ^{111}In is bound to the monoclonal antibody by linkage with the chelator DTPA (diethylene triamine pentaacetic acid). This compound retains the immunoreactivity of the original antibody. It localizes in primary and metastatic lesions from colorectal and ovarian cancer.[1,2]

Patient Preparation

No patient preparation is required before the injection of [111]In OncoScint. Before scanning, laxatives or enemas should be used to clear activity in the stool from the bowel, thus aiding in interpretation of abdominal activity. Instruct the patient in bowel cleansing if indicated by the nuclear medicine physician. For bowel cleansing, instruct the patient to drink one bottle of magnesium citrate or a half to one liter of a polyethylene glycol/electrolytic solution (GoLYTELY) on the night before imaging. A sodium phosphate (Fleet) enema may be given immediately before the imaging study.

Instrument Specifications

Gamma camera:	Planar views—any large field-of-view system may be used. SPECT—single-, dual-, or triple-head SPECT system.
Collimator:	Medium-energy collimator.
Energy setting:	20% energy window around the 173- and 247-keV photopeaks of [111]In.
Analog formatter:	Spot views—8 × 10 film, 70-mm (9-on-1) format.
Computer system:	Acquisition requirements—static (256 × 256 matrix). SPECT (64 × 64 word mode matrix). Processing requirements—SPECT reconstruction software.

Imaging Procedure

[111]In OncoScint should be injected slowly over a 5-minute period with a 21-gauge butterfly infusion set. Allergic reactions potentially can occur, including anaphylaxis. In such cases, discontinue the injection and immediately contact the nuclear medicine physician. Medications for the treatment of hypersensitivity reactions should be available during the administration of this agent, including IV fluids, diphenhydramine (Benadryl), and corticosteroids.

Note: After the injection, an adverse reaction occurs in 4% of patients. Serious reactions were not observed during the clinical trial for FDA approval. Reported reactions have been mild and include itching, fever, nausea, facial angioedema, and rash. About 40% of patients become positive for human anti-murine antibodies (HAMA) after administration of [111]In OncoScint.

Planar Imaging

At 72 and 96 hours after injection, acquire anterior and posterior spot views of the chest, liver and spleen, and pelvic region, for 10 minutes per view. Views of the pelvic region and chest should either exclude the liver and spleen, or these organs should be shielded with a lead apron. In a patient with a colostomy, mark the colostomy site with a [57]Co or ^{99m}Tc spot marker, and acquire an additional view of this region. Occasionally, additional marker views may be required of other areas of abnormal uptake.

SPECT Imaging

SPECT studies should be acquired using the following acquisition variables:

Single-head system: 360° body-contouring orbit, 64 × 64 word mode matrix, with 60–64 views every 6° at 40 seconds per view. No zoom for 40-cm field of view; use zoom of 1.2 for 50-cm or larger field-of-view systems.

Dual- or triple-head system: 360° body-contouring orbit, 64 × 64 word mode matrix, with 120–128 views every 3° at 15 seconds per view. No zoom for 40-cm field of view; use zoom of 1.2 for 50-cm or larger field-of-view systems.

Computer Analysis

No analysis is required for planar images. For SPECT studies, perform the following steps:

1. Apply uniformity and center-of-rotation correction to the data (on newer systems, this may be done automatically).
2. If possible, prefilter the planar data (possible filters are Butterworth, order 10, cutoff at 0.5 Nyquist, and a Hann filter, cutoff at 0.8–0.9 Nyquist).
3. Reconstruct 1-pixel-thick transaxial slices. The back-projection filter may be Ramp or Ramp-Butterworth with a cutoff at 0.6–0.8 Nyquist.

Information on Film

On each analog and computer film, ensure that the following information is recorded:

1. Patient name and clinic/hospital number
2. Type of scan and radiopharmaceutical
3. Date and time after injection
4. Orientation of each image (e.g., anterior, posterior)

Interpretation

[111]In OncoScint localizes in normal liver, spleen, and bone marrow. Activity may also be seen in the bowel, blood pool, kidneys, urinary bladder, male genitalia, and breast nipples of women.[3] It has also been reported that [111]In OncoScint may localize in colostomy sites, sites of degenerative joint disease, abdominal aneurysms, postoperative bowel adhesions, and local inflammatory lesions.[3] Hence, image interpretation requires a careful review of the patient's medical history. Optimal uptake in tumor occurs between 48 and 72 hours after injection.

Radiation Dosimetry

The estimated absorbed doses in organs and tissues of an average subject (70 kg) from an IV injection of 5 mCi (185 MBq) [111]In OncoScint are shown in Table 10-4.[3]

Table 10-4. Absorbed Radiation Dose Estimates in a 70-kg Adult From Intravenous Injection of 5 mCi (185 MBq) ^{111}In OncoScint

Tissue	Absorbed Radiation Dose	
	rad/5 mCi	mGy/185 MBq
Kidney	9.7	97.0
Liver	15.0	150
Bone marrow	12.0	120
Spleen	16.0	160
Lungs	4.9	49.0
Adrenal gland	4.5	45.0
Urinary bladder	2.8	28.0
Heart wall	3.2	32.0
Bone	3.3	33.0
Pancreas	3.7	37.0
Thyroid	1.5	15.0
Ovaries	2.9	29.0
Testes	1.4	14.0
Stomach wall	3.2	32.0
Small intestine	3.0	30.0
Upper large intestine	3.1	31.0
Lower large intestine	2.5	25.0
Total body	2.7	27.0

References

1. Collier BD, Abdel-Nabi H, Doerr RJ, et al. Immunoscintigraphy performed with In-111-labeled CYT-103 in the management of colorectal cancer: comparison with CT. Radiology 1992; 185: 179–186.
2. Neal CE, Baker MR, Hilgers RD, et al. In-111 CYT-103 immunoscintigraphy in the imaging of ovarian carcinoma. Clin Nucl Med 1993; 18: 472–476.
3. Kit for the preparation of Satumomab Pendetide, Oncoscint CR/OV. Cytogen Corporation, Princeton, NJ. Last revised December 30, 1992.

Special Imaging Procedures

Lee A. Forstrom

Lymphoscintigraphy of the Extremities

Summary Information

Radiopharmaceutical	^{99m}Tc antimony colloid is used in a volume of 0.1 ml per injection site. If ^{99m}Tc antimony colloid is not available, filtered ^{99m}Tc sulfur colloid can be used (see following section entitled "Radiopharmaceutical Preparation"). Maximum doses that can be injected follow:
Adults (older than 18 years):	Up to 1 mCi (37 MBq) per injection site, with 2 mCi or less (74 MBq) total.
Children (12–18 years):	Up to 500 μCi (18.5 MBq) per injection site, with 1 mCi or less (34 MBq) total.
Children (1–12 years):	Up to 250 μCi (9.25 MBq) per injection site, with 500 μCi or less (18.5 MBq) total.
Children (birth–1 year):	Up to 15 μCi (0.56 MBq) per injection site, with 30 μCi or less (1.11 MBq) total.
Contraindications	Lymphangiography performed within the previous week.
Dose/Scan Interval	Imaging begins immediately after injection.
Views Obtained	0–1 hour: Anterior view of the groin for foot injection or anterior view of the axillary nodes for hand injection. More than 1 hour: Anterior and posterior whole-body views.

Indications

Chronic lymphedema is a progressive, usually painless swelling of the extremity that develops because of decreased transport capacity of the lymphatic system. Lymphoscintigraphy is indicated in the diagnosis of primary or secondary lymphedema and in the differential diagnosis of the swollen extremity, when lymphedema, venous disease, or lipedema is considered.[1,2] Lymphoscintigraphy can also be used to identify viable lymph channels before lymphovenous anastomosis.[3]

Principle

^{99m}Tc-labeled colloidal particles, with a particle size less than 100 nm, are injected subcutaneously into the foot or hand. They are transported from the injection site to the liver through the lymphatic system.[4] Total or partial obstruction of the lymphatic system should be seen as a failure or a decrease in the number of radiolabeled colloidal particles to progress beyond the site of blockage.

Radiopharmaceutical Preparation

If ^{99m}Tc antimony colloid is not available, the following procedure can be used to generate colloidal particles of less than 100 nm in size.

1. Draw 1 ml of ^{99m}Tc sulfur colloid (25–30 mCi/925–1,110 MBq) into a lead-shielded 3-ml syringe.
2. Carefully remove the needle of the ^{99m}Tc sulfur colloid syringe, and aseptically attach the syringe to the female inlet of a sterile 0.1-µm filter (Millex-VV, Millipore Corp., Bedford, MA).
3. Attach a fresh 23-gauge needle to the male outlet end of the filter. Push the 1 ml of solution through the filter into a 5-ml sterile vial. This will give approximately 15 mCi (555 MBq) in 0.9 ml.
4. Add 2 ml of sterile saline to the vial to give a final concentration of approximately 5 mCi/ml (185 MBq/ml).
5. For each injection site, inject 0.1 ml of the filtered ^{99m}Tc sulfur colloid subcutaneously, using a 1-ml tuberculin syringe and a 27-gauge needle. This will give a dose of 400–500 µCi (14.8–18.5 MBq) ^{99m}Tc per injection.

Patient Preparation

The procedure should be explained fully to the patient. The patient needs to remove articles of clothing and any bandages that cover the injection site. If the patient wears elastic stockings, these generally should be removed 3–4 hours before the study. Occasionally, this cannot be done and the presence of elastic stockings should be considered in the interpretation. The injection itself is often associated with an intense stinging sensation that lasts for several seconds.

For studies of the legs, the patient should be encouraged to walk as much as possible in the time between the 1- and 3-hour images.

Instrument Specifications

Initial Images (0–I Hour)

Gamma camera:	Any large field-of-view system can be used.
Collimator:	Low-energy all-purpose collimator.
Energy setting:	140 keV, 15–20% energy window.
Analog formatter:	8 × 10 film, 70-mm (9 on 1) format.
Computer system:	Acquisition requirements—dynamic (64 × 64 word mode matrix).
	Processing requirements—dynamic display.

Delayed Images (More Than I Hour)

Gamma camera:	Single- or dual-head whole-body system.
Collimator:	Low-energy high-resolution collimator.
Energy setting:	140 keV, 15–20% energy window.
Analog formatter:	8 × 10 or 10 × 14 film, whole-body format.

Computer system: Acquisition requirements—whole-body (512 × 128 word mode matrix).
Processing requirements—none.

Additional items: Leg ergometer for lower extremity imaging or 2 squeeze balls for upper extremity imaging.

Imaging Procedure

1. Injections.
   a. *Foot injection*—If available, securely position the leg ergometer on the imaging table, as shown in Figure 11-1. Position the patient on the imaging table, with the gamma camera positioned over the groin and the feet placed in the leg ergometer, as shown in Figure 11-2.
   b. *Hand injection*—Position the patient supine on the imaging table. The patient should be given squeeze balls to hold in each hand. The gamma camera should be positioned over the axilla.
2. Check that the procedure has been explained to the patient.
3. The nuclear medicine physician will inject the ^{99m}Tc-labeled colloidal particle solution. The injection site should be cleaned 3 times with alcohol or povidone-iodine to prevent infection. The colloid solution is injected 1–3 mm deep subcutaneously into the webbing between the 2nd and 3rd toes or fingers, generally of both upper limbs or of both lower limbs.
4. Acquire 12 static images at 5 minutes per image on the analog formatter for 1 hour. Acquire a dynamic study on the computer (12 frames at 5 minutes per frame, 64 × 64 word mode matrix).
5. Immediately after the injection, instruct the patient to exercise the feet by alternate flexion and extension or to pedal the leg ergometer (foot injection) or to exercise the hand using the squeeze ball (hand injection). The patient initially should exercise for 5 minutes and, thereafter, for 1 minute every 10 minutes up to 1 hour.

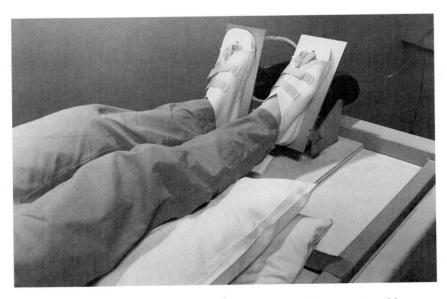

Figure 11-1. Leg ergometer in position at the end of the imaging table.

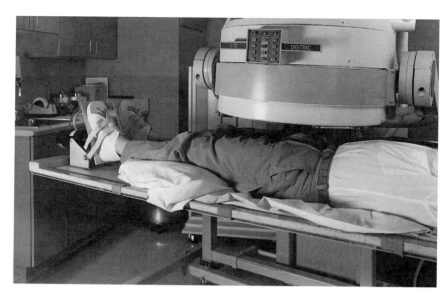

Figure 11-2. Patient with legs in ergometer and gamma camera positioned over the groin. A pillow may be placed under the knees for comfort.

6. At 1 and 3 hours after injection, acquire anterior and posterior whole-body images on the analog formatter and computer (512 × 128 word mode matrix). Images should be acquired at a scan speed of 15 cm/min. Occasionally, small ^{57}Co markers can be used to determine the location of tracer activity and/or to provide anatomic landmarks.
7. Occasionally, whole-body images may be required at 6 and 24 hours after injection.
8. For leg studies, encourage the patient to walk as much as possible between the 1-hour, 3-hour, and later images.

Computer Analysis

No analysis is required. The dynamic study can be viewed in cine mode to determine tracer movement into the region around the groin or thorax.

Information on film

On each analog and computer film, ensure that the following information is recorded:

1. Patient name and clinic/hospital number
2. Date and time of each image after injection
3. Type of scan and radiopharmaceutical dose injected
4. Orientation of each image

Interpretation

Normally, activity appears in the regional lymph nodes (groin or axilla) about 15–60 minutes after injection. Any appearance before 10–15 minutes suggests high-output lymphatic

Table 11-1. Absorbed Radiation Dose Estimates[a] in a 70-kg Adult
From 2 mCi (74 MBq) ^{99m}Tc Antimony Colloid

| | Absorbed Radiation Doses | | | |
| | Source in Liver | | Source in Bladder | |
Tissue	rad/2 mCi	mGy/74 MBq	rad/2 mCi	mGy/74 MBq
Urinary bladder wall	0.00	0.00	2.80	28.0
Bone (total)	0.00	0.02	0.02	0.16
Liver	0.80	8.00	0.00	0.00
Ovaries	0.01	0.08	0.12	1.20
Testes	0.00	0.01	0.08	0.80
Red marrow	0.00	0.03	0.04	0.40
Uterus	0.01	0.08	0.28	2.80
Blood	0.04	0.40	0.00	0.03
Total body	0.04	0.40	0.00	0.03

[a]Estimated dose to the skin at the injection site (assuming all activity remains at injection site): 66 rad/2 mCi (660 mGy/74 MBq). Estimated dose to lymph node (assuming uptake of 0.4% per node, with no clearance of activity from node): 40 rad/2 mCi (400 mGy/74 MBq).

failure. A transit time greater than 60 minutes indicates delayed lymphatic transport. Early liver uptake without activity in the abdominal nodes suggests IV injection. Uptake of the tracer in the lymph nodes is not always predictable, even in normal subjects. Nevertheless, abnormal patterns for nodes can be defined with respect to uptake intensity and the number of lymph nodes, such as (1) no lymph node uptake, (2) marked asymmetry, and (3) mild asymmetry. Quantitative evaluation of lymphatic transport does not appear to add additional information to this procedure.[5,6]

Additional Notes

The leg ergometer should give an exercise level similar to a very light setting on a stair-climbing machine. Squeeze balls should be similar to those commonly used in physiotherapy. Standardization of muscular exercise is thought to help in the reproducibility of this procedure.[6]

Radiation Dosimetry

Dosimetry for filtered ^{99m}Tc sulfur colloid and ^{99m}Tc antimony trisulfide colloid are similar, because the distribution of the activity, metabolism, and excretion are similar. The estimated absorbed doses in organs and tissues of an average subject (70 kg) from administration of 2 mCi (74 MBq) ^{99m}Tc antimony trisulfide colloid are shown in Table 11-1.[7]

References

1. Gloviczki P, Wahner HW. Clinical diagnosis and evaluation of lymphedema. In "Vascular Surgery," 4th Edition, ed RB Rutherford. W.B. Saunders, Philadelphia, 1995, pp 1899–1920.

2. Larcos G, Wahner HW. Lymphoscintigraphic abnormalities in venous thrombosis (clinical conference). J Nucl Med 1991; 32: 2144–2148.

3. Kleinhans E, Baumeister RG, Hahn D, et al. Evaluation of transport kinetics in lymphoscintigraphy: follow-up study in patients with transplanted lymphatic vessels. Eur J Nucl Med 1985; 10: 349–352.

4. Bergqvist L, Strand SE, Persson BR. Particle sizing and biokinetics of interstitial lymphoscintigraphic agents. Semin Nucl Med 1983; 13: 9–19.

5. Gloviczki P, Calcagno D, Schirger A, et al. Noninvasive evaluation of the swollen extremity: experiences with 190 lymphoscintigraphic examinations. J Vasc Surg 1989; 9: 683–689.

6. Vaqueiro M, Gloviczki P, Fisher J, et al. Lymphoscintigraphy in lymphedema: an aid to microsurgery. J Nucl Med 1986; 27: 1125–1130.

7. Technetium Tc-99m antimony trisulfide colloid kit. Package insert, Cadema Medical Products, Middletown, NY, October 1984.

Dacryoscintigraphy

Summary Information

Radiopharmaceutical

Adult dose: ^{99m}Tc sodium pertechnetate, 200 µCi (7.4 MBq [per drop] approximately 10 µl) for each eye.

Pediatric dose: Adjusted according to the patient's weight (see Appendix A-3).

Contraindications Note that marked epiphora (tearing) during the study can lead to contamination of the skin around the eye and hinder interpretation.

Dose/Scan Interval Imaging commences immediately after ^{99m}Tc sodium pertechnetate is placed in the eye.

Views Anterior views of each eye.

Indications

One of the most common causes of epiphora is obstruction in the lacrimal drainage apparatus. Common sites of obstruction are the sac–duct junction, canaliculus–sac junction, and individual canaliculi. Note that filling of the tear sac with debris, mucus, or pus can lead to misdiagnosis of a proximal obstruction.

Principle

A radioactive solution (similar to eye drops) is introduced into the conjunctival sac of the eye and follows the flow of the tear solution through the lacrimal drainage system. A comparable radiographic dacryocystogram is rather difficult and involves cannulation of the lacrimal canal.[1]

Patient Preparation

Have the patient remove his or her eyeglasses and wipe the eyes. If mucus or pus is present, the eyes should be cleaned and the tear sac should be massaged before starting dacryoscintigraphy. This is a high-resolution study; thus, the patient's head should be held firmly in place with a headrest such as that shown in Figure 11-3.

Instrument Specifications

Gamma camera: Any large field-of-view system can be used.

519

Collimators:	Pinhole collimator with 2–4-mm insert.
Energy setting:	140 keV, 15–20% energy window.
Analog formatter:	8 × 10 film, 70-mm (9-on-1) format.
Computer system:	Acquisition requirements—static (256 × 256 matrix).
	Processing requirements—none.
Additional item:	Headrest—adapted from a slit-lamp apparatus (see Fig. 11-3).

Imaging Procedure

1. Prepare a solution containing 15 mCi (555 MBq) ^{99m}Tc pertechnetate in 0.2 ml sterile saline.
2. Position the patient upright in a chair with the chin on the chin rest of the head holder. The pinhole collimator should be placed approximately 5 cm from the bridge of the nose, so both eyes are in the field of view, as shown in Figure 11-4. If only one eye is to be examined, place the collimator 2–3 cm in front of that eye. Figure 11-5 shows the normal distribution of the radiotracer relative to the eye and nose and illustrates the need for close patient-to-collimator distance to permit resolution of the radiotracer distribution in the lacrimal system.
3. The nuclear medicine physician should place 1 drop of sterile ^{99m}Tc pertechnetate solution into the lateral part of the conjunctival sac of the lower lid of each eye by means of a micropipette or tuberculin syringe equipped with a special beveled needle (blunt tip).
4. Acquire images of both eyes on the analog formatter at 1 and 5 minutes after the drop has been placed for 100 kct or 1 minute, whichever is shorter. *Note:* Even very slight head movement will blur the images of the eye; thus, the technologist may need to hold the

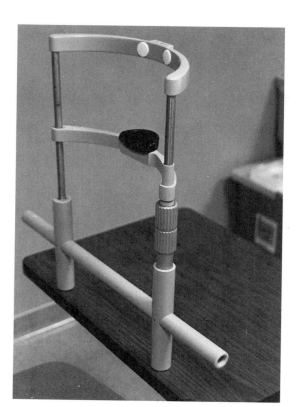

Figure 11-3. Headrest (modified from an ophthalmic slit-lamp apparatus) for dacryoscintigraphy.

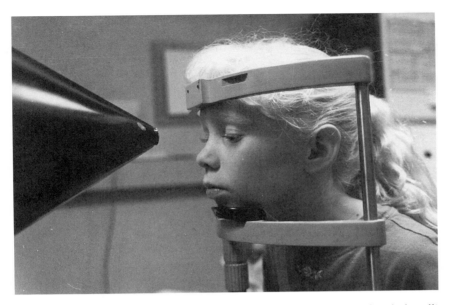

Figure 11-4. Patient in position with the bridge of the nose 5 cm in front of pinhole collimator.

patient's head for each picture. Additional images should be acquired at 10, 15, 20, 25, and 30 minutes for the same time as the 5-minute image.

5. Images should be acquired on a computer in a 256×256 matrix for 1 minute per image.
6. At the conclusion of the procedure, the eyes should be flushed with sterile water to reduce the absorbed radiation dose to the eyes.

Computer Analysis

None required.

Figure 11-5. Superposition of dacryoscintigram on view of eye, showing canaliculi, tear sac, and tear duct as well as functional stenosis at Hasner's valve (arrow). (From Denffer et al.,[1] with permission.)

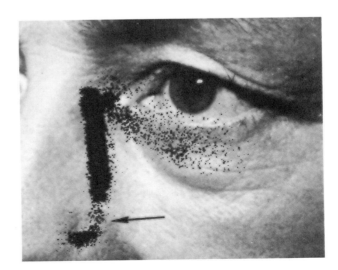

Information on Film

On each analog and computer film, ensure that the following information is recorded:

1. Patient name and clinic/hospital number
2. Date and time of each image after placement of the eye drops
3. Type of scan and radiopharmaceutical dose used
4. Orientation of each image (e.g., anterior)

Interpretation

Normal

In normal studies, drainage through the lacrimal apparatus to the nasal lacrimal duct is seen on the 5-minute view.

Abnormal

In cases of obstruction, delay of lacrimal flow may be unilateral or bilateral and can occur at the individual canaliculus, canaliculus–sac junction, sac–duct junction, within the lacrimal duct, or at Hasner's valve.[1-3]

Additional Notes

None.

Radiation Dosimetry

The estimated absorbed doses in organs and tissues of an average subject (70 kg) from the ophthalmic administration of 0.4 mCi (14.8 MBq) of ^{99m}Tc sodium pertechnetate are shown in Table 11-2.[4] These doses do not take into account any activity removed by washing the eyes after completion of the study.

Table 11-2. Absorbed Radiation Dose Estimates in a 70-kg Adult From Opthalmic Administration of 0.4 mCi (14.8 MBq) ^{99m}Tc Sodium Pertechnetate

Tissue	Absorbed Radiation Dose		
	rad/0.4 mCi	mGy/14.8 MBq	Comments
Eye lens	0.06	0.56	Lacrimal fluid turnover = 16%/min
	0.01	0.08	Lacrimal fluid turnover = 100%/min
	1.62	16.2	Drainage system is blocked
Ovaries	0.01	0.12	No blockage
Testes	0.00	0.04	No blockage
Thyroid	0.05	0.52	No blockage

References

1. Denffer NV, Dressler H, Pabst HW. Lacrimal dacryoscintigraphy. Semin Nucl Med 1984; 14: 8–15.
2. Amanat LA, Hiilditch TE, Kwok CS. Lacrimal scintigraphy. II. Its role in the diagnosis of epiphora. Br J Ophthalmol 1983; 67: 720–728.
3. Blanksma LJ, Schweitzer NMJ, Beekhuis H, Piers DA. Testing of lacrimal drainage with the aid of a gamma-ray emitting radiopharmaceutical (^{99m}Tc0$_4^-$). Doc Ophthalmol 1977; 42: 381–384.
4. Madsen MT, Ponto JL. "Medical Physics Handbook of Nuclear Medicine." Medical Physics Publishing, Madison WI, 1992, p 38.

LeVeen Shunt Patency

Summary Information

Radiopharmaceutical

Adult dose:
Shunt injection—500 µCi (18.5 MBq) ^{99m}Tc sulfur colloid.

Intraperitoneal injection—4 mCi (148 MBq) ^{99m}Tc macroaggregated albumin (MAA).

Pediatric dose:
Adjusted according to the patient's weight (see Appendix A-3).

Contraindications
Perfusion lung scan performed within 24 hours preceding the study.

Dose/Scan Interval

Shunt tubing injection:
Imaging commences immediately after injection.

Intraperitoneal injection:
Imaging commences about 10 minutes after injection.

Views Obtained

Shunt injection:
Anterior view of the injection site and liver.

Intraperitoneal injection:
Anterior view of the abdomen and lungs.

Indications

Peritoneovenous shunts, such as the LeVeen shunt, consist of tubing that runs subcutaneously along the chest wall and drains into a large central vein, such as the internal or external jugular vein. If abdominal pressure exceeds intrathoracic pressure by more than 3–5 cm H_2O, a one-way valve at the abdominal end of the shunt opens to drain ascites into the venous system.[1] LeVeen shunts generally are implanted in patients with intractable ascites. Evaluation of shunt patency is required in patients who have reaccumulation of excess ascitic fluid. This may be due to worsening of their medical condition or to valve malfunction or thrombosis of the shunt tubing.

Principle

The status of a peritoneovenous shunt can be evaluated by injecting a radiopharmaceutical either directly into the shunt tubing or into the peritoneal cavity. Some investigators prefer direct injection into the shunt tubing, because this provides a more rapid assessment of shunt function, with reduced radiation exposure to the patient.[2] Note that ^{99m}Tc MAA should not be used for direct injection, because of its tendency to precipitate and adhere to the wall of the tubing.[2] In cases in which a direct injection into the shunt tubing is not

525

possible, an intraperitoneal injection can be administered.[3] In a functioning shunt, intraperitoneal ^{99m}Tc MAA is transported through the shunt, enters the venous circulation, and becomes trapped in the lungs. Hence, shunt patency can be confirmed by the appearance of a lung image. This procedure only works if intra-abdominal pressure is sufficient to open the shunt.

Patient Preparation

None.

Instrument Specifications

Gamma camera:	Any large field-of-view system can be used.
Collimator:	Low-energy, all-purpose collimator.
Energy setting:	140 keV, 15–20% energy window.
Analog formatter:	8 × 10 film, 70-mm (9-on-1) format.
Computer system:	Acquisition requirements—static (256 × 256 matrix), dynamic (64 × 64 matrix). Processing requirements—region of interest (ROI) analysis curve generation for shunt tubing injection.

Imaging Procedure

Either procedure A or B, following, can be used.

A—Shunt Tubing Injection

1. Position the patient supine on the imaging table, and inject 500 μCi (18.5 MBq) ^{99m}Tc sulfur colloid directly into the shunt tubing.
2. The injected volume of ^{99m}Tc sulfur colloid should not exceed 0.2 ml, and the injection should be administered with a 26-gauge needle.
3. Immediately after the injection, position the gamma camera above the injection site, and acquire images on the analog formatter (9 images, at 3 minutes per image) and on computer (64 × 64 word mode matrix, 30 images at 1 minute per image).
4. If no significant clearance of activity from the tubing is seen by 30 minutes, acquire an additional image at 3 hours on the analog formatter (200 kct or 10 minutes) and on computer (64 × 64 word mode matrix, 5 minutes per image).

B—Intraperitoneal Injection

1. Position the patient supine on the imaging table. A paracentesis tray is required. The injection site should be prepared and covered with dressings. Leakage of the ascites may occur and require a change of dressing. The intraperitoneal injection of 4 mCi (148 MBq) ^{99m}Tc MAA should be administered by a nuclear medicine physician.
2. Immediately after the injection, roll the patient from side to side to mix the ^{99m}Tc MAA within the ascites.
3. At 10 minutes after injection, acquire an anterior image of the lungs on an analog formatter (300 kct) and on computer (256 × 256 word mode matrix, 300 kct per image).
4. Additional images should be acquired at 20, 30, and 60 minutes after injection.
5. If no activity is seen in the lungs by 1 hour, an additional image should be acquired at 6 hours after injection to confirm shunt obstruction.

Computer Analysis

Shunt tubing injection: Place a region of interest (ROI) around the injection site, and generate a time–activity curve to determine the movement of the ^{99m}Tc sulfur colloid from the injection site over the 30-minute scan period.

Information on Film

On each analog and computer film, ensure that the following information is recorded:

1. Patient name and clinic/hospital number
2. Date and time of each image after injection
3. Type of scan, radiopharmaceutical, and injection site
4. Orientation of each image (e.g., anterior)

Interpretation

Shunt tubing injection: Over the 30-minute period, clearance of activity from the injection site should be nearly complete, with visualization of the liver.

Intraperitoneal injection: With a patent shunt, activity should pass rapidly into the lungs, with clear visualization of lung activity at 10 minutes after injection. The shunt tubing may be visible as activity passes through it. Absence of lung activity or a delay in activity appearing in the lungs is indicative of total or partial occlusion of the shunt.

Radiation Dosimetry

The estimated absorbed doses in organs and tissues in an average subject (70 kg) from the intraperitoneal injection of 4 mCi (148 MBq) ^{99m}Tc MAA or from a direct shunt injection of 0.5 mCi (18.5 MBq) ^{99m}Tc sulfur colloid are shown in Tables 11-3 and 11-4, respectively.[4,5]

Table 11-3. Absorbed Radiation Dose Estimates in a 70-kg Adult From Intraperitoneal Injection of 4 mCi (148 MBq) ^{99m}Tc Macroaggregated Albumin

| | Absorbed Radiation Doses | | | |
| | Shunt Patent | | Shunt Occluded | |
Tissue	rad/4 mCi	mGy/148 MBq	rad/4 mCi	mGy/148 MBq
Lungs	0.92	9.20	0.22	2.20
Testes	0.02	0.20	0.22	2.20
Ovaries	0.04	0.40	0.22	2.20
Organs in the peritoneal cavity	—	—	0.22	2.20
Total body	0.05	0.50	0.08	0.80

Table 11-4. Absorbed Radiation Dose Estimates in a 70-kg Adult
From 0.5 mCi (18.5 MBq) ^{99m}Tc Sulfur Colloid

Tissue	Absorbed Radiation Dose	
	rad/0.5 mCi	mGy/18.5 MBq
Liver	0.17	1.70
Spleen	0.11	1.05
Bone marrow	0.01	0.14
Testes	0.00	0.01
Ovaries	0.00	0.03
Total body	0.01	0.09

References

1. Stewart CA, Sakimura IT, Applebaum DM, Siegel ME. Evaluation of peritoneovenous shunt patency by intraperitoneal Tc-99m macroaggregated albumin: clinical experience. AJR 1986; 147: 177–180.
2. Rosenthall L, Arzoumanian A, Hampson LG, Shennib H. Observations on the radionuclide assessment of peritoneovenous shunt patency. Clin Nucl Med 1984; 9: 227–235.
3. Algeo JH Jr, Powell M, Couacaud J. LeVeen shunt visualization without function using technetium-99m macroaggregated albumin. Clin Nucl Med 1987; 12: 741–743.
4. TechneScan MAA: Kit for the preparation of technetium Tc-99m albumin aggregated. Package insert Mallinckrodt Inc., St. Louis. Last revised June 1988.
5. MIRD dose estimate report no. 3. Summary of current radiation dose estimates to humans with various liver conditions from technetium 99m Tc-sulfur colloid. J Nucl Med 1975; 16: 108A–108B.

12

Therapy Procedures

Gregory A. Wiseman

^{131}I Therapy (Less Than 30 mCi)

Summary Information

Radiopharmaceutical
^{131}I sodium iodide: The administered dose is 3.0–29.9 mCi (111–1,106 MBq). The treatment dose is determined by the physician and may be either a fixed dose or a calculated dose to give a predetermined activity per gram of thyroid tissue (based on gland size and thyroid ^{131}I uptake).

Characteristics: ^{131}I sodium iodide is a clear colorless solution intended for oral administration. ^{131}I has a half-life of 8.08 days and emits both gamma particles (principal gamma ray energy = 364 keV) and beta particles (principal beta particle energy = 0.606 MeV). The beta particles have a maximal range of 2.1 mm in soft tissue.

Contraindications
1. The patient must not be pregnant or breast-feeding.
2. The patient must have had an ^{131}I thyroid scan or a thyroid uptake measurement within the last 2 weeks or approval from the nuclear medicine physician.
3. The patient must have stopped taking all antithyroid medications for at least 2 days.
4. The patient must not have received any iodinated IV contrast material within the last 3–4 weeks, because this will affect the uptake of ^{131}I.
5. Check that the patient is not taking any food or vitamins rich in iodine.

Indications

^{131}I therapy is indicated for patients who have an overactive thyroid gland (hyperthyroid). The principal disease conditions for which a well-defined therapy has been established are diffuse toxic goiter (Graves' disease) and toxic nodular goiter.[1-3] In addition, ^{131}I may be indicated for the ablation of residual thyroid tissue after subtotal thyroidectomy for thyroid cancer.[4,5]

Principle

Radioiodine (^{131}I) is taken up by functioning thyroid tissue and used in thyroid hormone synthesis. The 0.6-MeV beta particles emitted by ^{131}I travel only 1–2 mm in soft tissue and radiate the immediate local tissue around the area where the ^{131}I is concentrated, thus decreasing both the output of thyroid hormones and the size of the thyroid gland.

Patient Preparation

All premenopausal women 13–50 years old must have a serum pregnancy test performed within 80 hours and the test results available before the treatment. The only exception is if a patient has been sterilized surgically (hysterectomy or tubal ligation).

Therapy Procedure

1. The authorized nuclear medicine technologist should complete the radioisotope therapy form (written directive), as shown in Figure 12-1, based on the information obtained from the referring physician's notes and laboratory test results in the patient's medical history. The authorized nuclear medicine physician treating the patient should verify the information listed on the radioisotope therapy form and sign it. The nuclear medical technologist should not draw the dose to be administered until the information listed on the radioisotope therapy form has been verified and signed by the physician.
2. The authorized nuclear medicine physician and the referring physician will decide on the desired activity to be delivered to the thyroid gland, either in the form microcuries per gram of tissue or as a fixed dose. The microcurie per gram dose is generally in the range of

Radioisotope Therapy
MAYO CLINIC

Sheet No. ______
☐ RADIOIODINE Date ______

Diagnosis: ☐ Graves ☐ Toxic Nodular Goiter ☐ Remnant Ablation ☐ Metastatic Thyroid Cancer
Pregnancy Test: ☐ Positive ☐ Negative ☐ Not Needed
Breast Feeding: ☐ Yes ☐ No
Thyroid Size Estimate: ____ gm Endocrine Consultant: ______
Dose Requested (μCi/gm): ☐ Small (75) ☐ Mod (125) ☐ Large (200)
☐ Ablative (29.9 mCi)
☐ Cancer Therapy Dose ______ mCi
Diagnostic: ____ Hour ^{131}I Uptake ____ % Dose

Present Admission Lab Tests
T T_4 ___ T_3 ___ TBG ___ TSI ___
F T_4 ___ S TSH ___

Cancer Patients
Thyroglobulin ___
WBC ___

Previous ^{131}I Therapy Dose

Date	Dose (mCi)
1)	
2)	
3)	
4)	
5)	
6)	

Cumulative Dose ______ mCi

External Beam Therapy
Treatment Site: ______
Cumulative Dose: ______
Completion Date: ______

Comments ______

Physician's signature Date

RADIONUCLIDE DOSE ADMINISTERED: ____ mCi

TREATMENT DOSE CALCULATION

$$\frac{\text{Gland Size (\quad) gm} \times (\quad)\ \mu\text{Ci/gm}}{(\quad)\ \%\ \text{Uptake} \times 10} = ____\ \text{mCi}$$

Manufacturer ______ Control # ______
Calibration Date ______ Calibration Activity (mCi/ml) ______
Correction Factor ______ Route ______
Calculated Activity (mCi/ml) ______
ml to be Administered ______
Technologist ______ M.D. ______
Second Technologist to Confirm the Measured Dose ______

PATIENT MONITORING FOR CANCER TREATMENT

Date	Measured mR/hr at 1 meter	Calculated Remaining mCi

MC 670/R1292

Figure 12-1. Radioisotope therapy form. The equations for calculation of the patient's treatment dose are given in the upper right section of the form.

75–200 μCi/g of tissue. For a target dose (in terms of microcurie per gram of tissue), the amount of ^{131}I to be dispensed is based on the formula

$$\frac{\text{Gland Size (\quad) g} \times \text{(\quad) μCi/g}}{\text{(\quad) \% Uptake} \times 10} = \underline{\hspace{2cm}} \text{ mCi Administered Dose}$$

3. The prescribing physician will discuss the treatment and radiation precautions with the patient and will verify the dose calculations.

4. After the physician verifies the dose, draw the required dose of ^{131}I into a shielded specimen cup, as shown in Figure 12-2, under a vented fume hood. Assay the dose in the dose calibrator (**check that dose calibrator is set on** ^{131}**I**).

5. A dose verification must also be performed by a second staff technologist or the physician before the dose is administered. This second person must sign his or her initials to the radioisotope therapy form.

6. The required dose of ^{131}I in the small specimen vial should be diluted by adding 30 ml of water. Place the vial in a shielded lead cup (Fig. 12-2).

7. The patient should be asked to repeat his or her name and to provide a second form of identification (e.g., birth date, clinic number, driver's license, or confirmation by a second person such as a family member or accompanying nurse). The dose is then administered orally to the patient.

8. After the patient has swallowed the dose, refill the vial with 30 ml of water. Recap the vial, and swirl it to dilute any remaining ^{131}I sodium iodide. Have the patient drink the 30 ml of water. Repeat this process with another 30 ml of water to ensure that all the activity has been administered.

9. The dose should be administered in a therapy room, which should be a small room with nonabsorbent surfaces to permit easy containment and decontamination of any spills that may occur. A disposable absorbent sheet should be placed on the floor to contain any spilled droplets of liquid.

10. The patient should be instructed on radiation safety precautions as outlined later in "Additional Notes" and then should be dismissed. The therapy technologist must complete the information on the radioisotope therapy form and in the patient's medical record to ensure that all documentation is complete.

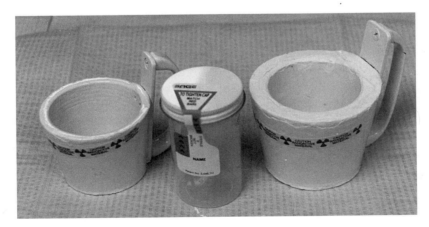

Figure 12-2. Specimen vial and lead cups used to contain patient dose of ^{131}I sodium iodide. The smaller lead cup is used for doses less than 30 mCi (1,110 MBq).

11. All waste should be discarded in the radioactive waste container. Monitor the therapy room after the patient is dismissed. Monitor the hands and feet of all medical personnel who were in the therapy room during the procedure.

Additional Notes

Radiation safety instructions for patients after therapy. Unless otherwise stated, these precautions should be followed for **2 days** after therapy.

1. Avoid prolonged contact with other people (closer than 3 feet).
2. Completely avoid contact with pregnant women and young children.
3. Sleep in a separate bed for 2 nights.
4. Do not have sexual relations.
5. If sexually active, men and women should prevent pregnancy for 6–12 months by using a reliable birth control method.
6. Women should stop breast-feeding before receiving ^{131}I therapy.
7. Wash hands well after using the toilet. If any urine is seen outside the toilet, clean it up with a disposable tissue and flush the tissue down the toilet. Flush the toilet twice after each use.
8. Drink 10 glasses (8 oz each) of liquid each day.
9. Rinse undergarments in a sink or tub before placing them in the washing machine with other laundry.
10. Separate eating utensils and cups should be used.

Radiation Dosimetry

The estimated absorbed doses in organs and tissues of an average, normally functioning thyroid subject (70 kg) from an oral dose of 10 mCi (370 MBq) ^{131}I sodium iodide are shown in Table 12-1.[6]

Table 12-1. Absorbed Radiation Dose Estimates in Organs and Tissues of an Average, Normally Functioning Thyroid Subject (70 kg) From an Oral Dose of 10 mCi (370 MBq) ^{131}I Sodium Iodide

	Absorbed Radiation Dose					
	rad/10 mCi			mGy/370 MBq		
	Thyroid Uptake					
Tissue	5%	15%	25%	5%	15%	25%
Thyroid	2,600	8,000	13,000	26,000	80,000	130,000
Stomach wall	17	16	14	170	160	140
Red marrow	1.4	2.0	2.6	14	20	26
Liver	2.0	3.5	4.8	20	35	48
Testes	0.8	0.9	0.9	8	9	9
Ovaries	1.4	1.4	1.4	14	14	14
Total body	2.4	4.7	7.1	24	47	71

References

1. Becker DV, Hurley JR. Current status of radioiodine (131-I) treatment of hyperthyroidism. In "Nuclear Medicine Annual," eds Freeman LM, Weissmann HS. Raven Press, New York, 1982, pp 265–290.
2. Pineda G, Clauria HJ, Rocha AFG, Harbert JC. The thyroid. In "Textbook of Nuclear Medicine: Clinical Applications," eds Rocha AFG, Harbert JC. Lea & Febiger, Philadelphia, 1979, pp 1–50.
3. Nordyke RA, Gilbert FI Jr. Optimal iodine-131 dose for eliminating hyperthyroidism in Graves' disease. J Nucl Med 1991; 32: 411–416.
4. Massin JP, Savoie JC, Garnier H, et al. Pulmonary metastases in differentiated thyroid carcinoma: study of 58 cases with implications for the primary tumor treatment. Cancer 1984; 53: 982–992.
5. Hurley JR, Becker DV. Treatment of thyroid carcinoma with radioiodine. In "Diagnostic Nuclear Medicine," eds Gottschalk A, Hoffer PB, Potchen EJ. Williams & Wilkins, Baltimore, 1988, pp 792–814.
6. Summary of current radiation dose estimates to humans from ^{123}I, ^{124}I, ^{125}I, ^{126}I, ^{130}I, ^{131}I, and ^{132}I as sodium iodide. J Nucl Med 1975; 16: 857–860.

^{131}I Therapy (30 mCi or More)

Summary Information

Radiopharmaceutical

^{131}I sodium iodide: The administered dose is 30–300 mCi (1.11–11.10 GBq). The treatment dose is determined by the nuclear medicine physician in consultation with the referring physician.

Characteristics: ^{131}I sodium iodide is a colorless solution intended for oral administration. ^{131}I has a half-life of 8.08 days and emits both gamma particles (principal gamma ray energy = 364 keV) and beta particles (principal beta particle energy = 0.606 MeV). The beta particles have a maximal range of 2.1 mm in soft tissue.

Contraindications

1. The patient must not be pregnant or breast-feeding.
2. A patient with thyroid cancer must have had an ^{131}I whole-body scan within the last 2 weeks.
3. A patient undergoing ablation of residual thyroid tissue must have had an ^{131}I scan showing a thyroid remnant within the 2 weeks preceding therapy.
4. The patient must have stopped taking all antithyroid medications for at least 2 days.
5. The patient must not have received any iodinated IV contrast material within the last 3–4 weeks, because this will affect the uptake of ^{131}I.

Indications

High-dose ^{131}I therapy (30 mCi or more) is indicated in patients who have residual thyroid cancer after thyroidectomy that shows iodine uptake.[1,2] ^{131}I may also be indicated for the ablation of residual thyroid tissue after subtotal thyroidectomy for thyroid cancer.[3,4]

Principle

Radioiodine (^{131}I) is taken up by normal functioning thyroid tissue and used in thyroid hormone synthesis. It is also taken up by most thyroid carcinomas, particularly well-differentiated ones. The 0.6-MeV beta particles emitted by ^{131}I travel only 1–2 mm in soft tissue and radiate the immediate local tissue around the area where the ^{131}I is concentrated, destroying both tumor cells and normal thyroid cells.

Patient Preparation

All premenopausal women 13–50 years old must have a serum pregnancy test performed within 80 hours and test results available before the treatment. The only exception is if a patient has been sterilized surgically (hysterectomy or tubal ligation).

Patients must be hospitalized for the administration of ^{131}I therapy doses of 30 mCi (1.11 GBq) or greater.

Therapy Procedure

1. The authorized nuclear medicine technologist should complete the radioisotope therapy form (written directive), as shown in Figure 12-1, based on the information obtained from the referring physician's notes and the laboratory test results in the patient's medical history. The authorized nuclear medicine physician treating the patient should verify the information listed on the radioisotope therapy form and sign it. The nuclear medicine technologist should not draw the dose to be administered until the information listed on the radioisotope therapy form has been verified and signed by the physician.

2. The prescribing physician will discuss the treatment with the patient and will verify the volume to be given, based on the prescribed dose and the specific activity of the ^{131}I.

3. After the physician verifies the dose, draw the required dose of ^{131}I into a shielded specimen cup, as shown in Figure 12-2. Assay the dose in the dose calibrator (**check that the dose calibrator is set on ^{131}I**).

4. A dose verification must be performed by a second staff technologist. This second technologist must sign his or her initials to the radioisotope therapy form.

5. The required dose of ^{131}I in the small specimen cup should be diluted with water up to a volume of 30 ml. Place the vial in a shielded lead cup (see Fig. 12-2). The vial and lead cup should then be placed in a lead cart and transported to the therapy procedure room.

6. After the physician has discussed the procedure fully with the patient, the patient should be asked to repeat his or her name and to provide a second form of identification (e.g., birth date, clinic number, driver's license, or confirmation by a second person such as a family member or accompanying nurse). Place a radioactive band on the patient's wrist. The dose is then administered orally to the patient.

7. After the patient has swallowed the dose, refill the vial with 30 ml of water. Recap the vial, and swirl it to dilute any remaining ^{131}I sodium iodide. Have the patient drink the 30 ml of water. Repeat this process with another 30 ml of water to ensure that all the activity has been administered.

8. Immediately after therapy, radioactive signs should be placed on the door to the therapy room. All the nurses attending the patient should wear a gown and gloves and have a radiation badge. Monitor the hands, feet, and laboratory coats of all medical personnel who were in the therapy room during the procedure.

9. After administration, the patient should be monitored with a radiation survey meter at a distance of 1 m to determine the exposure rate in milliroentgens per hour (mR/hr). The exposure rate should be divided by the administered activity to give a conversion factor in units of mR/hr per mCi administered or mR/hr per MBq administered.

10. The patient should be monitored on a daily basis. The measured exposure rate should be converted to millicuries (megabecquerels) ^{131}I remaining in the body by multiplying the milliroentgens per hour by the preceding conversion factor.

11. Document each daily reading on the radioisotope therapy form (see Fig. 12-1).

12. When the amount of ^{131}I remaining in the patient is calculated to be less than 30 mCi (1.11 GBq), the radioactive wrist band should be removed, and the patient should be dismissed from the hospital. Before dismissal, the patient should be instructed on radiation safety precautions, as outlined later in "Additional Notes."

    Note: The Nuclear Regulatory Commission requires that the activity in the patient be less than 30 mCi (1,110 MBq) or that the exposure rate be less than 5 mR/hr at 1 m before the patient can be dismissed.

13. The therapy technologist must complete the information on the radioisotope therapy form and master sheet of the patient's medical record to ensure that all documentation is complete.

14. The patient's room must be decontaminated and monitored before it is used in the treatment of another patient. All bedding and gowns must be monitored and stored for decay if contaminated.

15. If the patient has a medical emergency or dies before dismissal from the hospital, the radiation safety officer should be notified.

Additional Notes

The patient must be hospitalized in the designated therapy room for this procedure. This must be a private room, with a private toilet and shower. Family members are limited to 1 hr/day at 10 feet, unless special shielding is used, which may be required for pediatric patients. A leaded cart is required for transport of the dose to the therapy room.

The following list states the radiation safety instructions for the patient after dismissal from the hospital. Unless otherwise stated, these precautions should be followed for **2 days** after dismissal:

1. Avoid prolonged contact with other people (closer than 3 feet).
2. Completely avoid contact with pregnant women and young children.
3. Sleep in a separate bed for 2 nights.
4. Do not have sexual relations.
5. If sexually active, men and women should prevent pregnancy for 6–12 months by using a reliable birth control method.
6. Women should stop breast-feeding before ^{131}I therapy.
7. Wash hands well after using the toilet. If any urine is seen outside the toilet, clean it up with a disposable tissue, and flush the tissue down the toilet. Flush the toilet twice after each use.
8. Drink 10 glasses (8 oz each) of liquid each day.
9. Rinse undergarments in a sink or tub before placing them in the washing machine with other laundry.
10. Separate eating utensils and cups should be used.

Radiation Dosimetry

The estimated absorbed doses in organs and tissues of an average, normally functioning thyroid subject (70 kg) from an oral dose of 10 mCi (370 MBq) [131]I sodium iodide are shown in Table 12-1.[5]

References

1. Brown AP, Greening WP, McCready VR, Shaw HJ, Harmer CL. Radioiodine treatment of metastatic thyroid carcinoma: the Royal Marsden Hospital experience. Br J Radiol 1984; 57: 323–327.

2. Samaan NA, Maheshwari YK, Nader S, et al. Impact of therapy for differentiated carcinoma of the thyroid: an analysis of 706 cases. J Clin Endocrinol Metab 1983; 56: 1131–1138.

3. Massin JP, Savoie JC, Garnier H, et al. Pulmonary metastases in differentiated thyroid carcinoma: study of 58 cases with implications for the primary tumor treatment. Cancer 1984; 53: 982–992.

4. Hurley JR, Becker DV. Treatment of thyroid carcinoma with radioiodine. In "Diagnostic Nuclear Medicine," vol. 2, 2nd Edition, eds Gottschalk A, Hoffer PB, Potchen EJ. Williams & Wilkins, Baltimore, 1988, pp 792–814.

5. Summary of current radiation dose estimates to humans from ^{123}I, ^{124}I, ^{125}I, ^{126}I, ^{130}I, ^{131}I, and ^{132}I as sodium iodide. J Nucl Med 1975; 16: 857–860.

^{32}P Therapy for Polycythemia Vera

Summary Information

Radiopharmaceutical	^{32}P sodium phosphate: The administered dose is in the range of 1–15 mCi (37–555 MBq), usually 4–5 mCi (148–185 MBq). The exact dose will be determined by the prescribing physician.
	Characteristics: Sodium phosphate ^{32}P is a colorless liquid intended for IV administration (it should not be confused with chromic ^{32}P colloid, which is cloudy and blue). It has a half-life of 14.3 days and emits beta particles with a maximal energy of 1.7 MeV. These particles have a maximal range of 7.9 mm in tissue. Beta particles are effectively shielded by the glass vial or by a clear plastic syringe shield covering the syringe containing the ^{32}P. After the isotope is injected into the patient, external radiation hazard is minimal.
Contraindications	1. The patient should not be pregnant or breast-feeding.
	2. Low blood counts: Administration should be done with caution in patients with a leukocyte count less than $5,000/mm^3$ or a platelet count less than $150,000/mm^3$.

Indications

Phosphorus ^{32}P in the form of sodium phosphate can be used to treat myeloproliferative disorders such as polycythemia vera and essential thrombocythemia. Polycythemia vera is a disease characterized by an increased red blood cell mass, which results in an increased hematocrit. Patients with essential thrombocythemia have an increased platelet count. Patients with either of these diseases may have hyperplastic bone marrow.[1,2]

Principle

After IV administration of ^{32}P sodium phosphate, the isotope is incorporated into the actively dividing cells of the bone marrow and into trabecular and cortical bone, where it presumably is incorporated into hydroxyapatite crystal. The clearance from the blood is biexponential, with a rapid (2 days) and slow (20 days) component.[3] There appears to be considerable variability in the total radiation dose to the bone marrow, because it depends on the marrow and bone uptake as well as on its retention time in these sites. These vari-

541

ables make it difficult to predict an accurate radiation dose in each patient. Current estimates range from 20 to 50 rad/mCi (5.4–13.5 mGy/MBq) to the bone marrow.[4]

Patient Preparation

All women 13–50 years old must have a pregnancy test performed 80 hours before the treatment unless the patient has been sterilized surgically (hysterectomy or tubal ligation). The results of the pregnancy test must be available before the treatment begins.

Therapy Procedure

1. The authorized nuclear medicine technologist should complete the radioisotope therapy form (written directive), as shown in Figure 12-3, based on the information obtained from the referring physician's notes and the laboratory test results in the patient's medical history. The prescribing physician treating the patient should verify the information listed on the radioisotope therapy form (in particular, the radioisotope, administered dose, and date) and sign it. The authorized nuclear medicine technologist should not draw the dose to be administered until the information listed on the radioisotope therapy form has been verified and signed by the physician.
2. The treating physician will discuss the treatment and precautions with the patient. Radiation safety precautions involve careful hand washing after using the toilet and wearing gloves to handle any urine or contaminated clothing. This is recorded on the radioisotope therapy form (Fig. 12-3).
3. The dose should be drawn by an authorized nuclear medicine technologist. A dose verification should be performed by a second staff technologist at the time the dose is drawn. This

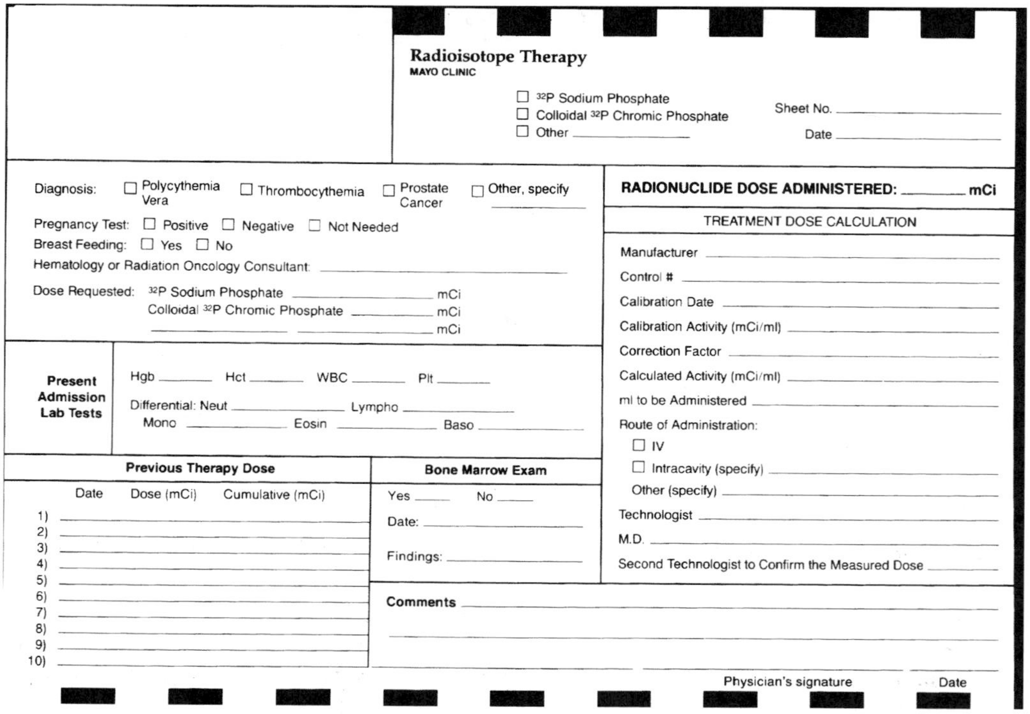

Radioisotope Therapy
MAYO CLINIC

☐ ^{32}P Sodium Phosphate
☐ Colloidal ^{32}P Chromic Phosphate
☐ Other ______

Sheet No. ______
Date ______

Diagnosis: ☐ Polycythemia Vera ☐ Thrombocythemia ☐ Prostate Cancer ☐ Other, specify ______

Pregnancy Test: ☐ Positive ☐ Negative ☐ Not Needed
Breast Feeding: ☐ Yes ☐ No
Hematology or Radiation Oncology Consultant ______

Dose Requested: ^{32}P Sodium Phosphate ______ mCi
Colloidal ^{32}P Chromic Phosphate ______ mCi
______ ______ mCi

Present Admission Lab Tests
Hgb ______ Hct ______ WBC ______ Plt ______
Differential: Neut ______ Lympho ______
Mono ______ Eosin ______ Baso ______

Previous Therapy Dose

	Date	Dose (mCi)	Cumulative (mCi)
1)			
2)			
3)			
4)			
5)			
6)			
7)			
8)			
9)			
10)			

Bone Marrow Exam
Yes ______ No ______
Date: ______
Findings: ______

RADIONUCLIDE DOSE ADMINISTERED: ______ mCi

TREATMENT DOSE CALCULATION

Manufacturer ______
Control # ______
Calibration Date ______
Calibration Activity (mCi/ml) ______
Correction Factor ______
Calculated Activity (mCi/ml) ______
ml to be Administered ______
Route of Administration:
☐ IV
☐ Intracavity (specify) ______
Other (specify) ______
Technologist ______
M.D. ______
Second Technologist to Confirm the Measured Dose ______

Comments ______

Physician's signature ______ Date ______

Figure 12-3. Radioisotope therapy form for radioisotopes other than radioiodine.

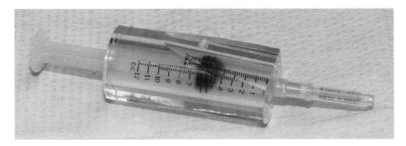

Figure 12-4. Clear plastic syringe shield used to reduce hand exposure with beta-emitting radionuclides.

second technologist should co-sign his or her initials on the radioisotope therapy form. A clear plastic syringe shield should be used to reduce hand exposure (Fig. 12-4).

4. Ask the patient to repeat his or her name and to provide a second form of identification (e.g., birth date, clinic number, driver's license, home address, or witness).
5. The IV dose should be administered only after both dose verifications have been performed, patient identification has been verified, and the physician has completed his or her discussion with the patient.
6. Great care should be taken to ensure that the dose is not extravasated, either by injecting it through a butterfly infusion set or by setting up an IV saline infusion and then injecting through the IV catheter.
7. After therapy, the patient can be dismissed and can carry out a normal daily routine.
8. The patient's blood cell counts should be checked at 4–6 weeks after therapy, or more frequently if necessary, to evaluate the response to treatment and to determine the need for further therapy doses. Therapy usually is not repeated within less than 3 months, to avoid prolonged suppression of the blood cell count.

Radiation Dosimetry

The estimated absorbed doses in organs and tissues of an average subject (70 kg) from IV injection of 4 mCi (148 MBq) ^{32}P sodium phosphate are shown in Table 12-2.[4,5]

Table 12-2. Absorbed Radiation Dose Estimates in a 70-kg Adult After Intravenous Injection of 4 mCi (148 MBq) ^{32}P Sodium Phosphate

	Absorbed Radiation Dose	
Tissue	rad/4 mCi	mGy/148 MBq
Skeleton	252.0	2,520
Liver	24.8	248
Spleen	29.3	293
Brain	12.0	120
Testes	4.0	40
Ovaries	3.3	33
Total Body	40.0	400

References

1. Berlin NI. Diagnosis and classification of polycythemias. Semin Hematol 1975; 12: 339–351.
2. Chandhuri TK. ^{32}P therapy in polycythemia vera. In "Radionuclides in Therapy," eds Spencer RP, Seevers RH Jr, Friedman AM. CRC Press, Boca Raton, FL, 1987, pp 103–110.
3. Spiers FW, Beddoe AH, King SD. The absorbed dose to bone marrow in the treatment of polycythemia by ^{32}P. Br J Radiol 1976; 49: 133–140.
4. International Commission on Radiological Protection. "Protection of the Patient in Radionuclide Investigations." ICRP Publication No. 17. Pergamon Press, Oxford, UK, 1971, p 64.
5. Sodium phosphate P-32 suspension kit, technical product data, product #461. Mallinckrodt Medical, Inc., St. Louis. Last revision August 1990.

^{32}P Intraperitoneal Therapy

Summary Information

Radiopharmaceutical ^{99m}Tc Sulfur colloid: 1 mCi (37 MBq) should be diluted into 250 ml 0.9% saline for infusion into the peritoneal cavity through an abdominal catheter. The infusion should be performed using a varistaltic pump.

^{32}P chromic phosphate: The administered dose is usually in the range of 10–15 mCi (370–555 MBq). The exact dose will be determined by the nuclear medicine physician.

Characteristics: ^{32}P chromic phosphate is a blue-green colloidal solution intended for intracavitary use only. It should not be confused with ^{32}P sodium phosphate, which is a colorless solution. ^{32}P has a half-life of 14.3 days and emits beta particles with a maximal energy of 1.7 MeV. These particles have a maximal range of 7.9 mm in soft tissue. Beta particles are effectively shielded by the glass vial or by a clear plastic syringe shield covering the syringe containing the ^{32}P. After the isotope is injected into the patient, external radiation hazard is minimal.

Contraindications   Although more than 95% of intraperitoneally administered ^{32}P chromic phosphate remains in the peritoneal cavity, some activity is present in the plasma, urine, and breast milk.[1] Thus, ^{32}P should not be administered to pregnant women or to women who are breast-feeding. The major contraindication to intracavitary ^{32}P chromic phosphate therapy is loculation of the material within the abdomen (i.e., incomplete distribution of material within the abdominal cavity, possibly because of adhesions). Hence, ^{99m}Tc sulfur colloid should be administered before intracavitary therapy to determine possible loculation.

^{99m}Tc Sulfur Colloid Dose/ Scan Interval   Imaging should commence after infusion of the ^{99m}Tc sulfur colloid and after appropriate patient maneuvers to ensure proper distribution (see following section entitled "Imaging Procedure").

Views Obtained   Anterior view of the abdomen.

Indications

^{32}P chromic phosphate colloid therapy may be used in the postoperative management of ovarian and endometrial carcinomas, because it is an effective method of destroying any malignant cells in the peritoneum.[2,3]

Principle

Within 24 hours after intracavitary administration, the distribution of ^{32}P colloidal chromic phosphate appears to be fixed, essentially with the colloidal particles adhering to the peritoneal surface either by absorption or by phagocytosis by macrophages on the surface of the serosa.[4] Less than 10% of ^{32}P chromic phosphate remains in the intracavitary fluid after 24 hours.[1] The ^{32}P delivers a high dose of radiation (several thousand rads) to the peritoneal surface, which eliminates or reduces the number of tumor cells on the peritoneal surface in the abdominal cavity.

Patient Preparation

1. All women 13–50 years old must have a pregnancy test performed within 80 hours before therapy unless the patient has been sterilized surgically (hysterectomy or tubal ligation). The results of the pregnancy test must be available before the treatment can commence.
2. Before the study, the patient should have an abdominal catheter in place. Generally, the surgeon will place one or two multiperforated catheters into the peritoneal cavity and suture them to the patient's skin (preferably using a loose purse-string suture around the site). In some instances, according to the surgeon's technique, a suture will not be placed.
3. A peritoneal distribution scan must be performed before the therapy. Administration of the ^{32}P chromic phosphate by the nuclear medicine physician or authorized nuclear medicine technologist should not proceed until the peritoneal distribution scan has shown satisfactory distribution of the ^{99m}Tc sulfur colloid.

Instrument Specifications

^{99m}Tc Sulfur Colloid Imaging

Gamma camera:	Any large field-of-view system can be used.
Collimator:	Low-energy all-purpose or low-energy high-resolution collimator.
Energy setting:	140 keV, 20% energy window for ^{99m}Tc.
Analog formatter:	8 × 10 film, 70-mm (9-on-1) format.
Computer system:	Acquisition requirements—static (256 × 256 matrix). Processing requirements—none.

Imaging Procedure

1. The technologist should move the patient into the imaging room, explain the test, and position the patient supine on the imaging table.
2. Attach a 96-inch IV solution set to a 250-ml bag of 0.9% normal saline.
3. Insert the tubing through the varistaltic pump, and flush the tubing with saline (Fig. 12-5).
4. With sterile technique, attach the solution set to the catheter injection port.
5. Inject 1 mCi (37 MBq) of ^{99m}Tc sulfur colloid into the saline bag. Flush the injection syringe 3 times.

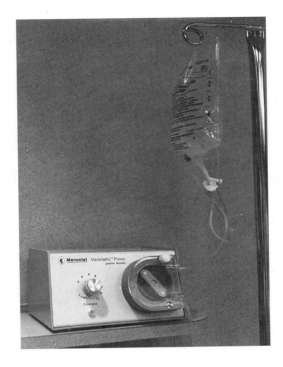

Figure 12-5. Arrangement of saline bag, infusion set, and varistaltic pump setup for ^{32}P intraperitoneal therapy.

6. Infuse the ^{99m}Tc sulfur colloid saline solution using the varistaltic pump.
7. After the infusion of ^{99m}Tc sulfur colloid, have the patient roll from side to side 1–2 times to aid distribution of the radiotracer.
8. An anterior image of the abdomen should then be acquired on analog formatter and on computer (256 × 256 matrix) for 200 kct.
9. If the nuclear medicine physician considers the distribution of the ^{99m}Tc sulfur colloid to be satisfactory, proceed with the therapy.

Computer Analysis

No analysis of the ^{99m}Tc sulfur colloid image is required.

Information on Film

On each analog and computer film, ensure that the following information is recorded:

1. Patient name and clinic/hospital number
2. Type of scan and radiopharmaceutical
3. Date and time of image after injection
4. Orientation of image (e.g., anterior)

Therapy Procedure

1. The authorized nuclear medicine technologist should complete the radioisotope therapy form (written directive), as shown in Figure 12-3, based on the information obtained from the referring physician's notes and laboratory test results in the patient's medical history. The prescribing nuclear medicine physician treating the patient should verify the information

listed on the radioisotope therapy form and sign and date it. The authorized nuclear medicine technologist should not draw the dose to be administered until the information listed on the radioisotope therapy form has been verified and signed by the physician treating the patient.

2. The dose should be drawn only by an authorized nuclear medicine technologist. A dose verification is done by a second authorized nuclear medicine technologist at the time of drawing the dose, and this second technologist should co-sign his or her initials on the radioisotope therapy form. A clear plastic syringe shield should be used to reduce hand exposure (see Fig. 12-4). After both dose verifications have been performed, the ^{32}P dose should be brought to the procedure room for injection.

3. If a purse-string suture has not been placed and the physician wishes to place it, the suture should be placed going from the inside of the wound to the outside to avoid damaging the catheter tube.

4. The physician personally should check that the correct dose of ^{32}P chromic phosphate has been drawn. By checking the label on the vial and confirming the blue color of the solution, the physician should also ensure that it is indeed chromic phosphate.

5. The injection procedure should be performed by either the nuclear medicine physician or a nuclear medicine technologist in the presence of the nuclear medicine physician.

6. Remove the empty 250-ml saline bag. Dilute 1.0 ml of methylene blue in 500 ml of 0.9% normal saline, and attach the 500-ml saline bag to the solution set.

7. Start the infusion into the peritoneal cavity using the varistaltic pump. If the solution flows without difficulty after the initial 50–100 ml, add 15 mCi (555 MBq) of chromic ^{32}P to the remaining solution. Massage the saline bag briefly to mix the chromic ^{32}P, and infuse it completely. The methylene blue will help identify any possible leakage by coloring the solution.

8. After step 7 is completed, infuse 250 ml of 0.9% normal saline into the peritoneal cavity to clear any remaining ^{32}P from the tubing. At the completion of this step, a total of 1,000 ml of 0.9% normal saline will have been infused into the patient's peritoneal cavity.

9. The physician should now remove the catheter and tie the purse-string suture tightly if present or apply a pressure dressing to the catheter site. If leakage persists, it may be necessary to suture the site or to apply a pressure dressing.

10. Apply a sterile dressing over the catheter site, and tape it to the patient's skin. The patient should be returned immediately to his or her hospital room.

11. After the patient has left the nuclear medicine laboratory, the dressings and linens should be cleaned up and put in the radioactive waste bins.

12. The nurses attending the patient should be instructed in adequate positioning of a patient after intraperitoneal administration of ^{32}P. The patient should be turned every 15 minutes for 2 hours as follows:
    a. In a 25° Trendelenburg position (head down, feet up): supine, right, left, and prone.
    b. In a reverse 25° Trendelenburg position (head up, feet down): repeat position changes as in step 12a.

13. Other nursing instructions:
    a. Wear gloves when changing dressings. Dispose of these in the ordinary trash. Check the dressings and linens for signs of leakage from the abdominal area. If leakage is present, change the linens and dressing, and place them in the ordinary trash. If significant leakage is present, contact the radiation safety officer.
    b. If the patient has a medical emergency or dies before dismissal from the hospital, the radiation safety officer should be notified.

Additional Notes

The following list of materials is required for the administration of ^{99m}Tc sulfur colloid and ^{32}P chromic phosphate:

^{99m}Tc Sulfur Colloid Administration

1. 1 mCi (37 MBq) ^{99m}Tc sulfur colloid
2. One 250-ml bag of 0.9% normal saline
3. One 96-inch solution set
4. Varistaltic pump

^{32}P Chromic Phosphate Administration

1. 1 ml of methylene blue (in a syringe)
2. One suture removal set
3. 3.0 or 4.0 silk sutures with a cutting needle
4. One 500-ml bag of 0.9% normal saline, and one 250-ml bag of 0.9% normal saline
5. Two 19-gauge needles
6. Sterile cotton swabs
7. Sterile gloves (small and large)
8. 4 × 4-inch gauze sterile dressing
9. Hypoallergenic tape
10. 15 mCi (555 MBq) of chromic ^{32}P (in a syringe)
11. Suture tray
12. Povidone-iodine packs

Radiation Dosimetry

The estimated absorbed doses in organs and tissues of an average subject (70 kg) from an intraperitoneal injection of 1 mCi (37 MBq) of ^{99m}Tc sulfur colloid are shown in Table 12-3.[5]

The estimated absorbed doses in organs and tissues of an average subject (70 kg) from an intraperitoneal injection of 15 mCi (555 MBq) of ^{32}P chromic phosphate are shown in Table 12-4.[1,6]

Table 12-3. Absorbed Radiation Dose Estimates in a 70-kg Adult
From Intraperitoneal Injection of 1 mCi (37 MBq) of ^{99m}Tc Sulfur Colloid

Tissue	Absorbed Radiation Dose	
	rad/1 mCi	mGy/37 MBq
Liver	0.06	0.56
Organs in the peritoneal cavity	0.06	0.56
Testes	0.06	0.56
Ovaries	0.06	0.56
Total body	0.02	0.19

Table 12-4. Absorbed Radiation Dose Estimates in a 70-kg Adult From Intraperitoneal Injection of 15 mCi (555 MBq) of ^{32}P Chromic Phosphate

Tissue	Absorbed Radiation Doses		
	rad/15 mCi	Gy/555 MBq	Tissue Depth From Organ Surface, cm
Peritoneal cavity	13,500	135.0	0.004
	11,250	112.5	0.008
	10,500	105.0	0.012
	9,000	90.0	0.016
	8,250	82.5	0.020
	3,225	32.3	0.10
	1,275	12.8	0.20
Liver	165	1.65	
Spleen	150	1.50	
Kidney	30	0.30	

References

1. Boye E, Lindegaard MW, Paus E, et al. Whole-body distribution of radioactivity after intraperitoneal administration of ^{32}P colloids. Br J Radiol 1984; 57: 395–402.
2. Croll MN, Brady LW. Intracavitary uses of colloids. Semin Nucl Med 1979; 9: 108–113.
3. Karimeddini MK, Spitznagle LA. Intracavitary treatment with radiocolloid ^{32}P chromic phosphate. In "Radionuclides in Therapy," eds Spencer RP, Seevers RH Jr, Friedman AM. CRC Press, Boca Raton, FL, 1987, pp 74–81.
4. Harbert JC. "Nuclear Medicine Therapy." Thieme Medical Publishers, New York, 1987.
5. Kit for the preparation of technetium Tc-99m sulfur colloid. CIS-US, Inc., Bedford, MA. Last revision December 1988.
6. Phosphocol P-32, chromic phosphate P-32 suspension kit, product #470. Mallinckrodt Medical, Inc., St. Louis. Last revision August 1990.

⁸⁹Sr Bone Therapy

Summary Information

Radiopharmaceutical

⁸⁹Sr strontium chloride: The administered dose is generally 4 mCi (148 MBq), although a lower dose may be given.

Characteristics: Strontium chloride is a clear solution intended for IV administration. It has a half-life of 50.6 days and emits beta particles with a maximum energy of 1.46 MeV. These particles have a maximum range of 6.6 mm in tissue. Beta particles are effectively shielded by the glass vial or by a clear plastic syringe shield covering the syringe containing the ⁸⁹Sr. After injection into the patient, external radiation hazard is minimal.

Contraindications

⁸⁹Sr should not be administered unless there is documented evidence of bony metastasis from a recent radionuclide bone scan. Other causes of pain, including nerve invasion, spinal cord compression, and muscular sources, should be excluded.

⁸⁹Sr should not be administered to pregnant women or women who are breast-feeding. Use of ⁸⁹Sr in patients with evidence of seriously compromised bone marrow, which is due to previous therapy or to tumor infiltration into the bone marrow, is not recommended unless the potential benefit of the treatment outweighs its risks. In general, ⁸⁹Sr should be used with caution in patients with platelet counts less than 60,000/mm^3 and white blood cell counts less than 2,400/mm^3. Patients with impaired renal function may have delayed excretion of ⁸⁹Sr and should be treated with caution. If the patient is has urinary incontinence, a Foley catheter should be placed for the first 4 days after treatment.

Indications

⁸⁹Sr therapy is indicated in the management of patients with intractable bone pain from bone metastases. Metastases to the skeleton occur in more than 50% of patients with breast, lung, or prostrate cancer in the end stages of the disease. Pain management becomes very important in these patients.[1] Because bone metastases are widespread in the body, the administration of systemic radiation with ⁸⁹Sr is effective in the relief of bone pain.[2]

Principle

[89]Sr is essentially a pure beta emitter with a physical half-life of 50.6 days. Strontium in the form of strontium chloride is a calcium analog that is rapidly cleared from the blood and localizes in sites of osteoblastic skeletal metastases. Because of its high uptake (2–25 times that of normal bone) and very long retention time in bone, it can deliver high radiation doses to osteoblastic lesions over a long period of time. It may improve (80% of patients) or eliminate (16% of patients) pain.[3,4]

Patient Preparation

All women 13–50 years old must have a pregnancy test done within 80 hours before therapy unless the patient has been sterilized surgically (hysterectomy or tubal ligation). The results of the pregnancy test must be available before the treatment can commence.

Therapy Procedure

1. The authorized nuclear medicine technologist should complete the radioisotope therapy form (written directive), as shown in Figure 12-3, based on the information obtained from the referring physician's notes and laboratory test results in the patient's medical history. The prescribing physician treating the patient should verify the information listed on the radioisotope therapy form (in particular, the radioisotope, the administered dose, and the date) and sign it. The authorized nuclear medicine technologist should not administer the dose until the information listed on the radioisotope therapy form (see Fig. 12-3) has been verified and signed by the physician treating the patient.

2. The dose should be drawn from the vial only by an authorized nuclear medicine technologist. A dose verification is done by a second nuclear medicine technologist at the time of drawing the dose, and this second technologist should co-sign his or her initials on the radioisotope therapy form (see Fig. 12-3).

3. [89]Sr generally is supplied in 4 mCi (148 MBq) unit dose vials. In such cases, the dose can be verified from the drug label or measured in a beta counter (if available). Doses less than 4 mCi can be calculated volumetrically. A clear plastic syringe shield should be used to reduce hand exposure (see Fig. 12-4).

4. After both dose verifications have been performed, the ^{89}Sr dose should be brought to the procedure room for injection. Great care should be taken to ensure that the dose is not extravasated by setting up an IV saline infusion and then injecting through the IV line.

5. The ^{89}Sr should be administered by slow IV injection (over 5 minutes). Repeated administrations of ^{89}Sr generally are not recommended at intervals of less than 90 days.

6. Nursing instructions:
    a. Gloves and a gown should be worn when changing bed linen and dressings for 4 days after treatment. [89]Sr is excreted in the urine (80%) and feces (20%), mostly over the first 4 days. Hence, soiled bed linen and clothes may need to be stored to allow for decay of the [89]Sr. Contact the institution radiation safety officer for guidance on management of contaminated linen.
    b. If the patient has a medical emergency or dies before dismissal from the hospital, notify the radiation safety officer.

7. After the patient has left the nuclear medicine laboratory, the syringe and any associated tubing should be wrapped in absorbent paper, labeled with the date and isotope, and allowed to decay 10 half-lives (approximately 17 months) in storage.

Follow-Up Guidelines

1. Aside from mild myelosuppression, an occasional "flare response" has been observed in the first week after treatment. This may involve a transient worsening of bone pain. No other significant side effects have been reported. Pain improvement is generally not seen for 7–21 days after treatment.
2. Bone marrow toxicity is expected to follow the administration of ^{89}Sr, particularly white blood cells and platelets. It is recommended that the peripheral blood counts of the patient be monitored every 2 weeks. The nadir of the depression of platelet counts generally occurs around 6 weeks (range, 4–16 weeks) after treatment. Platelets typically will be depressed by 30% at the nadir. Recovery occurs slowly, and may take up to 6 months to return to near pretreatment levels.
3. Generally, treatment can be repeated at 3-month intervals, but it should be based on the patient's response to therapy, current symptoms, and hematologic status.

Radiation Dosimetry

The estimated absorbed doses in organs and tissues of an average subject (70 kg) from an IV injection of 4 mCi (148 MBq) ^{89}Sr strontium chloride are shown in Table 12-5.[5] However, it should be noted that considerable variation exists in the predicted dosimetry of ^{89}Sr, particularly to bone metastases.[4]

Table 12-5. Absorbed Radiation Dose Estimates in an Average Subject (70 kg) From Intravenous Injection of 4 mCi (148 MBq) ^{89}Sr Strontium Chloride

Tissue	Absorbed Radiation Dose	
	rad/4 mCi	mGy/148 MBq
Bone surface	252.0	2,520
Red bone marrow	162.8	1,628
Lower bowel wall	69.2	692
Bladder wall	19.2	190
Testes	11.6	116
Ovaries	11.6	116
Uterine wall	11.6	116
Kidneys	11.6	116
Bone metastases (estimated)	3,000–30,000	30,000–300,000

References

1. Wilson JD, Braunwald E, Isselbacher KJ, et al. "Harrison's Principles of Internal Medicine," 12th Edition. McGraw-Hill, New York, 1991, p 1945.
2. Robinson RG, Preston DF, Spicer JA, Baxter KG. Radionuclide therapy of intractable bone pain: emphasis on strontium-89. Semin Nucl Med 1992; 22: 28–32.
3. Dickinson CZ, Hendrix NS. Strontium-89 therapy in painful bony metastases. J Nucl Med Tech 1993; 21: 133–137.
4. Breen SL, Powe JE, Porter AT. Dose estimation in strontium-89 radiotherapy of metastatic prostatic carcinoma. J Nucl Med 1992; 33: 1316–1323.
5. Radiation dose to patients from radiopharmaceuticals, ICRP #53, vol. 18, No. 1–4. Pergamon Press, London, 1988, p 171.

Appendices

Michael K. O'Connor
Joseph C. Hung

General Policy for Patient Identification in Nuclear Medicine

Introduction

The procedures described apply to all nuclear medicine and nuclear cardiology studies except those involving blood products. For any study involving reinjection of labeled blood components (e.g., ^{111}In- or ^{99m}Tc-labeled white blood cell scan, ^{99m}Tc-labeled red blood cells with the use of the UltraTag RBC kit for gastrointestinal bleeding, spleen imaging, or radionuclide angiographic study), please follow the instructions stated in the "Policy for Patient Identification During Radiolabeled Blood Product Procedures" (Appendix A-2).

Procedures Requiring a Written Directive

For procedures requiring a written directive (i.e., for any administration of quantities greater than 30 μCi [1.11 MBq] of either NaI ^{125}I or ^{131}I) and for therapeutic administration of a radiopharmaceutical other than NaI ^{125}I or ^{131}I:

1. Before each administration, the nuclear medicine technologist should ask the patient to state his or her **full name** (first and last name) and **birth date**. The patient's name and birth date should then be confirmed with the information printed on the request form for either the nuclear medicine procedure or the radioisotope therapy.
2. If the patient cannot comply with both of the identification methods, i.e., stating his or her full name and birth date, do **NOT** perform the procedure; instead, contact the prescribing physician for further instructions.

Diagnostic Procedures

For all diagnostic procedures other than studies requiring administration of activity greater than 30 μCi (1.11 MBq) of NaI ^{125}I or ^{131}I, and/or studies involving radiolabeled blood products:

1. Before a patient is administered a radiopharmaceutical, the nuclear medicine technologist must always ask the patient to state his or her full name (first and last name), making sure that the name as stated corresponds to the name listed on the nuclear medicine request form. The name verification procedure should be conducted **immediately** before the administration of the radiopharmaceutical by the person who is administering the radiopharmaceutical dosage to the patient. The only exception to this is with stress myocardial perfusion studies using ^{201}Tl or ^{99m}Tc sestamibi, in which case the patient identification can be conducted before the initiation of exercise or pharmacologic stress.
   Note: If there is a name-alert sticker (i.e., the patient's name is similar to that of another patient scheduled for a nuclear medicine study that day), the technologist should also ask

the patient the state his or her birth date and then verify this information with the information listed on the nuclear medicine request form or in the patient's medical chart.

2. If a patient is unable to speak, the patient's hospital wrist band may be used for patient identification, or a mediator should be consulted to confirm the patient's identification.

3. If no wrist band is present and a mediator cannot be found, do **NOT** perform the study; instead, contact the nuclear medicine/nuclear cardiology physician for further instructions.

Policy for Patient Identification During Radiolabeled Blood Product Procedures

Introduction

For any study requiring the withdrawal of blood from a patient and reinjection of labeled blood components (e.g., ^{111}In- or ^{99m}Tc-labeled white blood cell scan, ^{99m}Tc-labeled red blood cells with the use of the UltraTag RBC kit for gastrointestinal bleeding, spleen imaging, or radionuclide angiographic study), the following procedures should be performed. Two procedures are outlined. The primary procedure is designed for use with a portable bar-coding system. In the event that the bar-code system is unavailable or malfunctions, the secondary procedure should be followed. Strict adherence to the hospital/clinic control plan for blood-borne pathogen exposure is required during any radiolabeled blood procedure.

Primary Procedure

The primary procedure requires a combination bar-code scanner and printer with the appropriate software for the generation of labels and subsequent scanning of these labels to confirm the identification of the blood products.[1]

Instrumentation

Bar-code scanner and printer: Pathfinder Ultra (Monarch Marking Systems; Dayton, OH). This is a fully programmable and portable combination bar-code scanner and printer (Fig. A-1). The system has an RS-232C port for communication with a desktop PC.

Principle

Whereas conventional bar-code scanners allow for blood matching in the nuclear pharmacy, they generally are interfaced to a desktop computer and are not designed for transport to a patient's bedside. Therefore, they provide only partial verification, because they cannot be used for initial patient identification or reinjection. A portable bar-code scanner and printer provide a complete verification of the entire blood-labeling process. The portable system performs the following functions:

1. Checks, validates, and records all blood transfers between patient, syringes, and test tubes via bar code.
2. Generates unique bar-code labels for each syringe and test tube that is used.
3. Provides step-by-step instruction for the technologist throughout the blood-labeling procedure.
4. Provides a visual and audible alert when items are scanned out of order or when items belonging to a different patient are detected.
5. Uses time delays between steps to control pace of verification.
6. Generates report of all entries with a time stamp.

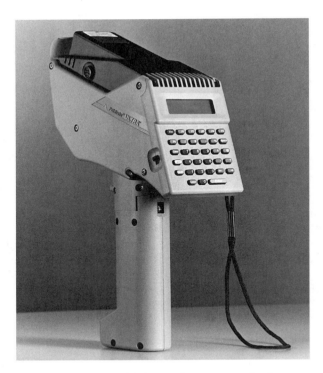

Figure A-1. Portable bar-code scanner and printer.

Procedure

1. After the study is scheduled, a bar-coded wrist band should be generated for the patient by the hospital/clinic appointment system. This contains the patient's name and clinic number. Also, before the procedure and before meeting the patient, enter the patient's name and clinic number into the bar-code scanner.

2. When the patient arrives for the study, the technologist should make sure that **no empty, used, or loaded syringes are in the blood withdrawal/reinjection area other than the one to be used for withdrawing blood from the patient.**

3. When blood is drawn from more than one patient, each patient's blood should be transported in separate containers so as not to mix up the patients' blood.

4. When ready to draw blood, adhere to the following procedures for verifying patient identification:

   a. Ask the patient to state his or her full name.

   b. Attach the bar-coded wrist band to the patient (Fig. A-2). The technologist should explain to the patient that the wrist band, with bar-coding, is required for identification purposes.

   c. Scan the patient's wrist band (Fig. A-3). The scanner compares the manually entered patient clinic number with the number on the wrist band and confirms the patient's identity. The scanner then generates labels for the blood drawing and the reinjection syringes (Fig. A-4).

   d. Ask the patient to sign his or her name on both the nuclear medicine report form (this form will contain the scan report and will be included in the scan jacket) and on the bar-

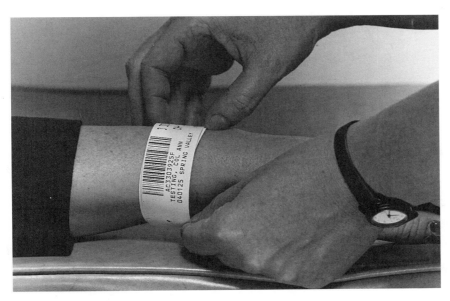

Figure A-2. Wrist band attached to patient's wrist. The bar code on the wrist band contains the patient's name and hospital/clinic number.

code label for the reinjection syringe. The technologist should explain to the patient that the signatures are required for identification purposes. If the patient is unable to sign his or her name, a second person is asked to verify the patient's identification. This verification is documented on the nuclear medicine report form.

5. The bar-code label should be placed **immediately** on the syringe for reinjection.

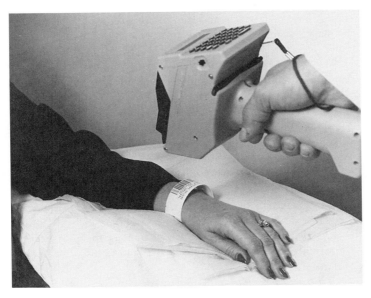

Figure A-3. Scanning wrist band to verify patient identity.

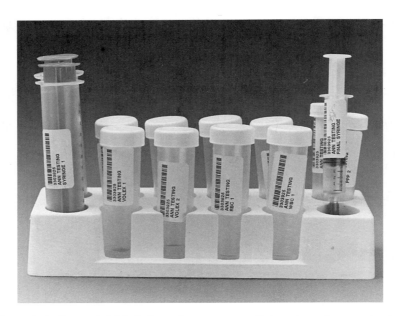

Figure A-4. Bar-coded labels from the scanner applied to the syringes and tubes.

6. During the labeling procedure, the bar code labels must be scanned with the bar-code scanner when blood products are transferred to a new set of tubes, vials, or syringes. The scanner provides complete instructions on the blood-labeling steps and notifies the technologist of any error or mismatch. The technologist should perform only **one** radiolabeling procedure on **one** patient's blood at a time. **Never** place blood products from two different patients in the same centrifuge or laminar flow hood.

7. The patient and dosage information should be documented in the nuclear pharmacy computer system. A dose prescription and label are then generated. The label generated by the nuclear pharmacy system contains the patient's name, the radiopharmaceutical, and a unique study number for that patient's study. This label should be applied to the dose syringe used for reinjection.

8. If more than one dose syringe is transported, each one should be carried in a separate container so as not to mix up the syringes.

9. Before bringing the patient into the blood withdrawal/reinjection area for reinjection, the technologist should check the area to ensure that **no used or loaded syringes, other than the one to be used for reinjection, are lying in the open area of the room.**

10. Before reinjection, patient identification should be verified by the following steps:
    a. Ask the patient to state his or her full name.
    b. Ask the patient to sign his or her name on the nuclear medicine report form. Check that the patient's signature matches that obtained in step 4d. If the patient is unable to sign his or her name, a second person is asked to verify the patient's identification.
    c. Use the bar-code scanner to scan the bar code on the patient's wrist band and on the final reinjection syringe. Reinject the radiolabeled blood cells when the scanner confirms a successful match.

11. The initials of the person who administered the dose, the dose activity, and the exact time of administration should be recorded on the nuclear medicine report form.

12. After the reinjection is completed, the technologist **immediately** should discard all used syringes into a biohazard container.

13. Any error in administration (e.g., administration involving the wrong patient or radiopharmaceutical) should be reported immediately to the supervisor and to the prescribing physician. The prescribing physician should then contact the referring physician, so that possible options can be discussed. The recommendation from the Centers for Disease Control and Prevention for the management of persons after exposure to blood in the health care setting will be followed.[2-4] All administration errors and narrowly avoided errors in administration should be evaluated carefully in a nuclear medicine staff meeting to determine whether additional precautions are necessary to prevent similar potential errors in administration.

Secondary Procedure

This procedure should be used in the event that the portable bar-code scanner is not available or malfunctions.

1. After a study is scheduled, patient identification labels with the patient's name and hospital/clinic number for syringes, vials, and tubes should be generated.

2. Place these labels on the syringes, vials, and tubes for the radiolabeled blood procedure.

3. When the patient arrives for the study, the technologist should make sure that **no empty, used, or loaded syringes are in the blood withdrawal/reinjection room other than the one to be used for withdrawing blood from the patient.**

4. When blood is drawn from more than one patient, each patient's blood should be transported in a separate container so as not to mix up the patients' blood.

5. When ready to draw blood, adhere to the following procedures for verifying patient identification:

    a. Ask the patient to state his or her full name. If the patient is unable to say his or her name, check the wrist band and then proceed to step 5b. If the patient is not wearing a wrist band, do not initiate the study; instead, contact the prescribing physician (i.e., nuclear medicine physician) for further instructions.

    b. Ask the patient to sign his or her name on both the nuclear medicine report form (this form will contain the scan report and will be included in the scan jacket) and on a preprinted label that contains the patient's name and hospital/clinic number. The technologist should explain to the patient that the signatures are required for identification purposes. If the patient is unable to write his or her name, a mediator should be consulted to confirm patient identification and to sign the patient's name with their own initials. If a mediator cannot be found, do not perform the study; instead, contact the nuclear medicine physician or the patient's referring physician for further instructions.

6. The preprinted label with the patient's signature or mediator's signature and initials should immediately be placed on the final dose syringe for reinjection.

7. During the labeling procedure, the stickers that contain the patient's name and hospital/clinic number (from step 1) should be checked carefully when the blood products must be transferred to a new set of syringes, vials, or tubes. The technologist should perform only one radiolabeling procedure on one patient's blood and blood products in each laminar flow hood and should never place any blood products from any other patient in the same centrifuge.

8. The patient and dosage information should be entered into the nuclear pharmacy computer system. A dose prescription and label are then generated. The label generated by the nuclear

pharmacy system contains the patient's name, the name of the radiopharmaceutical, and a unique study number for that patient's study. This label is then applied to the dose syringe.

9. If more than one dose syringe is transported, then each one should be carried in a separate container so as not to mix up the syringes.

10. Before bringing the patient into the blood withdrawal/reinjection area for reinjection, the technologist should check the area to ensure that **no used or loaded syringes other than the one to be used for reinjection are lying in the open area of the room.**

11. Before reinjection, the patient's identification should be verified according to the procedures listed in steps 5a and b. A second healthcare worker (e.g., nurse, nuclear medicine technologist, bone mineral technologist) must be present to cross-check syringe labeling, the nuclear medicine request form, and the patient's signature or mediator's initials (i.e., the signature/initials on the nuclear medicine report form and another set of signature/initials on the final dose syringe label) to ensure consistency in all aspects of the procedure. If these requirements are fulfilled, the labeled blood product may be injected. If the patient is unable to comply with the requirements stated in steps 5a and b or a second healthcare worker cannot be found, do not perform the reinjection. Consult the nuclear medicine physician or the patient's referring physician for further instructions.

12. The initials of the person who administered the dose and the exact time of administration should be recorded in the nuclear medicine report form.

13. After the reinjection is completed, the technologist should **immediately** discard the used syringes into a biohazard container.

14. Any error in administration (e.g., administration involving the wrong patient or radiopharmaceutical) should be reported immediately both to the supervisor and to the prescribing physician. The prescribing physician should then contact the referring physician so that possible options can be discussed. The recommendations from the Centers for Disease Control and Prevention for the management of persons after exposure to blood in the healthcare setting should be followed.[2–4] All administration errors and narrowly avoided errors in administration should be evaluated carefully in nuclear medicine staff meetings to determine whether additional precautions are necessary to prevent similar potential errors in administration.

References

1. Porter DV, Hung JC. Portable bar-code scanners/printers for matching patients to radiolabeled blood in nuclear medicine. Proceedings of the American Pharmaceutical Association 142nd Annual Meeting, Orlando, FL, 1995, p 98.

2. Recommendations for prevention of HIV transmission in health-care settings. MMWR 1987; 36(Suppl. 2): 1S–18S.

3. Public Health Service statement on management of occupational exposure to human immunodeficiency virus, including considerations regarding zidovudine postexposure use. MMWR 1990; 39 (RR-1): 1–14.

4. Hepatitis B virus: a comprehensive strategy for eliminating transmission in the United States through universal childhood vaccination. Recommendations of the Immunization Practices Advisory Committee (ACIIP). MMWR 1991; 40 (RR-13): 1–25.

Pediatric Dose Chart for Radiopharmaceuticals (Children Less Than 18 Years of Age)

Introduction

The following tables and charts permit calculation of the appropriate radiopharmaceutical doses for pediatric studies (older than 1 month). The tables are based on the relative body surface areas of children to adults.[1] However, earlier studies have shown that strict application of this technique results in insufficient counts for satisfactory studies in very young children.[2] Hence, a minimal administered activity has been set to ensure adequate image quality in small children.

Radiopharmaceutical Doses

Table A-1 lists the minimal doses that can be administered for various nuclear medicine procedures.[3–10] Table A-2 illustrates how the pediatric dose can be calculated as a fraction of the adult dose. If this results in a calculated pediatric dose outside the minimal limit in Table A-1, use the dose value in Table A-1. The nuclear medicine physician may increase the dose depending on the clinical situation, e.g., an uncooperative or critically ill child, to expedite the study and to ensure adequate image quality.

Table A-1. Minimal Doses for Various Nuclear Medicine Procedures

Procedure	Radiopharmaceutical	Minimal Dose	Reference
Central nervous system			
Brain imaging—SPECT study	99mTc HMPAO or ECD	2 mCi (74 MBq)	5
CSF imaging—cisternography/ventriculography	111In DTPA	100 µCi (3.7 MBq)	5
201Tl scan for recurrent brain tumor	201Tl thallous chloride	50 µCi (1.85 MBq)	—
Confirmation of brain death	99mTc HMPAO	2 mCi (74 MBq)	5
Cardiovascular system			
Cardiac left-to-right shunt	99mTc DTPA	2 mCi (74 MBq)	4
Radionuclide angiography	99mTc modified in vivo red blood cell labeling	5 mCi (185 MBq)	8
99mTc sestamibi myocardial perfusion study	99mTc sestamibi	3 mCi (111 MBq)	—
201Tl myocardial perfusion study	201Tl thallous chloride	300 µCi (11.1 MBq)	5
Myocardial infarct study	99mTc PYP	4 mCi (148 MBq)	3
Endocrine system			
131I/123I substernal thyroid scan	131I sodium iodide	20 µCi (740 kBq)	—
	123I sodium iodide	30 µCi (1.11 MBq)	4
99mTc pertechnetate thyroid scan	99mTc sodium pertechnetate	1 mCi (37 MBq)	3
131I thyroid uptake measurement	131I sodium iodide	2 µCi (74 kBq)	3
131I neck scan	131I sodium iodide	150 µCi (5.55 MBq)	—
131I total body scan	131I sodium iodide	150 µCi (5.55 MBq)	—
99mTc sestamibi parathyroid scan	99mTc sodium pertechnetate	250 µCi (9.25 MBq)	—
	99mTc sestamibi	3 mCi (111 MBq)	—
131I MIBG adrenal medulla scan	131I mIBG	500 µCi (18.5 MBq)	9
123I MIBG adrenal medulla scan	123I mIBG	2 mCi (74 MBq)	10
131I NP-59 adrenal cortex scan	131I NP-59	500 µCi (18.5 MBq)	—
111In pentetreotide scan	111In pentetreotide	None established	—

Gastrointestinal system

Salivary gland scan	99mTc pertechnetate	1 mCi (37 MBq)	3
Esophageal scintigraphy	99mTc sulfur colloid	150 μCi (5.55 MBq)	7
Gastroesophageal reflux study—children	99mTc sulfur colloid	500 μCi (18.5 MBq)	4
Gastric emptying (solid/liquid phases)	99mTc sulfur colloid	500 μCi (18.5 MBq)	4,5
	111In DTPA	250 μCi (9.25 MBq)	—
Detection of gastrointestinal bleeding	99mTc-labeled red blood cells (UltraTag)	2 mCi (74 MBq)	6
Detection of Meckel's diverticulum	99mTc pertechnetate	2 mCi (74 MBq)	4, 6
Protein-losing enteropathy	99mTc human serum albumin	2 mCi (74 MBq)	—
Liver/spleen scan	99mTc sulfur colloid	500 μCi (18.5 MBq)	3, 8
Liver hemangioma study	99mTc-labeled red blood cells (UltraTag)	2 mCi (74 MBq)	6
Hepatobiliary scan	99mTc disofenin	1 mCi (37 MBq)	4, 5

Genitourinary system

Dynamic renal scan	99mTc MAG3	1 mCi (37 MBq)	5, 9
	99mTc DTPA	2.5 mCi (92.5 MBq)	3
99mTc DMSA renal scan	99mTc DMSA	500 μCi (18.5 MBq)	—
Voiding cystography	99mTc DTPA		
Age 0–1 year		1 mCi (37 MBq)	3
Age more than 1 year		2 mCi (74 MBq)	3
Determination of residual urine	99mTc DTPA	500 μCi (18.5 MBq)	—
Testicular scan	99mTc pertechnetate	2 mCi (74 MBq)	5

Infection/bone

111In white blood cell scan	111In-labeled white blood cells	50 μCi (1.85 MBq)	—
99mTc HMPAO white blood cell scan	99mTc HMPAO	1 mCi (37 MBq)	10
67Ga gallium scan	67Ga gallium citrate	1 mCi (37 MBq)	6

Continues

567

Table A-1. (Continued)

Procedure	Radiopharmaceutical	Minimal Dose	Reference
Bone marrow scan	99mTc sulfur colloid	500 µCi (18.5 MBq)	3, 8
Bone scan	99mTc MDP	4 mCi (148 MBq)	3
Joint scan	99mTc sodium pertechnetate	1 mCi (37 MBq)	3, 5
Respiratory system			
133Xe lung ventilation scan	133Xe gas	1 mCi (37 MBq)	5
99mTc DTPA lung aerosol scan	99mTc DTPA aerosol	100 µCi (3.7 MBq)	5
99mTc pertechnegas ventilation scan	99mTc pertechnegas	None established	—
99mTc MAA lung perfusion scan	99mTc MAA	500 µCi (18.5 MBq)	8
Tumor imaging			
67Ga gallium scan	67Ga gallium citrate	1 mCi (37 MBq)	6
111In OncoScint	111In OncoScint	None established	—
Special imaging procedures			
Dacryoscintigraphy	99mTc pertechnetate	200 µCi (7.4 MBq)/eye	8
LeVeen shunt patency	99mTc MAA (injection into shunt tubing)	100 µCi (3.7 MBq)	—
	99mTc MAA (intraperitoneal injection)	1 mCi (37 MBq)	—

Table A-2. Pediatric Dose as a Fraction of the Adult Dose Based on Relative Body Surface Area[a]

Patient Weight (kg)	Body Surface Area (m^2)	Fraction of Adult Dose	Patient Weight (kg)	Body Surface Area (m^2)	Fraction of Adult Dose
2	0.15	0.08	13	0.55	0.31
3	0.20	0.11	14	0.58	0.32
4	0.24	0.13	15	0.61	0.34
5	0.28	0.16	20	0.74	0.42
6	0.32	0.18	25	0.87	0.49
7	0.35	0.20	30	0.98	0.55
8	0.39	0.22	35	1.10	0.62
9	0.42	0.24	40	1.20	0.68
10	0.46	0.26	45	1.31	0.73
11	0.49	0.27	50	1.41	0.79
12	0.52	0.29	55	1.50	0.84

[a]Body surface area (BSA) = (body weight)$^{0.7}$/11.
For 70-kg adult, BSA = 1.779 m^2.
Fraction of adult dose = BSA / 1.779.

References

1. Goetz WA, Hendee WR, Gilday DL. In vivo diagnostic nuclear medicine. Pediatric experience. Clin Nucl Med 1983; 8: 434–439.
2. Webster EW, Alpert NM, Brownell GL. Radiation doses in pediatric nuclear medicine and diagnostic x-ray procedures—symposium on nuclear medicine. Johns Hopkins Medical Institutions, Baltimore, February 18–19, 1972.
3. Weiss S. Pediatric considerations. In "CRC Manual of Nuclear Medicine Procedures," eds Carey JE Jr, Kline RC, Keyes JW. CRC Press, Boca Raton, FL, 1983, pp 211–214.
4. Mettler FA Jr, Guiberteau MJ. "Essentials of Nuclear Medicine Imaging." Grune & Stratton, New York, 1983, pp 302–304.
5. Eggli DF. Appendix 2: Pediatric radiopharmaceutical dosages. In "Clinical Practice of Nuclear Medicine," eds Taylor A Jr, Datz FL. Churchill Livingstone, New York, 1991, pp 449–450.
6. Siddiqui AR. Pediatric applications. In "Radionuclide Imaging of the GI Tract," ed Mettler FA Jr. Churchill Livingstone, New York, 1986, pp 247–286.
7. Klein HA, Wald A. Esophageal transit scintigraphy. In "Nuclear Medicine Annual 1988," eds Freeman LM, Weissmann HS. Raven Press, New York, 1988, pp 79–124.
8. Conway JJ. Practical considerations in radionuclide imaging of pediatric patients. In "Freeman and Johnson's Clinical Radionuclide Imaging," ed Freeman LH. Grune & Stratton, Orlando, FL, 1988, pp 329–359.
9. Weiss SC, Conway JJ. Pediatrics. In "Nuclear Medicine, Technology and Techniques," eds Bernier DR, Christian PE, Langan JK. Mosby Year Book, St. Louis, 1994, pp 418–437.
10. Piepsz A, Hahn K, Roca I, et al. A radiopharmaceuticals schedule for imaging in paediatrics. Paediatric Task Group European Association Nuclear Medicine. Eur J Nucl Med 1990; 17: 127–129.

Emergency Procedures for Radiation Spills/Contamination

Personal and Room Contamination Guidelines

Each laboratory must have a Geiger-Muller (GM) meter for monitoring purposes. In addition, a logbook, disposable gloves, and shoe covers should be kept adjacent to the meter.

The trigger level for personal contamination is **500 cpm measured with a GM meter.** This level applies to skin, clothing, and shoes. A similar trigger level is defined for all areas or surfaces in a restricted area. An area or surface must be decontaminated if the detected activity exceeds **500 cpm measured at 12 inches** from the contaminated surface with a GM meter. If the detected activity exceeds **50,000 cpm measured at 12 inches** from the contaminated area with a GM meter, the Radiation Safety Officer should be called immediately to deal with the contamination.

If any contamination is detected on any area or surface in an unrestricted area, contact the Radiation Safety Officer immediately to deal with the contamination.

Guidelines for Personal Decontamination

1. When leaving the nuclear medicine laboratory to go to an unrestricted area (e.g., cafeteria, break room, home), always remove your lab coat and monitor your hands and feet before leaving the area.

2. If your hands are contaminated, decontaminate them by washing with soap and water or with a suitable decontaminant. Monitor your hands again to check whether the decontamination was successful. Repeat the decontamination procedure until the contamination levels are below the trigger levels specified previously. If the decontamination process does not decrease the contamination level below 500 cpm on the GM meter, contact the Radiation Safety Officer or nuclear medicine supervisor. **The initial and final contamination readings should be documented in the logbook kept next to the GM meters.**

3. If the contamination is on your shoes, remove the shoes, and put on disposable shoe covers located next to the GM meters. The contaminated shoes should be cleaned with soap and water and monitored again. If the level of contamination is still above 500 cpm on the GM meter, place the shoes in a plastic bag and store them in the laboratory until the contamination has decayed below the stated trigger level. If there are any concerns with the decontamination process, contact the Radiation Safety Officer or nuclear medicine supervisor for further assistance.

4. If the contamination is on your lab coat, remove the coat and place it in a plastic bag. The plastic bag should be stored in the laboratory until the contamination has decayed below 500 cpm on the GM meter. Monitor clothing again to ensure that the contamination did not penetrate through the lab coat. If your clothing is still contaminated with activity greater than 500 cpm on the GM meter, contact the Radiation Safety Officer or nuclear medicine supervisor for further assistance.

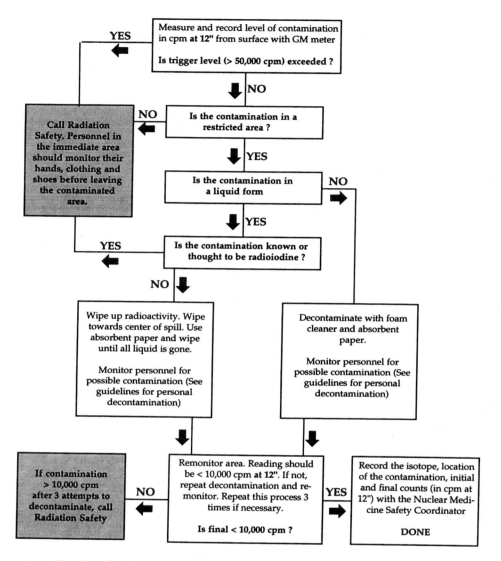

Figure A-5. Flowchart for the management of a radiation spill or contamination of a room or area.

Guidelines for Room Decontamination

Guidelines for the decontamination of areas or surfaces in a restricted area are given in the flowchart in Figure A-5. Note that restricted areas are generally limited to the nuclear pharmacy, imaging rooms, and immediate connecting hallways and corridors. All other areas are generally classified as unrestricted.

Infection Control Procedures for Nuclear Medicine

Introduction

Special precautions are required when studies are performed on patients who are under isolation. Isolation is designed either to protect the patient from outside contamination or to prevent the patient from infecting other patients, relatives, or healthcare workers. Extensive details of the procedures to be followed with patients under isolation should be obtained from the hospital/clinic infection control procedure manual. The procedures outlined here should be used to supplement the hospital/clinic infection control procedures.

The Isolated Patient

Patients are isolated for two reasons:

1. To prevent the infected patient from transmitting that infection to other patients, relatives, or healthcare workers.
2. To protect the patient from outside infections. The immune system may be severely compromised in some patients, making them susceptible to infection. In such patients, even minor infections can be fatal.

The Isolation System

A card or notice is usually placed on the door or window of the room of an isolated patient. The card describes what type of isolation the patient is under and what precautions must be taken by those coming in contact with the patient. There are five types of isolation:

1. Strict isolation—designed to prevent transmission of highly contagious or virulent infections spread by airborne and contact routes.
2. Respiratory isolation—designed to prevent infections transmitted by the airborne route through droplet nuclei, e.g., tuberculosis.
3. Wound and contact isolation—designed to prevent infections spread by direct or indirect contact with infected material or by close contact with large droplet particles. This includes patients with wounds or abscesses in which drainage cannot be easily contained or confined and microorganisms of epidemiologic importance that are involved in infection or colonization, e.g., resistant strains of bacteria.
4. Enteric isolation—designed to prevent infections transmitted by the fecal-oral route.
5. Blood and body fluids isolation—designed to prevent infections transmitted by direct contact with blood or mucus products. This includes patients with suspected hepatitis B and C, acquired immune deficiency syndrome (AIDS), AIDS-related complex, human immunodeficiency virus (HIV), etc. Infection Precaution ("IP" designation) denotes the presence of a confirmed or suspected blood-borne illness.

Technologists are required to wear gloves, gowns, and masks when dealing with an isolated patient. These items should be kept in a clean area.

Imaging Studies

1. Before starting the study, read the isolation sign accompanying the patient. It will explain the type of isolation, what you must wear, and what precautions are to be taken.
2. Before coming into contact with the patient, wash your hands and put on a gown or clean lab coat, mask, and/or gloves, as designated on the isolation card.
3. After the imaging study, perform the following procedures:
   a. All gowns and bedding from the examination tables should be placed in the laundry. If any of these items are soiled excessively with body fluids, they should be disposed of as biohazardous waste.
   b. All nonradioactive masks, gloves, paper sheets, and other disposable wastes should be disposed of in the proper waste container.
   c. All syringes and needles used for the injection of radiopharmaceuticals should be disposed of in the containers prescribed for radioactive materials.
   d. All equipment that came in direct contact with the patient should be cleaned and wiped with a surface disinfectant. Any areas contaminated with body fluids should be cleaned with a 10% bleach solution. The bleach solution should be used only on the day it was prepared and then disposed of.
   e. All personnel having contact with the patient should wash their hands according to the instructions on the isolation card.

Physical Data for Commonly Used Radionuclides

Table A-3. Physical Characteristics of the Most Commonly Used Radionuclides and Radionuclidic Contaminants in Nuclear Medicine

Nuclide	Half-Life	Principal Emissions, keV	Abundance, %
^{11}C	20.3 min	970 (β)	100
		511 (γ)	200
^{13}N	10.0 min	1,200 (β)	100
		511 (γ)	200
^{15}O	124 sec	1,740 (β)	100
		511 (γ)	200
^{18}F	109 min	635 (β)	100
		511 (γ)	200
^{32}P	14.3 days	1,710 (β)	100
^{56}Co	77.3 days	1,490 (β)	20
		3,260 (γ)	13
		2,600 (γ)	17
		2,020 (γ)	11
		1,760 (γ)	15
		1,240 (γ)	66
		1,040 (γ)	15
		847 (γ)	100
		511 (γ)	40
^{57}Co	271.8 days	136 (γ)	10
		122 (γ)	87
^{58}Co	70.9 days	470 (β)	15
		810 (γ)	99
		511 (γ)	30
^{60}Co	5.27 years	310 (β)	99
		1,332 (γ)	100
		1,173 (γ)	100
^{67}Ga	77.9 hr	388 (γ)	7
		296 (γ)	22
		184 (γ)	24
		93 (γ)	40
^{68}Ga	68.3 min	1,898 (β)	88

Continues

Table A-3. (Continued)

Nuclide	Half-Life	Principal Emissions, keV	Abundance, %
^{68}Ga (continued)		511 (γ)	176
^{81m}Kr	13 sec	191 (γ)	65
^{82}Rb	75 sec	3,150 (β)	96
		777 (γ)	9
		511 (γ)	192
^{89}Sr	50.6 days	1,463 (β)	100
^{99}Mo	66.7 hr	1,230 (β)	82
		450 (β)	17
		740 (γ)	14
		188 (γ)	7
^{99}Tc	2×10^5 years	292 (β)	100
^{99m}Tc	6.05 hr	141 (γ)	90
^{111}In	67.4 hr	247 (γ)	94
		173 (γ)	89
		23 (x)	71
^{113m}In	1.66 hr	392 (γ)	62
		24 (x)	19
^{114m}In	50.0 days	393 (γ)	64
^{123}I	13 hr	159 (γ)	97
		27 (x)	71
^{124}I	4.2 days	2,149 (β)	12
		1,543 (β)	13
		1,691 (γ)	10
		603 (γ)	62
^{125}I	60.2 days	36 (γ)	7
		27 (x)	93
^{131}I	8.04 days	610 (β)	90
		637 (γ)	7
		364 (γ)	83
		284 (γ)	5
^{127}Xe	36.4 days	375 (γ)	20
		203 (γ)	65
		172 (γ)	22
^{133}Xe	5.25 days	346 (β)	100
		81 (γ)	37
		80 (γ)	6

Continues

Table A-3. (Continued)

Nuclide	Half-Life	Principal Emissions, keV	Abundance, %
^{133}Xe (continued)		35 (x)	7
		31 (x)	39
^{133}Ba	10.54 years	384 (γ)	8
		356 (γ)	69
		302 (γ)	14
		276 (γ)	7
		80 (γ)	36
		35 (x)	22
		30 (x)	98
^{137}Cs	30.0 years	1,176 (β)	7
		514 (β)	95
		662 (γ)	85
^{153}Gd	241.6 days	103 (γ)	20
		97 (γ)	28
		47 (γ)	18
		41 (γ)	96
^{201}Tl	73 hours	167 (γ)	10
		80 (x)	21
		71 (x)	47
		69 (x)	27
^{226}Ra	1,604 years	4,800 (α)	95
		4,600 (α)	6
		186 (γ)	4

Nuclear Cardiology Crash Cart

Introduction

A crash cart must be available in the nuclear cardiology laboratory at all times during exercise and pharmacologic stress procedures. This appendix lists the essential contents of a crash cart. Additional drugs may be added to the cart at the discretion of the cardiologist.

Contents

As the arrangement of drugs may vary between crash carts, an inventory list specifying the location of each drug should be kept in each cart. In the following list are the drugs and ancillary equipment that should be present in each cart.

Item	Approx. Quantity
Adenosine, 6-mg vial	1
Airway tubing	3
Albuterol inhaler	1
Aminophylline, 250 mg	2
Atropine, 1-mg syringe	6
Blood gas kit	2
Bretylium tosylate, 500-mg syringe	6
Calcium chloride	4
Defibrillator paddle pads (1 set)	1
Dextrose 5% in water (500 ml)	1
Dextrose 5% in water (250 ml)	3
Dextrose 5% in 0.9% NaCl (250 ml)	1
Dextrose 50% (50 ml)	2
Diazepam, 10-mg syringe	2
Digoxin, 0.5-mg ampule	2
Diphenhydramine, 50-mg syringe	2
Dopamine, 200-mg/5 ml	4
Esmolol, 100-mg vial	1
ECG electrodes (packet)	1
ECG paper (1 roll)	1
Epinephrine, 1:10,000 syringe	6
Epinephrine, 1:10,000 ampule	10
Furosemide, 100 mg	2
Glucagon emergency kit	1
Heparin, 1,000 U/ml, 10-ml vial	1
Insulin syringe	1
Isoproterenol, 1 mg/ml	6
IV catheter placement unit, 16 gauge	2
IV catheter placement unit, 18 gauge	2

Item	Approx. Quantity
IV catheter placement unit, 20 gauge	2
Lactated Ringer's, 1,000 ml	1
Norepinephrine bitartrate, 4-ml ampule	4
Lidocaine, 1 g in 250 ml D5W	1
Lidocaine, 100 mg/10-ml syringe	4
Lidocaine, 1 g/5-ml syringe	1
Metaproterenol sulfate inhaler	1
Methylprednisolone, 125-mg vial	2
Methylprednisolone, 1-g vial	1
Midazolam, 1 mg/ml	2
Nasal cannula with tubing	1
Needles—assorted sizes	—
Nifedipine capsules, 10 mg	5
Nitroglycerin, 0.4-mg tablets	1
Oxygen mask with tubing	1
Oxygen tubing	3
Pacing electrodes (external)	1
Phenylephrine, 10 mg/ml	1
Phenytoin sodium, 100-mg syringe	2
Povidone-iodine solution	1
Potassium chloride, 40-mEq vial	1
Procainamide, 100 mg/ml, 10-ml vial	2
Propranolol, 1-mg ampule	4
Propranolol tablets, 10 mg	5
Sodium bicarbonate, 50-mEq syringe	6
Sodium chloride, 0.9%, 1,000 ml	1
Syringes—assorted sizes	—
Tape adhesive	1
Thiopental sodium, 500-mg/ml syringe	1
Verapamil, 5-mg syringe	4

Index

Page numbers followed by *f* indicate figures; those followed by *t* indicate tables.